Population Health, Communities and Health Promotion

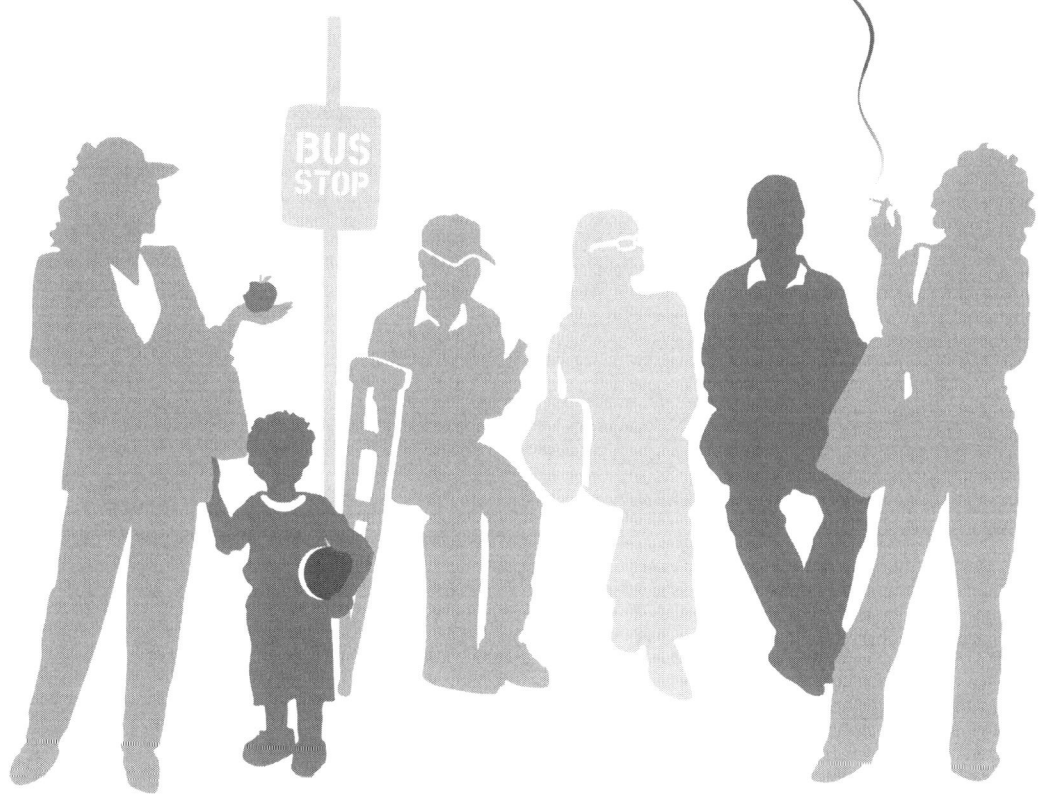

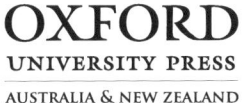

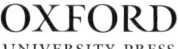

Oxford University Press is a department of the University of Oxford.
It furthers the University's objective of excellence in research,
scholarship, and education by publishing worldwide. Oxford is a registered
trademark of Oxford University Press in the UK and in certain other
countries.

Published in Australia by
Oxford University Press
253 Normanby Road, South Melbourne, Victoria 3205, Australia

© Sansnee Jirojwong and Pranee Liamputtong 2009

The moral rights of the authors have been asserted.

First published 2009
Reprinted 2011, 2012

All rights reserved. No part of this publication may be reproduced, stored in a retrieval system, or transmitted, in any form or by any means, without the prior permission in writing of Oxford University Press, or as expressly permitted by law, by licence, or under terms agreed with the appropriate reprographics rights organisation. Enquiries concerning reproduction outside the scope of the above should be sent to the Rights Department, Oxford University Press, at the address above.

You must not circulate this work in any other form and you must impose this same condition on any acquirer.

National Library of Australia Cataloguing-in-Publication data

Jirojwong, Sansnee.

Population health, communities and health promotion / Sansnee Jirojwong,
Pranee Liamputtong.

978 0 19 556055 8 (pbk.)

Includes index.
Bibliography.

Health education.
Public health.

Liamputtong, Pranee, 1955-

Community health and population

362.1

Reproduction and communication for educational purposes
The Australian *Copyright Act 1968* (the Act) allows a maximum of one chapter or 10% of the pages of this work, whichever is the greater, to be reproduced and/or communicated by any educational institution for its educational purposes provided that the educational institution (or the body that administers it) has given a remuneration notice to Copyright Agency Limited (CAL) under the Act.

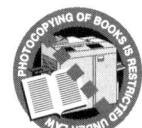

For details of the CAL licence for educational institutions contact:

Copyright Agency Limited
Level 15, 233 Castlereagh Street
Sydney NSW 2000
Telephone: (02) 9394 7600
Facsimile: (02) 9394 7601
Email: info@copyright.com.au

Edited by Elaine Cochrane
Cover design by studio overture
Text design and typeset by Kerry Cooke, eggplant communications
Proofread by Bruce Gillespie
Indexed by Russell Brooks
Printed and bound in Australia by Ligare Book Printers, Pty Ltd.

Links to third party websites are provided by Oxford in good faith and for information only. Oxford disclaims any responsibility for the materials contained in any third party website referenced in this work.

Brief Contents

List of Figures — xvii
List of Tables — xviii
Preface — xix
About the Editors — xxi
About the Contributors — xxiii
Acknowledgments — xxx
List of Abbreviations and Acronyms — xxxi

PART 1 Theory and Concepts — 1

Chapter 1 Introduction: Population Health and Health Promotion — 3
Chapter 2 Primary Health Care and Health Promotion — 26

PART 2 Needs Assessment — 43

Chapter 3 Health Needs Assessment of Communities and Populations — 45
Chapter 4 Health of Indigenous Australians and Health Promotion — 69
Chapter 5 Emerging Population Health Issues and Health Promotion — 92
Chapter 6 Assessing the Needs of Health Professionals and Stakeholders — 104

PART 3 Planning — 121

Chapter 7 Project Planning: Projects and Protocols — 123
Chapter 8 Project Planning Using the PRECEDE–PROCEED Model — 134
Chapter 9 Planning Human Resources — 159
Chapter 10 Planning for Policy Advocacy for Health Promotion — 173

PART 4 Implementation — 193

Chapter 11 Health Promotion: How to Build Community Capacity — 195
Chapter 12 Community Development and Empowerment — 215

Chapter 13	Health Promotion and Health Education for a Multicultural Community	232

PART 5 Evaluation 251

Chapter 14	Frameworks of Project Evaluation	253
Chapter 15	Levels of Project Evaluation and Evaluation Study Designs	267

Appendices

Appendix 1	Selected theories, models, and frameworks used in health promotion	286
Appendix 2	Example of project planning and protocol	288
Appendix 3	Applications of PRECEDE–PROCEED	295

Glossary	299
References	308
Index	345

Expanded Contents

List of Figures	xvii
List of Tables	xviii
Preface	xix
About the Editors	xxi
About the Contributors	xxiii
Acknowledgments	xxx
List of Abbreviations and Acronyms	xxxi

PART 1   Theory and Concepts — 1

Chapter 1 Introduction: Population Health and Health Promotion — 3
Sansnee Jirojwong & Pranee Liamputtong

Introduction	4
What is health?	5
Definitions of disease and illness	5
Models of health	6
What are the determinants of health?	9
Health measurement: From illness to wellness	10
Measurements of ill health	11
Measurements of wellness	11
Health education and health promotion	12
Evolution of population health: International, national and state levels	14
Population health in Australia	16
Characteristics of communities and their relationships with population health	17
Focusing on Australia	17
Social characteristics and population health	17
Physical characteristics and population health	19

	Demographic characteristics and population health	19
	Geographic characteristics and population health	20
	Cultural characteristics and population health	21
	Characteristics of communities and their relationships with health promotion	22
	Current issues in population health and health promotion	23
	Conclusion	24

Chapter 2 Primary Health Care and Health Promotion 46
Sansnee Jirojwong & Pranee Liamputtong

Primary health care and its development in developed and developing countries	27
Primary health care in developing countries	28
Primary health care in developed countries	28
The Ottawa Charter of Health Promotion	29
Building healthy public policy	30
Creating supportive environments	30
Strengthening community actions	30
Developing personal skills	30
Reorientating health services	31
Health promotion: International, national, and local levels	31
Health promotion: Healthy settings	32
Health promotion: Healthy population groups	33
Health promotion: Theories and models	34
Behaviour change theories: Individual level	36
Behaviour change theories: Group level	37
Behaviour change theories: Population level	39
Conclusion	41

PART 2 Needs Assessment 43

Chapter 3 Health Needs Assessment of Communities and Populations 45
Pranee Liamputtong & Sansnee Jirojwong

Needs assessment in health: An introduction	46
Why do we need to conduct a needs assessment?	48
Needs assessment processes	49
Strategies for needs assessment: What methods?	50
The use of existing data	52
Survey and questionnaire method	53
Delphi method	54

	Observation	55
	In-depth interviewing method	57
	Focus group interview	57
	Nominal group technique	59
	Rapid appraisal method	60
	Community-based methods	61
	Characteristics of the population for needs assessment	62
	Disadvantaged and vulnerable groups as the target population	62
	Prioritising identified health needs of population	63
	Case study 1: Health needs assessment—St Ives, Sydney	64
	Case study 2: Reproductive and sexual health initiative—The Photovoice Project and Indigenous Australians	65
	Conclusion	66
Chapter 4	Health of Indigenous Australians and Health Promotion *Janya McCalman, Komla Tsey, Teresa Gibson & Bradley Baird*	69
	Disclaimer	70
	Introduction	70
	Historical context of Indigenous Australians' health	71
	The diversity of Indigenous Australians	73
	Indigenous Australians and their health indicators	75
	What do Indigenous health promotion practitioners say?	77
	What does the literature say?	79
	What is Indigenous health promotion?	79
	What is working well?	80
	What is difficult?	84
	Learnings for the future	86
	Conclusion	87
	Acknowledgment	88
Chapter 5	Emerging Population Health Issues and Health Promotion *Diane Goldsworthy, Sansnee Jirojwong & Pranee Liamputtong*	92
	Introduction	93
	Travel, health issues, and health promotion	93
	Population Mobility and Health	95
	Emerging and re-emerging infectious diseases	96
	Society and health	97
	Environment and health	99
	Conclusion	102

Chapter 6	Assessing the Needs of Health Professionals and Stakeholders *Omar Ha-Redeye*	104
	Introduction: Identifying health professionals and stakeholders	105
	Assessing the needs of health professionals and stakeholders	106
	Disadvantaged and vulnerable groups as stakeholders	108
	Managing competing interest groups	109
	Prioritising identified needs	111
	Case study 1: MPHPs in the state of Victoria	114
	Case study 2: Turf wars in rural Australia	116
	Background	116
	Tensions within the hospitals	117
	Challenges to dominance	117
	Conclusion	117
PART 3	**Planning**	**121**
Chapter 7	Project Planning: Projects and Protocols *Robert MacLennan*	123
	Introduction	124
	Setting program goals and project objectives	124
	Program goals	124
	Project objectives	124
	Prerequisites for developing projects	125
	Identifying a problem	125
	Feasibility	125
	Significance of the problem	125
	Is the problem soluble?	126
	Induction or intuition?	126
	Project design	127
	The project protocol	128
	The project manual	128
	Quality control and monitoring	130
	Check list prior to implementation and collection of data	130
	Case study: Fast foods, exercise and body weight in primary school children in Brisbane	131
	Background	131
	Objectives of the baseline prevalence project	131
	Comment	131
	Conclusion	132

Chapter 8	Project Planning Using the PRECEDE–PROCEED Model *Peter Howat, Graham Brown, Sharyn Burns & Alexandra McManus*	134
	Introduction	135
	The PRECEDE–PROCEED model	135
	Program planning and the PRECEDE–PROCEED model	137
	Epidemiological assessment	139
	Identification of etiological factors	140
	Types of factors	142
	Case study 1: The Child Pedestrian Injury Prevention Program (CPIPP)	144
	Phase 1: Social assessment	144
	Phase 2, Step 1: Epidemiological assessment	144
	Phase 2, Step 2: Behavioural and environmental assessment	145
	Phase 3: Educational and ecological assessment	146
	Phase 4: Administrative and policy assessment and intervention alignment	146
	Re-defining the target group	148
	Determining goals and objectives	149
	Setting goals	149
	Setting objectives	150
	Case study 2: The Seniors Pedestrian Injury Prevention Program (SIPP)	152
	Program goal	152
	Behavioural objectives	152
	Sub-objectives	152
	Environmental objectives	153
	Strategies	153
	Intervention alignment, administrative and policy assessment	154
	Implementation	156
	Conclusion	157
	Acknowledgments	158
Chapter 9	Planning Human Resources *Lee Stewart, Rusioli Taukei & Kim Usher*	159
	Introduction: Leadership	160
	Local champions, key stakeholders	161
	Partnership, collaboration, and sponsors	163
	Roles and responsibilities	164
	Training	165

	Mentoring and supervising	166
	Sustainability	167
	Examples and case studies	168
	Case study 1: Introducing clinical governance in Fiji	169
	Case study 2: Development of human resources in rural Australia	170
	Conclusion	171

Chapter 10 Planning for Policy Advocacy for Health Promotion 173
Vivian Lin & Prue Bagley

Introduction	174
Key concepts	174
Basis for health advocacy	175
Principles for policy advocacy for health	176
Defining the desired policy objectives	177
Where should the policy advocacy effort go?	178
Planning advocacy	179
How to get started	179
Making contacts and assessing climate for change	180
Targeting and framing the messages	182
Choosing the advocacy approach and the tools	182
Advocacy toolkit	183
Lobbying and government relations	183
Media	185
Coalition building	187
Critical factors for success	188
Case study: The Penrith Food Project	190
Conclusion	191

PART 4   Implementation   193

Chapter 11 Health Promotion: How to Build Community Capacity 195
Glenn Laverack

Introduction	196
The definition of community capacity	196
The 'domains' of community capacity	196
Improving stakeholder participation	197
Developing local leadership	198
Building organisational structures	198
Increasing problem-assessment capacities	199
Enhancing the ability of the community to ask 'why?'	199
Improving resource mobilisation	199

Strengthening links to other organisations and people	200
Creating an equitable relationship with the outside agent	200
Increasing stakeholder control over program management	201
Building and measuring community capacity	201
How is the 'tool' implemented?	201
The visual representation of community capacity	205
Case study 1: Building community capacity in Fiji	207
Case study 2: Building community capacity in a remote Aboriginal community in Northern Australia	209
Participation	209
Leadership	210
Problem assessment	210
Asking why	210
Organisational structures	211
Resource mobilisation	211
Links to others	211
Outside agents	212
Program management	212
Conclusion	212

Chapter 12 Community Development and Empowerment — 215
Komla Tsey

Introduction	216
Empowerment and health	216
Where to start. Balancing principles and approaches with narrative	219
Community development in Indigenous Australian communities	220
Case study: The Family Wellbeing (FWB) empowerment program	222
Monitoring and evaluating empowerment	224
Personal or psychological domain of empowerment	225
Group or organisational domain of empowerment	226
Community or structural domain of empowerment	226
Conclusion	227
Acknowledgments	228

Chapter 13 Health Promotion and Health Education for a Multicultural Community — 232
Myna Hua & Chris Rissel

Introduction	233
The migration context	233
Definition of cross-cultural communication	234

Services available in helping health professionals to communicate with people from CALD backgrounds	235
Government services	235
Community-based services	236
Engaging with people from CALD backgrounds	237
Familiarity with the culture and conducting culturally inclusive health assessment	237
Demonstrating willingness and openness	238
Developing awareness of and sensitivity to cultural diversity	238
Enhancing skills through cross-cultural competency training	238
Planning and implementing a cross-cultural population-based health promotion program	239
Theories, principles, models, and frameworks related to health promotion	239
Obtaining relevant data to assist you in defining a health issue	240
Literature searches and needs assessments to plan for health promotion interventions	240
The concept of acculturation	240
Formative investigation to inform project design	241
Forming a project team	242
Tips for developing promotional resources	242
Disseminating messages and promotional materials	243
Cultural relevance in planning and conducting an evaluation	243
Budgetary planning	244
Case study 1: 'First Aid for Scalds' campaign	244
Reaching Sydney's Chinese, Vietnamese, and Arabic-speaking communities	244
Case study 2: 'Health is Gold'	246
An intervention to reduce tobacco use in the Vietnamese community in Sydney	246
Conclusion	248

PART 5   Evaluation   251

Chapter 14   Frameworks of Project Evaluation   253
Margaret Dykeman & Kathleen Cruttenden

Evaluation	254
Philosophy	254
Paradigms	255

	Critical thinking	256
	Evidence-informed practice	257
	Evidence-informed policy	257
	Planning an evaluation	258
	Evaluation models	259
	Four models relevant to social science program evaluation	259
	Types of evaluation	261
	Steps in evaluation	261
	Case study: Evaluating a housing project	262
	Conclusion	264
Chapter 15	Levels of Project Evaluation and Evaluation Study Designs	267
	David Dunt	
	Introduction	268
	Overview of evaluation in health promotion	268
	Differences between evaluation study designs and traditional scientific study designs	268
	Program cycle and evaluation strategy	269
	Evaluation study design	271
	Stakeholders	278
	Integrating utilisation into the evaluative process	278
	Behaviour change theory and program logic models	279
	Suchman's outcomes hierarchy	281
	Smith's 'if–then' approach	281
	Funnell's program logic matrix	281
	Case study: Evaluation of a school-based stop-smoking program	282
	Conclusion	283
	Acknowledgment	284
Appendix 1	Selected theories, models, and frameworks used in health promotion	286
	Focus on the individual	286
	Focus on groups	286
	Focus on the community	286
	Other important models	287
Appendix 2	Example of project planning and protocol	288
	Letter to Director of Education in Queensland state government	288
	Letter to schools to gain participation in the project	289
	Information sheet for participants and their parents	290

        Excerpt from plan of action: Proposed time schedule
            for Townsville Mole Survey   292
        Excerpts from Project Manual (Townsville Mole Survey 1990)   293

Appendix 3   Applications of PRECEDE–PROCEED   295

Glossary   299
References   308
Index   345

List of Figures

1.1	The modified social skeleton: health, illness, and structure–agency	8
1.2	The conceptual framework for the determinants of health	10
2.1	Health promotion approaches at different organisational levels	35
4.1	Population pyramid of Indigenous and non-Indigenous populations—2001	74
4.2	Cultural attachment by remoteness, 2002	75
4.3	Selected sources of support in time of crisis by remoteness area—2002	82
5.1	Flowchart of the World Health Organization's alert and verification activities	98
5.2	Effects of climate change on health through the changes to environment and associated impacts on infectious diseases, food production, and communities	101
6.1	Bioethical model for decision-making	112
6.2	Stakeholder input for Municipal Public Health Plans	116
8.1	PRECEDE–PROCEED model	137
8.2	Phase 1 of PRECEDE: social assessment and situational analysis	138
8.3	Phases 1 to 2 of PRECEDE: epidemiological assessment	139
8.4	Phases 1 to 3 of PRECEDE: educational and ecological assessment	142
8.5	Phases 1 to 4 of PRECEDE: intervention alignment, administrative and policy assessment	155
10.1	Factors affecting advocacy	178
10.2	The advocacy process	179
11.1	The design of the 'tool' to build and measure community capacit	202
11.2	Measurements for the Tokbai-Talaa village	206
11.3	Spider graph for Naivicula community	207
15.1	A community trial quasi-experimental study design	273
15.2	An interrupted time series trial quasi-experimental study design	274
15.3	Example of an evaluation using Suchman's outcomes hierarchy	280
15.4	Program logic matrix	282

List of Tables

1.1	Self-assessed health status by number of long term conditions, 2004–05 Australian Bureau of Statistics National Health Survey	12
1.2	Levels of health promotion interventions, with examples	14
6.1	Bioethical analysis guidelines	113
8.1	Research questions related to the PRECEDE–PROCEED model	136
8.2	Factors that may contribute to a person quitting smoking	143
8.3	Exploring reasons why people continue to smoke	143
10.1	A stakeholder management strategy	181
10.2	Examples of key stakeholders to consider for common health promotion action areas	181
10.3	Legislative process	184
10.4	Media advocacy planning	186
12.1	Spectrum of empowerment	218
12.2	Areas of basic human needs	229
12.3	Some inner qualities	230
15.1	Program cycle and evaluation strategies	270
A3.1	PRECEDE–PROCEED applied to child pedestrian injuries	295

Preface

This book focuses on the principles of population health, communities, health promotion, and disease prevention, and on emerging issues at local, national, and international levels. It is intended for use by undergraduate students who are studying community and population health and health promotion disciplines as a part of their course of study. The book is of particular interest to lecturers who teach community health nursing, public health, health promotion, primary health care, health management, and the sociology of health and illness behaviours.

In the current environment, where people are expected to be responsible for their own health and health care, undergraduate students are required to have the requisite knowledge and later work as a team member who can provide health services that meet local needs. It is desirable that students understand the concepts and steps required to assess these needs and the service outcomes. As such, the application of the basic concepts to a variety of population groups at a local community level is included. International examples are also provided in order to provide context to some particular concepts.

Our overall approach is on the principles used in conducting a health promotion project, beginning with assessing the needs of communities, including target population and key stakeholders. Included are the concepts of health promotion targeting a population by using the information from the community needs assessment to plan a project, implement it, and evaluate it according to the project's purposes, with examples or case studies from communities in developed and developing countries.

We also discuss the history of health promotion. Specific principles, concepts, methods, and strategies used in each stage of health promotion projects are provided. The discussion deals with principles relating to four major steps in health promotion projects—needs assessment, planning, implementation, and evaluation—so that the project can be sustained/continued, revised, or discontinued.

Each chapter presents the following features individually: chapter objectives, key terms, concepts relevant to the chapter, and critical thinking exercises. When possible, examples or case studies are provided, based on a range of communities mainly in Australia. Examples in Canada and Pacific Oceanic countries are also included.

Resources and tools that have been used in the community are mentioned. Information relating to additional resources is provided so that readers can gain access to these, if needed. Questions are then posed for self-assessment.

The book is divided into five major sections. In the first section, we present theories and framework applicable to community and population health, and the importance of health promotion at global, national, and local levels. We also include discussions on the foundation of population health and the evolution of population health at national and international levels, as well as health promotion and disease prevention at individual, group, and population levels. Chapters in the second section discuss principles and issues relating to the need assessments of a population group. The third section provides various components of the planning stage of a project, and the fourth section focuses on the implementation of the project. The fifth section describes the issues to be considered for the evaluation of the project. We believe that this book provides comprehensive information applicable to a range of population groups and communities.

Sansnee Jirojwong & Pranee Liamputtong
November 2007

About the Editors

Sansnee Jirojwong is a Senior Lecturer at the School of Nursing, University of Western Sydney. Prior to moving to University of Western Sydney, Sansnee was a Senior Lecturer at the School of Nursing and Health Studies at Central Queensland University for more than ten years. Sansnee also taught at a Faculty of Nursing in Thailand and Brunei. Sansnee's earlier research projects focused on migrants' health and their behaviours while they are in a host country or returning to their home country. Over the past six years, Sansnee has been involved in a number of projects in Queensland rural communities and worked closely with local health practitioners. Sansnee has worked with local communities and disadvantaged groups including migrants and people in rural areas to increase the accessibility of health and social services to the migrants. Sansnee's research articles are published in *Women and Health*, *Transcultural Psychiatry*, *Australian Journal of Rural Health*, *Health and Social Care in the Community*, *Southeast Asian Journal of Tropical Medicine & Public Health* and *Journal of Advanced Nursing*.

Pranee Liamputtong is a Professor at the School of Public Health, La Trobe University, Melbourne, Australia. Pranee has previously taught in the School of Sociology and Anthropology and worked as a public health research fellow at the Centre for the Study of Mothers' and Children's Health, La Trobe University.

Pranee's book *Qualitative Research Methods: A Health Focus* (with Douglas Ezzy, Oxford University Press, 1999) has been reprinted in 2000, 2001, 2002, 2003, and 2004, and the second edition of this book is titled *Qualitative Research Methods* (2005). Pranee's new focus is on the use of the internet in qualitative research, and she has recently completed an edited book on *Health Research in Cyberspace: Methodological, Practical and Personal Issues*, which was published by Nova Science Publishers, New York, in 2006. Her new book, *Researching the Vulnerable: A Guide to Sensitive Research Methods*, was published by Sage, London, in 2007. Her books *Undertaking Sensitive Research: Managing Boundaries, Emotions and Risk* (with Virginia Dickson-Swift and Erica James), Cambridge University Press, and *Knowing Differently: Arts-Based and Collaborative Research Methods* (with Jean Rumbold), Nova Science Publishers, will both be published in 2008. She is now working on *Doing Cross-Cultural Research* (Springer),

Performing Qualitative Cross-Cultural Research (Cambridge University Press), and *Focus Group Methodology: Principles and Practices in the Health and Social Sciences* (Sage).

In her own research, Pranee has a particular interest in issues related to cultural and social influences on childbearing, childrearing and women's reproductive and sexual health. She has published a large number of papers in these areas, and her three books on these issues have been used widely in the health field: *My 40 Days: A Cross-Cultural Resource Book for Health Care Professionals in Birthing Services* (The Vietnamese Antenatal/Postnatal Support Project, 1993); *Asian Mothers, Australian Birth* (editor, Ausmed Publications, 1994); *Maternity and Reproductive Health in Asian Societies* (editor, with Lenore Manderson, Harwood Academic Press, 1996). Other recent books include: *Asian Mothers, Western Birth* (new edition of *Asian Mothers, Australian Birth*, Ausmed Publications, 1999); *Living in a New Country: Understanding Migrants' Health* (editor, Ausmed Publications, 1999); *Hmong Women and Reproduction* (Bergin & Garvey, 2000); *Coming of Age in South and Southeast Asia: Youth, Courtship and Sexuality* (editor, with Lenore Manderson, Curzon Press and Nordic Institute of Asian Studies (NIAS), 2002); and *Health, Social Change and Communities* (editor, with Heather Gardner, Oxford University Press, 2003). She published two books for Nova Science Publishers in 2007: *Reproduction, Childbearing and Motherhood: A Cross-Cultural Perspective*, and *Childrearing and Infant Care Issues: A Cross-Cultural Perspective*. Her most recent book on *The Journey of Becoming a Mother amongst Thai Women in Northern Thailand* was published by Lexington Books, Lanham, Maryland, in 2007.

About the Contributors

Prue Bagley MA (Hons) is a lecturer in the School of Public Health at La Trobe University. She is currently completing her PhD on infrastructure and capacity in public health. Her research interests include public health systems research (PHSR) and the sociology of food and nutrition.

Bradley Baird is a Gunghangi man from Yarrabah. He is currently the Coordinator of the Yaba Bimbie Men's Group at Gurriny Yealamucka Health Service in Yarrabah. Bradley has a Graduate Diploma in Indigenous Health Promotion from the University of Sydney, 2007. The focus of his work with Yarrabah men is to address the 'loss of spirit' experienced in this stolen generation community and to help rebuild family values and family unity. Bradley uses the principles derived from his Christian faith and his involvement with the Family Wellbeing Program to guide his work with Yarrabah men. He is also a cultural dancer and uses dance as a tool to speak to community members and others about health and well-being issues. Bradley has co-authored research publications based on his work in communities.

Graham Brown (BBus, PGradDip (Health Promotion), PhD) is a Senior Lecturer with the School of Public Health, Curtin University and Co-director of the Western Australian Centre for Health Promotion Research. Graham managed health promotion programs and initiatives in non-government community-based organisations for ten years before moving to Curtin University. Graham now conducts intervention research in the areas of HIV prevention, sexuality, and youth mental health, and peer-based interventions in collaboration with government and non-government organisations. Graham also writes and teaches a range of undergraduate and postgraduate health promotion units in Health Promotion Methods and Health Promotion Planning.

Sharyn Burns (PhD, MPH, PGDipHealthProm, BEd, DipTch) is a Senior Lecturer and Coordinator of the Health Promotion Postgraduate Program in the School of Public Health, Curtin University in Western Australia, and a Co-Director of the Western Australian Centre for Health Promotion Research (Curtin University). She has a broad range of expertise in the field of education, health promotion, and public health. Sharyn has expensive experience in the implementation of state-wide multimedia campaigns and school and community-based interventions. Sharyn's research interests include bullying, school health promotion, youth health, and obesity prevention.

Kathleen Cruttenden (RN, PhD) has a BScN from University of Toronto, a MHSc (A) in Geriatrics from McMaster University, and a PhD in Regional Planning and Resource Development (Health) from the University of Waterloo. She has practised in the community, long-term care, and in acute care. Her research focus is care for older adults, including her doctoral research undertaking policy analysis of Ontario's Long-Term Care Reform. Her planning study of the strengths and learning needs of nursing staff in long-term care was published in 2006. Currently, she is a co-applicant / co-investigator of the Atlantic Seniors' Housing Research Alliance (www.ashra.ca) and member of the research evaluation team using Program Logic to assess the process and outcomes of the five-year study that involves forty community partners/stakeholder groups and five researchers. Dr Cruttenden is the Director at the School of Nursing, Laurentian University in Northern Ontario.

David Dunt, an Associate Professor, is a public health specialist and epidemiologist with major interests in health program evaluation and health services research. He is Head of the Program Evaluation Unit in the School of Population Health at the University of Melbourne, and was previously a co-Director of the Centre for Health Program Evaluation. His main current interests are in the integration of health services, particularly in the primary care sector, and community-based health promotion projects. He has published around 160 academic papers and other reports. He is a medical graduate of the University of Melbourne, with a PhD in Public Health, and is a Fellow of the Faculty of Public Health (of the Royal College of Physicians, UK). Significant research projects recently carried out under David's supervision have included: Statewide Evaluation of Best Start the Victorian State Government's Early Childhood Development Initiative; National Evaluation of the After Hours Primary Medical Care Trials; Integration of the General Practitioner into the Wider Healthcare System; Evaluation of the Southern Health Care Network Coordinated Care Trial.

Margaret Dykeman is a Professor in the Faculty of Nursing, University of New Brunswick in Canada. Clinically she is a nurse practitioner with experience working in marginalised communities. Since 2004 she has been nurse manager in a community health clinic that was established by the Faculty of Nursing to provide service for the homeless, low-income and addicted populations in a small city (population less than 50,000) and its surrounding rural areas. In addition to providing service, the facility provides interesting opportunities for students of multiple faculties and institutions to learn about primary health care and interdisciplinary care provision. Currently Margaret is involved in a number of community-based research projects that are interlinked with the services being provided at the Clinic. She has previously published in a number of peer-reviewed journals, including the *Journal of Nurses in AIDS Care* and the *Journal of AIDS Care*.

Teresa Gibson is a Bulgoone and Ankamuthi clan member from Hope Vale with seven years of work/life experience working in the seventeen communities across Cape York. She has a Graduate Diploma in Indigenous Health Promotion from the University of Sydney, 2006, and currently works as a Research Officer for the School of Indigenous Australian Studies at James Cook University. The focus of her research is towards the development of a social and emotional well-being framework for Cape York communities. Teresa has a passion and commitment for assisting community and service providers to utilise the Family Wellbeing Program as a holistic empowerment tool for health promotion. She sees Family Wellbeing as a tool to bring groups of people together, and create a safe environment for them to ask important questions about themselves and their place in society.

Diane Goldsworthy is a Lecturer at Central Queensland University, Rockhampton, Australia. Coming originally from the UK, Diane has experience in many nursing disciplines, from acute to community care. As a qualified registered nurse teacher, community health teacher, and district nurse, Diane practised as a community nurse in rural and industrial areas for a number of years before returning to acute care. It was her community background that motivated Diane to begin her PhD studies into the relationship between *Parthenium hysterophorus*, an introduced weed, and its allergic responses in a Queensland rural community. Diane has received a grant to conduct this study, and is currently completing her research work. While continuing in her academic role, Diane has recently written a new subject for third-year undergraduate nursing students, Population Health. With Diane's continuing involvement with communities, she intends to extend her research in community health further in combination with her teaching position.

Omar Ha-Redeye began his health care career in Nuclear Medicine Technology. After training and practising in several institutions in the American Mid-West, he completed a BHA in Health Services Management from Ryerson University in Toronto, Canada, the only accredited program of its type in the nation. Serving on the HSM Alumni Council and the Program Evaluation Committee for the Ryerson program allowed him to participate in promoting policy relevant to the Canadian health care system. He developed a specialty and interest in disaster preparedness and emergency response, and found himself working in settings such as rural Aceh, Indonesia, following the 2004 tsunami. Using his familiarity with cutting-edge telecommunications technology with an administrative focus led to an interest in the delivery of health services in rural and remote settings. He currently has returned to school at McMaster University to complete a MSc (PT) at McMaster University while doing fieldwork in small community placements in Ontario, Canada.

Peter Howat is a Professor and former Head of the Department of Health Promotion in the School of Public Health at Curtin University in Perth, Western Australia. He is also Associate Director of the Western Australian Centre for Health Promotion Research, and a Senior Research Fellow with the Centre for Research into Aged Care Services. He has worked in health promotion for almost three decades in several countries, including New Zealand, the USA, Australia, and the Asia–Pacific region. He has taken an active role in many community organisations involving community development programs. His early work was in rural towns in New Zealand, where he was involved in community and school-based programs as well as in community, political, and media advocacy. As well as over 100 refereed journal articles, book chapters and conference proceedings, he is the author or co-author of more than 100 other reports and policy documents. His undergraduate education was in New Zealand at Canterbury University and the University of Otago, and he completed an MSc and PhD at the University of Illinois. In 2001, he spent a period as a Visiting Research Scientist in the Centers for Disease Control and Prevention in Atlanta, USA.

Myna Hua has over ten years' experience in health promotion, especially in tobacco control programs. As a senior health promotion officer in the Health Promotion Unit of the Central Sydney Area Health Service in New South Wales, she has been one of the principal authors of the Second Central Sydney Tobacco Action Plan 1999–2004. She was responsible for the provision of high-level expertise for the strategic direction and coordination of the Tobacco Control Action Team in the Health Promotion Unit. She has extensive experience in developing, implementing and evaluating tobacco control programs for culturally and linguistically diverse communities, which include the Arabic Tobacco and Health Project, the Vietnamese anti-smoking project Health is Gold, and the Chinese Tobacco and Health Project. During 2004–05, she served as Deputy Director of the Health Promotion Unit, Sydney South West Area Health Service. At various times, Myna has been invited to provide expertise in providing advice on planning and developing media campaigns targeting Vietnamese, Chinese, and Arabic-speaking communities. Currently, she is a member of the Environmental Tobacco and Children Taskforce.

Glenn Laverack is the newly appointed Director of Health Promotion at the School of Population Health, University of Auckland. He is committed to empowerment strategies, having a strong practice background internationally in health promotion and public health, including Africa, Asia, and the Pacific region. His PhD investigated the accommodation of community empowerment within top-down health promotion programming in Fiji. He also holds a Masters degree in Health Promotion. His current research interests are in the link between empowerment and improved health outcomes, especially within Pacific communities. He has a wide range of publications on health promotion in international settings.

Vivian Lin is the Professor of Public Health at La Trobe University and was Head of School from 2000 to 2005. She was previously the Executive Officer for the National Public Health Partnership. She has held senior positions within the New South Wales Health Department, the National Occupational Health and Safety Commission, and the Victorian Health Department (and its successors), where she had responsibility for policy, planning, and program development across a wide range of health issues. Vivian is the President of the Chinese Medicine Registration Board of Victoria and consults for the World Bank, UK Department for International Development, World Health Organization, and the Australian Agency for International Development (AusAID). Her research interests are in the political economy of health, health system development, and policy implementation. Her recent books include: *Health Planning: Australian Perspectives* (with Eagar and Garrett) and *Evidence-Based Health Policy: Problems and Possibilities* (co-edited with Gibson). Vivian received her educational qualifications at Yale (BA) and the University of California Berkeley (MPH and DrPH).

Janya McCalman is a Senior Research Officer with the Empowerment Research Program at the School of Indigenous Australian Studies at James Cook University in Cairns. This research program aims to explore how the concepts of empowerment and control might contribute to a better understanding of the social determinants of Indigenous Australian health and well-being. Janya has a Masters degree in Public Health from Sydney University, and many years' experience working in the health promotion field. She is currently enrolled in a PhD, using participatory action research to support organisational change and improvement of health and well-being outcomes in one Aboriginal community-controlled health service. Her areas of interest/experience have included Indigenous health, alcohol and drugs, sexual health, and HIV prevention. She has worked to develop and implement both 'top-down' and 'bottom-up' health promotion strategies, but is currently enjoying supporting 'bottom-up' approaches from North Queensland and Central Australian Aboriginal organisations.

Robert MacLennan (MB BS, MS, DCH, DTM&H, MRCP, FRACP) is an Honorary Professor and Senior Principal Research Fellow, Queensland Institute of Medical Research, Brisbane since 1982, Professor in the Joint Tropical Health Program with the University of Queensland, and Visiting Professor, James Cook University. In addition to Australia, he has conducted epidemiological fieldwork in developed and developing countries, including Papua New Guinea, Colombia, Ecuador, Kenya, Uganda, Denmark, Finland, Hong Kong, Singapore, and Thailand. His interests are in cancer epidemiology, field epidemiology, and tropical health. He had previous appointments at Tulane School of Public Health and Tropical Medicine, New Orleans; the International Agency for Research on Cancer, World Health Organization, Lyon, France; and the Commonwealth Institute of Health, University of Sydney. Current interests include cancer epidemiology and control in tropical populations; cancer registration in developing countries; and diet and neoplasia. Bob has more than 180 research articles published in international refereed journals and as book chapters.

Alexandra McManus (PhD, MPH, PGradDipPH, BScHP (H.Biol)) is an Associate Director and Senior Research Fellow with the Western Australia Centre for Health Promotion Research at Curtin University. Previous appointments include Biostatistician, Curtin University (2003) and Senior Research Fellow with the University of Western Australia (2000–03). She has extensive experience in project management and intervention research, and has been an investigator on 17 interventions, twice won the Award for Excellence in Research and Teaching, presented at 44 national/international conferences, and published 26 articles and reports since 2002. Alexandra has spent considerable time working in community-based research, injury prevention, workplace health, and child health, and with Indigenous populations. Alexandra is currently Co-Investigator on several grants, including a grant from the National Institutes of Health in the USA ($1 million) investigating brain injury in sport. Other recent projects include: positional specificity in Australian football and field hockey and netball, and how this impacts on training and competition.

Chris Rissel, an Associate Professor, has worked in community-based health promotion for more than twenty years. This has included a variety of roles, including program planning and implementation, social marketing, policy development, and organisational change, as well as a strong emphasis on research and evaluation. This work has benefited from exposure to the health services of Sydney, as well as those of the USA and Germany, where Chris completed doctoral and postdoctoral research around the themes of community, participation, and empowerment in health promotion. He has published widely on a range of topics, including migrant health, tobacco control, and sexual health. Chris's personal interests now are focused on active transport to encourage physical activity, particularly cycling.

Lee Stewart (RN, RM, DipTeach (Nurs), B.HealthSc. (Nursing), PostgradCertEd, M Dispute Resolution, MRCNA) is currently a Lecturer at the School of Nursing Sciences, James Cook University. She is a registered nurse and midwife who has worked in both Australia and Fiji. Her experience includes acute hospital, community health, nursing education, and health management in Australia; and World Health Organization and Australian Agency for International Development (AusAID) consultancies in Fiji. Lee has recently completed her PhD project, investigating the impact of introducing a clinical governance framework on nursing leadership in Fiji.

Rusieli Taukei (RN, RM, BHealthSc (Nursing), CertTeach, Dip Frontline Management, CertPublic Health, Adv DipNursing (Public Health)) currently is National Clinical Governance Coordinator for the Fiji Ministry of Health. She is a registered nurse who has worked and managed in a number of areas throughout Fiji, including acute major and subdivisional hospitals, community health services, nursing education, and the Fiji Ministry of Health Head Office. Her qualifications have been obtained in Fiji, Australia, and New Zealand, and include nursing, community health, and management tertiary qualifications.

Komla Tsey is Associate Professor and National Health and Medical Research Council (NH&MRC) Principal Research Fellow at James Cook University's School of Indigenous Australian Studies and School of Public Health and Tropical Medicine in Cairns. His research interests include: the social determinants of health; empowerment and community development; participatory action research; traditional healing systems; and program planning and evaluation. Since 2001, Komla has been a lead investigator in a ten-year collaborative research program examining the contribution that concepts of empowerment and control can make towards understanding and addressing the social determinants of Indigenous Australian health.

Kim Usher, a Professor, is an experienced researcher and educator, and a consultant for the World Health Organization and the Australian Agency for International Development (AusAID). She has conducted ten projects in the South-West Pacific Region, including the reform of nurse education in the Fiji School of Nursing and the Mapping of Nurse Education Standards project in the Pacific Islands, within her overall research portfolio of fifteen projects and $460,000 in funding over five years from 2002. She has supervised doctoral, masters and honours research students. Kim's publications include thirty refereed papers and eight books/book chapters since 2002. Professor Usher's research interests are in the areas of Indigenous students in nursing, psychotropic and PRN medications, reflective practice, and qualitative methodologies. Kim Usher is a Professor of Nursing in the School of Nursing, Midwifery & Nutrition at James Cook University, Townsville.

Acknowledgments

In bringing this book to life, we owe our gratitude to many people. Throughout the major part of editing this book, Sansnee was working at the School of Nursing and Health Studies, Central Queensland University. She would like to acknowledge in-kind support provided to her. Staff at the CQU—Publishing Unit, Library Services and Public Relations—assisted with the administrative aspects of the project. Emeritus Professor Amy Zelmer provided encouragement and intellectual stimulation to the development of this book.

The important motivation to write this book was based on Sansnee's health promotion work in four small rural communities in Queensland. Lessons learnt from the field were the driving force to complete this book. The generosity and kindness of rural people was much appreciated by Sansnee. She also would like to acknowledge the support provided by Professor Bob MacLennan throughout the project process.

We also would like to thank Sally Schukking and Rosemary Oaks, who assisted with the English grammar of few chapters, and Chrislyn Apellado-Hunn and Nguyet Vi (Rose) Truong, who undauntedly checked references of all chapters. It was a big task appreciated by all contributors. We also thank Jennifer Heumiller, who helped draw the figures for Chapter 2. We are grateful to Debra James, the Higher Education Publishing Manager of the Oxford University Press, who provided professional support and encouragement throughout the project. Her understanding and collegiality are much appreciated by both of us. Last but not least, we want to express our thanks to all contributors who have their chapters included in this book. It is only with your help that this book has come to life.

List of Abbreviations and Acronyms

ABS	Australian Bureau of Statistics
ACCHS	Aboriginal Community Controlled Health Services
AEDB	Aboriginal Education Development Branch
AIHW	Australian Institute of Health and Welfare
ASHRA	Atlantic Seniors' Housing Research Alliance
ATSIC	Aboriginal and Torres Strait Islander Commission
BSE	bovine spongiform encephalopathy
CALD	culturally and linguistically diverse backgrounds
CCAHP	Collaborative Centre for Aboriginal Health Promotion
CDC	Centers for Disease Control and Prevention
CDEP	Community Development Employment Projects
CHD	coronary heart disease
CHIP	Community Health Improvement Process model
CPIPP	Child Pedestrian Injury Prevention Project
DALY	disability-adjusted life year
DHBs	District Health Boards, New Zealand
DIMA	Department of Immigration and Multicultural Affairs
ETS	environmental tobacco smoke
FWB	Family Wellbeing empowerment program
GOTME	goal, objective, target, message, evaluation
HALE	health adjusted life expectancy
HBM	health belief model
HILDA	Household, Income and Labour Dynamics in Australia
HIV/AIDS	human immunodeficiency virus/acquired immune deficiency syndrome
HREOC	Human Rights and Equal Opportunity Commission
ICN	International Council of Nurses
ISRD	Index of Relative Socio-Economic Status
KSAs	knowledge, skills and attitudes
LCF	Leadership for Change program

LGA	local government area
MAPP	Mobilising Action through Planning and Partnership
MMHA	Multicultural Mental Health Australia
MPHP	Municipal Public Health Plan
MRFIT	Multiple Risk Factor Intervention Trial
NAATI	National Accreditation Authority for Translators and Interpreters
NACCHO	National Aboriginal Community Controlled Health Organisation
NH&MRC	National Health and Medical Research Council
NPHPSP	National Public Health Performance Standards Program
NSW	New South Wales
OCHNA	Orange County Health Needs Assessment
OECD	Organisation for Economic Co-operation and Development
PATCH	Planned Approach to Community Health model
PBS	Pharmaceutical Benefits Scheme
PHC	Primary Health Care
PHWQ	Public Health Workforce Questionnaire
PLA	Participatory Learning Action
PRECEDE	predisposing, reinforcing and enabling constructs in ecological diagnosis and evaluation (planning and developmental phases of the PRECEDE–PROCEED model)
PROCEED	policy, regulatory and organisational constructs in education and environmental development (implementation of strategies and evaluation phases of the PRECEDE–PROCEED model)
QOL	quality of life
RCT	randomised controlled trial
SARS	severe acute respiratory syndrome
SLLPC	Sustainable Livelihoods for Livestock Producing Communities Project
SWOT analysis	Strengths, Weaknesses, Opportunities and Threats analysis
TIS	Translating and Interpreting Service
TTM	transtheoretical model of change
U3A	University of the Third Age
UNICEF	United Nations Children's Fund
VACCHO	Victorian Aboriginal Community Controlled Health Organisation
WHO	World Health Organization

PART 1

Theory and Concepts

Chapter 1   Introduction: Population Health and Health Promotion   3
Chapter 2   Primary Health Care and Health Promotion   26

Introduction: Population Health and Health Promotion

Sansnee Jirojwong
& Pranee Liamputtong

Objectives

After reading this chapter, readers will be able to:

- Understand definitions of key terms in population health and health promotion
- Explain the development of models of health and evaluate the application of these models in different settings and contexts
- Relate the evolution of population health at international and national levels
- Apply information relating to characteristics of a community and health status of its population and relevant health promotion programs.

Key terms

community
culture
health
health education
health promotion
population health
public health

Introduction

Over the last hundred years, there has been much improvement in the health and life expectancy of the Australian population. Leading causes of death have changed from infectious and parasitic diseases to chronic diseases. Australians now live longer, and their risk of developing cardiovascular diseases, cancer, and diabetes has increased over the years (AIHW, 2006). There have been on-going changes in the social, economic and political environment, and these have had an impact on individuals' health behaviours and their life styles. Medical and therapeutic technologies for the diagnosis and treatment of diseases have also improved significantly, while at the same time the cost of health care has increased markedly.

The symptoms of many chronic diseases take a long time to develop. However, once these diseases are diagnosed, treatments and changes in behaviour and life style are required, generally for a number of years. Health planners, health professionals, and health academics have agreed that disease prevention and health promotion are necessary to reduce the impacts of chronic diseases in the twenty-first century. Different strategies in the provision of health promotion services have to target specific individuals, groups, and society. A strong collaborative effort across different sectors, including the public health, economic, and education sectors, will be required to reduce these growing health problems. In the past three decades, the contributions of health promotion to community and public health services have been increasing. Despite this, increased evidence has also shown that there is a gap of health status between different population groups.

This chapter serves as an introduction to issues discussed in this volume. Hence, the topics we discuss in the chapter will be general in scope. The chapter is divided into three major sections. In the first section, we provide general information about health, disease, and illness. The development of models of health and how health is measured are included in this section. In the second section, we briefly describe the roles of health education and health promotion at different levels of health. The third section explains the development of public health and population health at international, national, and local levels. We outline some examples of an increasing interest in population health among practitioners, researchers, and policy makers. The relationship between population health, characteristics of communities and health promotion programs is included in this third section.

The chapter attempts to fill in the gaps in the literature on population health, health promotion, and communities. Terms used in health, public health, population health, and health promotion will be defined.

What is health?

Health means different things to different people. Individuals who have a physical disability may say that they are 'healthy' when they are able to function independently. Health also can be freedom from disease, feeling happy, or being satisfied with one's current situation (Kleinman, 1980; AIHW, 2000). A person's health is never static, and it can vary according to the context and environment in which the individual lives. For example, individuals who are well in the morning may experience anxiety because of work pressure in the afternoon. Many cultural groups perceive health and illness as the results of an individual's long-term relationships with family, community, and environment. A dysfunctional relationship may influence that individual's health status (Kleinman, 1980; Landrine & Klonoff, 1992).

In 1946, the World Health Organization (WHO, 1946, 1978: 2) defined health as 'a state of complete physical, mental and social well-being and not merely the absence of disease or infirmity'. The continuum of health and illness has been considered in this definition. Disease and infirmity have been used as health status measurements for more than two decades. However, the term 'well-being' is increasingly used to describe the health of populations (Jones, 2003). Well-being is a subjective sense that there is nothing wrong and can be completely independent of our objectively measured health or disease status. This definition of health has been used for more than 60 years. In the 1980s, the World Health Oganization emphasised that the ability to function normally in a person's social setting should be integrated into the definition of health (Beaglehole & Bonita, 2004). An attempt to include spiritual aspects as a part of the definition of health has not eventuated (WHO, 1998).

Health: a state of complete physical, mental and social well-being and not merely the absence of disease or infirmity.

Definitions of disease and illness

When individuals experience symptoms because of changes in their usual physical, mental, or social condition, they interpret these symptoms. Two terms, 'disease' and 'illness', are used to describe the sickness. Disease is a malfunctioning of biological and/or psychological processes, while illness refers to the psychosocial experience and meaning of perceived disease. Illness includes personal, social, and cultural responses to a disease. Illness contains responses to disease to provide it with a meaningful form and explanation as well as control. Disease affects single individuals, even when it attacks a population, but illness most often affects others, including family and the social network (Kleinman, 1980). In some Australian

Sansnee Jirojwong & Pranee Liamputtong

Aboriginal and migrant cultures, the illness is believed to be constituted by the affected persons, their family or their supporters (Huff & Kline, 1999; McCalman et al., Chapter 4 this volume).

An example can be demonstrated by two women's interpretation of, and responses to, having cervical cancer in situ. Both have the same pathological change to cells. The majority of cervical cancers are caused by human papillomavirus infection (Bosch et al., 1995). However, one of the women perceives that the disease is caused by heredity, as her mother and three of her female relations also had the disease. The occurrence of the disease cannot be controlled and she projects her anger towards her mother. Another woman thinks that the disease is caused by an earlier abortion, which later caused 'damage' to her reproductive organs, including cervix. Having cervical cancer is the punishment for her killing her unborn baby. She is angry with herself and the father of the baby. Different perceptions of the 'illness' by both women may influence their behaviours in seeking help and having the disease treated. Their illness may also influence their emotions and the support they receive from family.

Models of health

Many models of health have been developed to explain the health status of individuals, communities, and populations. These models help provide a better understanding of the health of an individual and a population, and act as a guide as to how their health can be maintained or improved. The development of different models of health has been based on the complexity of disease and illness patterns, changes in health behaviours, increasing knowledge about an individual's health behaviours, and the growth and development of health professions. Selected frequently used health models are presented below (Baum, 2008; Germov, 2005a).

Until the early twentieth century, infectious diseases, including cholera and plague, were major causes of death in many European countries. The contagion and germ theories were used to explain the causes of these diseases. The discovery of micro-organisms, made possible with the invention of the microscope in 1683, supported the use of the biomedical model of health with its emphasis on diseases and pathology (Beaglehole & Bonita, 2004; Germov, 2005a, 2005b). The focus was on disease, which was explained as a malfunction of one of the body's biological systems.

Later, during the industrial revolution of the eighteenth century, various social and psychological factors were identified as underlying causes of disease. These biological, psychological and social factors are taken into consideration in the development of the biopsychosocial model. Individuals or families who were exposed to an infectious agent typically also lived in a neighbourhood with poor sanitation. Many worked in an environment hazardous to health, and lived in crowded households with poor sanitation. People subject to these multiple factors were also more likely to be made sick than those who lived and worked in a better social and economic environment. A biopsychosocial model focused on disease prevention and aimed at improving the conditions of the poor and disadvantaged. Good health was seen as an absence of illness. The evidence of the use of this biopsychosocial model was in the improvement of sanitation and public health infrastructure that controlled many infectious diseases (Beaglehole & Bonita, 2004; Baum, 2008).

Since the early twentieth century, there have been social, economic, and political changes at the global level as well as at a national level. People have an increasing risk of developing chronic diseases, with complex relationships between various factors including their life styles. Many social models of health have been developed to explain an individual's health and the complexity of the individual's personal, family, society, and environmental factors. Two of the social models of health, the *new public health model* and the *social skeleton: health, illness and structure–agency model* are described briefly below because they are applied in various chapters of this book.

The new public health model links the 'traditional' psychosocial model of health with the social, cultural, behavioural, and politico-economic factors that affect people's health. It directs attention to the prevention of illness through community participation and social reforms that address living and working conditions. The model has its clearly defined aim of health equity. Some of the model's major components are an intersectional action and the sustainability and viability of environments for health and well-being of individuals and communities (see also Germov, 2005b; Baum, 2008). It is a very useful model for disease prevention and health promotion at individual, social, and community levels.

Germov (2005b: 14–21) has discussed another social model of health, the social skeleton: health, illness and structure–agency. This has three major dimensions. The first is the social production and distribution of health and illness. The occurrence of many illnesses is related to social factors. For example, poor health among Aborigines and the long-term unemployed can be explained in a historical, social, and cultural context of an individual or a group. The second is the social construction of health and illness. Symptoms of an illness may be defined differently in different cultures and times. For example, an increasing recognition of mental illnesses by society has helped sufferers identify themselves as being sick and to seek care. The third dimension is the social organisation of health care. Generally, health care services are influenced by the characteristics of the society they serve, allocated resources, and the interest of health professionals in health issues. Within a health professional sector, the power imbalance of medical practitioner, nurse, and allied health workers influences the organisation of health care. The social organisation of health care has a direct impact on prioritisation of the population groups it serves. A good example is the child abuse in Aboriginal communities, which has made it as a high priority health and social problem. This could be compared to the 2005 abolition of the Aboriginal and Torres Strait Islander Commission (ATSIC), which led to decreased attention to health issues among Aboriginal and Torres Strait Islander people. Schwartz and colleagues (1999) confirm that the historical context is another dimension which would influence health, and it has been incorporated in the social model proposed by Germov (2005b) as shown in Figure 1.1.

FIGURE 1.1 The modified social skeleton: health, illness and structure-agency

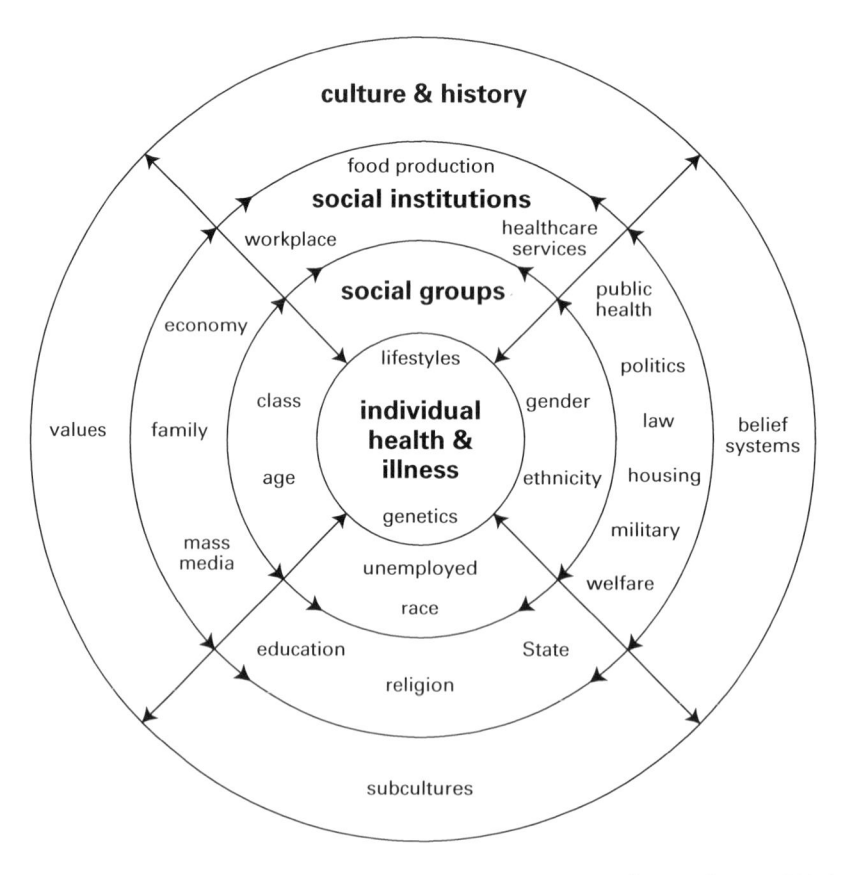

Source: Germov, 2005b: 19

The social skeleton model provides for the concept that individuals have different characteristics such as genetics and intelligence. They may behave or act differently in different social groups. The characteristics of social groups also range widely. Shown in Figure 1.1 are some of these characteristics, such as employment status, ethnicity, and gender. Power positioning of a group in a society can be an inherent factor of a social group.

Public health, law, and politics are examples of social institutions that are associated with the individual's health and illness status. Workers who are working in a non-supportive working environment with no law or legislation enforcement are at risk of physical or psychological illnesses.

Culture is a dynamic template or framework that a society uses to view, understand, behave, and pass on its culture to each succeeding generation (Huff & Kline, 1999). Culture helps to specify what behaviours are acceptable in a given society, when they are acceptable, and what is not acceptable. Differences in beliefs and practices influencing life styles and health behaviours have significant importance to Australia because 22 per cent of the population were born overseas and more than half of these people were born in a non-English speaking country (ABS, 2007a). Culture and history also have significant importance for Australian Aborigines, who, as a group, have poor health similar to the health of people in developing countries.

Culture: a learned, non-random, systematic behaviour that is transmitted from person to person and from generation to generation.

What are the determinants of health?

Another conceptual framework used to guide health care services is that of the determinants of health. The Australian Institute of Health and Welfare (AIHW, 2006: 143) proposes a conceptual framework for determinants of health. There are three levels—'upstream', 'intermediate', and 'downstream' determinants—which range from general background factors to specific health behaviours. The general background factors or the 'upstream factors' (Garrard et al., 2004: 4) are comparable to the social institution and social group levels shown in Figure 1.1; they include housing and the social environment. Knowledge and attitude are considered to be intermediate determinants of health, while specific health behaviours or the 'downstream' factors include smoking and lack of physical activity, which have direct effects on health (AIHW, 2006: 143; Keleher, 2007: 43). Health determinants also include biomedical and genetic factors, human behaviours, socio-economic factors, and environmental factors. Figure 1.2 is a diagram which displays the complex relationships of determinants of health. This conceptual framework is somewhat similar to the modified social skeleton: health, illness, and structure–agency (Figure 1.1).

Sansnee Jirojwong & Pranee Liamputtong

FIGURE 1.2 The conceptual framework for the determinants of health

Upstream ⟷ Downstream

General background factors
- Culture
- Resources
- Systems
- Policies
- Wealth
- Social cohesion
- Media
- Other

Environmental factors
- Landscape
- Climate
- Chemical
- Human-made

Socio-economic characteristics
- Education
- Employment
- Income
- Family, neighbourhood
- Access to services
- Other

Knowledge and attitudes

Health behaviours
- Dietary behaviour
- Physical activity
- Tobacco use
- Alcohol consumption
- Use of illicit drugs
- Vaccination
- Sexual practices
- Other

Psychological effects

Safety factors

Biomedical factors
- Body weight
- Blood pressure
- Blood cholesterol
- Immune status
- Other

Individual and population health

Individual makeup: physical and psychological (genetics, intergenerational, ageing and life course influences)

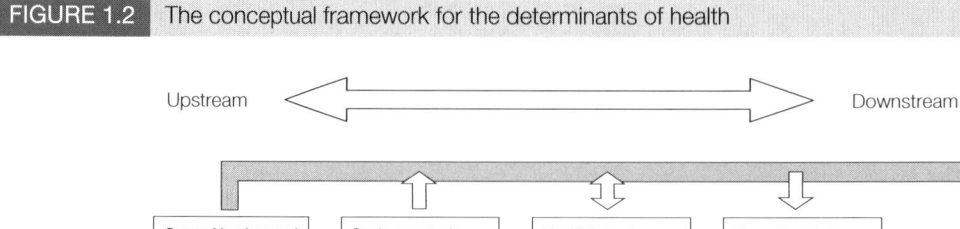

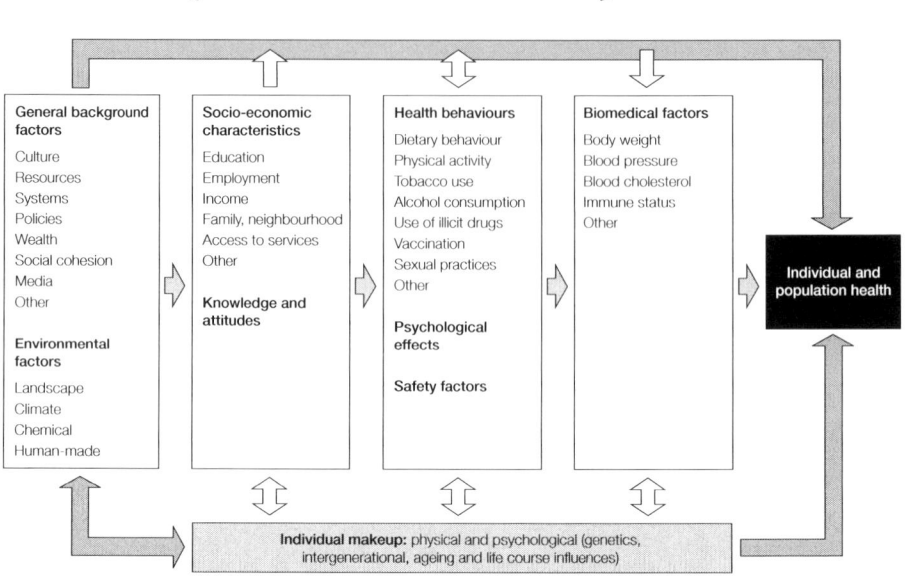

Source: Australian Institute of Health and Welfare (2006: 143)

Health measurement: From illness to wellness

We often come across reports of accidents, deaths, and disease occurrences within a community. Although there may be some reports of how people are happy with their lives or the extent to which people can return to their day-to-day activities after having surgery, these are less common. Morbidity and mortality rates are the traditional measurements of the levels of sickness and deaths, and they present the ill-health of a community.

Over the past 20 years, many health indicators, such as disability-adjusted life year (DALY), health adjusted life expectancy (HALE), and self-assessed health statuses (SF-36 or SF-12), have been developed to measure the population's wellness (WHO, 2004). Other wellness indicators include the quality of life (QOL) index and the Personal Wellbeing Index (International Wellbeing Group, 2006). Standardisation of these measurements is required as they need to be used across different cultures. These measurements are also useful for assessing the outcomes of health promotion programs.

Since 1988, the Australian Institute of Health and Welfare has published *Australia's Health* biennially as a reference source with information about Australian health status and health services. Data and the findings of many studies are integrated in the publications and made widely available (AIHW, 1994) from the Institute website, http://www.aihw.gov.au/.

Measurements of ill health

As in many other developed countries, the mortality rates of Australians have declined over the past eight decades. The improvement in Australians' health is supported by a number of health indicators. In 1907, the first national statistics showed that the crude death rate was 1200 per 100,000 population. In 2005, the crude death rate decreased to less than half—598 per 100,000 population (AIHW, 1994; ABS, 2007b). Compared with 14 selected OECD countries, the 2003 Australian male standardised death rate ranked third lowest, while the female standardised death rate ranked the fifth lowest (AIHW, 2006: 24).

In 2005, the top two major underlying causes of deaths were malignant neoplasms (cancer), and ischaemic heart disease. The cancer standardised death rate was 178 deaths per 100,000 population, and contributed 29.4 per cent of all deaths. The ischaemic heart disease standardised death rate was 106 deaths per 100,000 population, and contributed 18.0 per cent of all deaths (ABS, 2007b: 3303.0). Other diseases that are considered to be disease priorities because of their major contribution to the burden of illness and injury in the community include arthritis and musculoskeletal conditions, diabetes, injury, mental illnesses, and communicable diseases (Department of Health and Ageing, 2007).

Measurements of wellness

Life expectancy has been used as a wellness indicator for more than 60 years. It is defined as the average number of years of life remaining to a person, and is usually calculated using age-specific death rates for a particular period. In 1920–22, life expectancy at birth in Australia was 59.2 years for males and 63.3 years for females. In 2000–02, life expectancy in Australia at birth had increased to 77.4 years for males and 82.6 years for females (AIHW, 1998, 2000, 2006).

Since the late 1990s, other wellness indicators, including self-assessment of health and the satisfaction with life, have been reported as a part of health measurements (AIHW, 1998; Turrell et al., 1999; WHO, 2004). The use of these indicators helps better understand how well each group in the population is. The following selected information uses wellness indicators to present Australians' health overall.

In 2004, Australians enjoyed good health for about 90 per cent of their life span, with the remaining 10 per cent of their time spent with illness or disability. This information is based on the health adjusted life expectancy (HALE) to indicate the expected number of years that people can live without reduced functioning (WHO, 2004).

Self-reported health status is commonly used as an indicator of general health and well-being. It refers to how individuals assess their own health at a given point in time according to their values. It has been found to be a good indicator of future health care use and mortality, particularly in older Australians. Table 1.1 presents self-assessed health status by number of long-term conditions, based on the 2004–05 National Health Survey. Both measures of ill health and wellness are used to present the health status of those who have a range of long-term conditions compared with those without any condition. Both measures indicate that the more long-term conditions people have, the worse health status they perceive.

TABLE 1.1 Self-assessed health status by number of long-term conditions, 2004–05 Australian Bureau of Statistics National Health Survey

Self-assessed health status	Number of long-term conditions					
	None	One	Two	Three	Four	Five or more
Excellent/very good	74	71	63	55	49	30
Good	22	24	29	32	33	31
Fair/poor	4	5	8	13	18	39
Total	100	100	100	100	100	100

Source: Australian Institute of Health and Welfare, 2006: 27

Other health measurements include incidence, prevalence, disability, activity limitations, potential years of life lost, and specific mortality for a specific cause. Quality data are required so they can be used to assess changes in a population's health through time.

Health education and health promotion

Governments are the major provider of health care services to their citizens, including treatments, rehabilitation, palliation, disease prevention, health education, and health promotion. Health education is a structured discipline that provides learning opportunities about health through interactions between educators and learners using a variety of learning experiences. The learning process can enable people to change conditions or modify behaviour voluntarily for health enhancement. Health education includes those experiences and skills that affect the way people think and feel about their health, and it motivates them to put information into practice (Modeste & Tamayose, 2004: 58). In the early 1970s, health education was recognised as having potentially important roles in reducing the impact of chronic diseases and increased health care costs in the Australian health care system. By 1973, the Community Health Programme was initiated and funded by the Commonwealth government. One of its aims was to revive community health centres. Health education in wider communities was included as a part of the Community Health Programme activities. Community health staff delivered health education to prevent diseases in communities and health care units. Most of the health education was on a one-to-one basis. A range of health education programs and activities were delivered under the Community Health Programme through many health care organisations, including immunisation, family planning, and cervical cancer screening. In 1978, the financial support from the Federal government to the Community Health Programme ceased.

Following an increasing focus on health promotion in its broadest sense (Chapter 2) and the widely adopted Ottawa Charter of Health Promotion, the term 'health promotion' has been increasingly used in public discourse. Health promotion has aimed at helping people change to healthier life styles through various efforts to enhance awareness and create environments that support positive health practices that may result in reducing health risks in a population. Tasks include needs assessment, problem identification, development of an appropriate plan including goals and objectives, creation of interventions, implementation of interventions, and evaluation of outcomes or results.

Health promotion uses a combination of health education and specific interventions at the primary level of prevention, such as anti-smoking campaigns, designed to facilitate behavioural and environmental changes conducive to health enhancement and harm reduction. One major component of health promotion is supporting policy to assist the introduction of changes. Benefits of health promotion include changes in attitudes, increased awareness and knowledge, lowered risk of certain health problems, better health status, and improved quality of life (Modeste & Tamayose, 2004: 68–69).

Health promotion interventions can occur at three levels of organisation: individual, group, and society, and they can help people at three different levels of the health and illness continuum (Jones, 2003). These levels of health promotion intervention, with examples, are shown in Table 1.2.

Health education: an educational process concerned with providing a combination of approaches to lifestyle change that can assist individuals, families, and communities to make informed decisions on matters that affect the restoration, achievement, and maintenance of health.

Health promotion: any combination of educational, political, regulatory, and organisational supports for actions and conditions of living conducive to the health of individuals, groups, or communities.

TABLE 1.2 Levels of health promotion interventions, with examples

Level of health and illness	Level of organisation		
	Individual	Group	Society
Being well or primary level of having a disease	Teaching a child to eat fruit and vegetables	Communication skills training for students to prevent bullying in a school	Mass media campaign for regular mammograms
At risk of having a disease or secondary level of having a disease	Individual coping skills: training for the spouse of a terminal cancer sufferer	Stress management workshop for workers who were offered a redundancy package	'Meals on Wheels' program to improve nutrition for the elderly
Having a disease or tertiary level of having a disease	Developing an asthma management plan for a patient	Support and self-help group for patients with diabetes	Working with patients and families to lobby for services to personnel with post-traumatic stress disorder.

Modified from: Jones, 2003: 197

Population health: the health of groups, families, and communities. Populations may be defined by locality, biological criteria such as age and gender, social criteria such as socio-economic status, or cultural criteria.

Public health: the art and science of preventing disease, promoting health, and prolonging life through the organised efforts of society.

Evolution of population health: International, national, and state levels

Wide gaps in health status between population groups from different social, economic, and cultural backgrounds have been identified (see Syme et al., 1965; Marmot & Syme, 1976; Berkman & Kawachi, 2000; Wilkinson & Marmot, 2003). The overall goal of a population health approach is to maintain and improve the health of the entire population, and to reduce inequalities in health between population groups (WHO, 2004). Population health may be seen as the advancement of public health and health promotion. In this section, we briefly outline the evolution of population health from both disciplines.

Public health aims to reduce disease and maintain and promote the health of the whole population. The Committee for Inquiry into the Future Development of the Public Health Function (1988: 1) defined public health as:

> the art and science of preventing disease, promoting health, and prolonging life through organised efforts of society.

In the nineteenth century, public health was effective in reducing mortality and morbidity from infectious diseases in two main phases. The first was the environmental sanitation phase, approximately 1840–1890. The second phase was the period of the scientific control of communicable disease, based on bacteriological discoveries and the germ theory, between 1890 and 1910 (Beaglehole & Bonita, 2004).

Since the early twentieth century, public health has focused on the contribution of individual behaviours to non-communicable diseases and premature death (Kickbusch, 2003: 386). The relationship between an individual's life style, biological, psychosocial factors, and health behaviour and illness has been the underlying concept of public health activities.

Over the past five decades, globalisation and environmental issues have had significant impacts on the health of populations. Major international hallmarks of the growth of health promotion and population health are the Primary Health Care, the Declaration of Health for All by the Year 2000 and the Ottawa Charter of Health Promotion (WHO, 1978, 1986). Following studies by leading researchers in social epidemiology, including Syme et al. (1965) and Marmot and Syme (1976) (see also Berkman & Kawachi, 2000; Wilkinson & Marmot, 2003), one of the population health concerns has been the health inequality of different population groups. Another is environmental changes, which have major impact on population health. The inclusive term 'population health' has been increasingly used.

Beaglehole and Bonita (2004) indicate that current public health action is primarily on the determinants of health that lie outside the control of individuals. The essential elements of modern public health theory and practice are the collective responsibility for health and the significant role of the state in protecting and promoting the public's health, with its focus on whole populations and their working partnership with various multidisciplinary sectors. Other elements are prevention, especially the population strategy for primary prevention with a primary concern on the underlying socio-economic determinants of health and disease, as well as proximal risk factors. Both quantitative and qualitative methods are needed as appropriate (Chapter 3).

The goals of public health aim at population-wide health improvement, implying a concern to reduce health inequalities. The United States Association of Schools of Public Health stipulates that populations can be as small as a local neighbourhood or as big as the entire world (Association of Schools of Public Health, 2007).

In order to highlight social environment and policy, the context and meaning of health actions and the determinants of health actions have been included in our discussion. This helps orientate the positive aspects of what keeps people healthy (Kickbusch, 2003: 383). There are a number of countries, including Canada,

Sweden, the United Kingdom, Australia, and Germany, adopting the population health approach to address health issues. Healthy settings, increased access to effective health care services, and improving the opportunity of health through the life course are examples of population health programs.

Population health in Australia

In 1973, the Commonwealth government launched the Community Health Programme, with allocated funds. The structure of the program aimed to allow increased preventive health services, used more providers, and increased user participation in the organisation of services. It expected to revive Australian community health programs (Milio, 1983).

Over the past four decades, a number of initiatives addressing population health were founded. These initiatives have undergone changes following changes in health issues, research findings, and government policies, and the influence of professional bodies (Duckett, 2007). These initiatives have had various levels of success. Selected programs are listed below to outline their relevance to population health. Some are national programs; some are state-based with similar programs conducted in other states and territories. Some programs, such as installation of fire alarms and restrictions on smoking in public places, have legislation to enforce their adoption by individuals and groups.

- ➤ The National Health and Medical Research Council (NH&MRC) founded in 1936, universal national health insurance (Medicare) introduced in 1983, and the Australian government's Pharmaceutical Benefits Scheme (PBS) introduced in 1986
- ➤ Mass immunisation programs and initiatives: immunisations for infants, children, and high-risk groups including elderly people and people with low immunity
- ➤ Services for specific gender, age or ethnic groups (for example, services through women's health centres, breast cancer screening, men's health services, Queensland's 60 and Better Program, migrant health services, Aboriginal community-controlled health services)
- ➤ Research focusing on health and wellness issues (Women's Health Australia: the Australian Longitudinal Study on Women's Health, Australian Centre on Quality of Life, the Australian Longitudinal Study of Ageing, the Household, Income and Labour Dynamics in Australia (HILDA), Growing Up in Australia: The Longitudinal Study of Australian Children, Healthy Cities Project)

▸ Projects focusing on life styles and illness issues (10000 STEPS, Heart Foundation 'Just Walk It', healthy eating campaigns, Chronic Disease Self-Management Program, Accident Prevention Program, National Youth Suicide Prevention Strategy, National Tobacco Strategy, water fluoridation, fencing of swimming pools, and installation of fire alarms).

Characteristics of communities and their relationships with population health

Focusing on Australia

As mentioned earlier, a number of Australian population subgroups do not enjoy the same level of good health as the general population (AIHW, 2006; ABS, 2007b). Some groups have poorer health and health behaviour than others. It is important to understand the relationships between the diseases and health behaviours of population subgroups and their social, physical, demographic, and cultural characteristics. These characteristics certainly have direct or indirect impacts on their health.

Higgs and Gustafson (1985) defined a community as a group of people with a common identity or perspective, occupying space during a given period of time, and functioning through a social system to meet its needs within a social environment. People, place, and social interaction, including common interests or goals, are three critical characteristics of a community. In this volume, the terms 'population group' or 'aggregate' are synonyms for population.

Community: a group of people with a common identity or perspective, occupying space during a given period of time, and functioning through a social system to meet its needs within a social environment.

Social characteristics and population health

The major concept of social determinants of health has been widely supported by public health professionals, researchers, and academics. The concept has been based on a number of international and Australian studies (Ginzberg, 1999; Turrell et al., 1999; WHO, 1999; 2004). Income, employment, work, and education are some social characteristics related to the health of population groups.

In industrialised countries, having a good or adequate income helps individuals to gain resources to meet social and physical needs. Poverty in the form of an inadequate diet, overcrowding, poor sanitation, and lack of protection from risk factors can harm humans and cause disease (Le Fanu, 1999; Fitzpatrick, 2001).

At national and community levels, Ross (2004) reviewed data pertaining to 528 cities in the USA, United Kingdom, Australia, Sweden, and Canada, and found a strong association between income distribution and mortality. Lack of income is related to social isolation from opportunities to improve life through employment. People who live in many poor communities tend to distrust people of different groups, and have limited social connection to the community. However, an association between income inequality and mortality was not evident in the more egalitarian countries of Australia, Sweden, and Canada. Ross concluded that income inequality might have to reach a certain level to affect health.

Another measure of socio-economic status of a residential area is the Index of Relative Socio-Economic Status (ISRD). Information on education, occupation, income, family structure, race, ethnicity, and housing of different areas is used to compute the index, which indicates the relative socio-economic disadvantage of the area. In Australia, the percentage of people who live in the most disadvantaged areas who report poor health is higher than in the relatively more advantaged ISRD areas. Compared with people in more advantaged areas, those in disadvantaged areas have a higher rate of hospital admission, premature deaths, and death from avoidable causes (Glover & Tennant, 1999; Korda et al., 2007).

There is extensive literature linking unemployment with poor health outcomes in individuals. Bartley's review outlines a number of mechanisms that might account for the consistent relationship between unemployment and health, and these are very similar to the types of explanations often offered linking income inequality to poor health; the role of relative poverty, social isolation, loss of self-esteem, and the cultures of poor health behaviours (Wilkinson & Marmot, 2003).

Occupation is another frequently used indicator of socio-economic status. There are occupation-related diseases. For example, workers in an abattoir are at risk of having Q fever. The 2004–05 National Health Survey reported that adults who worked in the construction industry and tradespersons had a higher rate of having work related injuries than other occupations (ABS, 2006a).

At a population level, mortality data for Australian men and women aged 25–54 years for the period of 1998–2000 found that male blue-collar workers had an all-cause mortality rate of 234 deaths per 100,000 persons. The rate was higher than for males employed in managerial, administrative and professional occupations (115 deaths per 100,000 persons). A similar pattern was found among females (Draper et al., 2004).

It has been found that types of employment (Wilkinson & Marmot, 2003) that entail a lack of control over one's work are strongly related to an increased risk of low back pain, sickness-related absences, and cardiovascular disease. Stress in the workplace also increases sickness-related absences and premature death.

Education is another important indicator of socio-economic status, as it provides an opportunity for employment and various types of work. Education also helps an individual to gain and understand information relating to health. Women's education has an impact on health by changing women's expectations, raising awareness, and improving health behaviours. Educated women have better nutrition and use appropriate health services (Fitzpatrick, 2001).

Physical characteristics and population health

Physical characteristics can include roads, the built environment, and the availability of walkways or bicycles. The term 'built environment' has been used to explain how town and city designs and available roads and public transport influence the health of a population. These elements of the built environment determine the ability of individuals to move around to conduct their daily activities (Cohen et al., 2003; Wilkinson & Marmot, 2003; Hodgens, 2005).

Poor housing conditions, poor sanitation, poor neighbourhoods, and crowded households are some physical characteristics of areas with low socio-economic status. People living in crowded households are more likely to transmit parasitic and infectious diseases such as flu, colds, and lice (Cohen et al., 2003). Lack of public playgrounds and places for social interaction limit the opportunities for people to meet socially. The lack of social meetings has an impact on social isolation and poor psychological health, particularly with elderly people (Christchurch Community Mapping Project, 2004; Department of Communities, 2004).

Demographic characteristics and population health

In general, women live longer than men. The Australian male life expectancy in 2003 was 78 years, and the female life expectancy was 83 years. Compared to men, women generally tend to seek care when they are sick, have a healthy bodyweight, and eat foods with recommended nutrition levels, and they are less likely to smoke, drink alcohol, and use illicit drugs. Women are less likely to die from accidents, injuries, and self-harm while they are of working age (25–64 years). In recent years, more adolescent females (9.1 per cent) smoked daily than males (7.3 per cent). If there is no change in this behaviour, by 2025 the mortality rate due to lung cancer among women will increase (McDermott et al., 2002).

The variations in health of the population of different age groups can be caused by differences in immunity, developmental stage, and the ageing process. A high death rate during the perinatal period (0–28 days after birth) is related to the immaturity and low immunity of an infant (AIHW, 2006; Mohsin et al., 2006).

During adolescence, the death rate is relatively low compared to other age groups, but their developmental period is an underlying factor in their risk-taking behaviours. There has been an increasing number of young people using alcohol and illicit drugs recreationally. There is also an increasing proportion of overweight or obese children, and children with Type 1 diabetes (AIHW, 2006). Studies also indicate that slow growth and poor emotional support for young children increases their lifetime risk of poor physical health and reduced physical, cognitive, and emotional functioning in adulthood (Wilkinson & Marmot, 2003). The leading causes of deaths for adolescents are injuries, accidents, and self-harm.

Adults and working-age groups are people aged 25–64 years. This group includes the 'baby boomers', or those who were born between the end of World War II and the early 1960s. About one in five (19 per cent) of people of this age group live with a disability. Young adults, particularly young men, may have had spinal cord and brain injuries from vehicle accidents. Alcohol and work-related activities also contribute to injuries among adults. Premature deaths and a high rate of chronic diseases are observed among Indigenous Australians and Australians from groups with low socio-economic status.

Increasing age is related to long-term health conditions, higher rates of disability, and poorer reported health status among older people, defined as people aged 65 years and over. Population ageing and the health of older people are likely to have an impact on overall health resources. Older people often have one or more chronic illnesses, including mental health problem (AIHW, 2006; ABS, 2007b).

In 2004, the number of people aged 65 years or more in Australia was estimated to be 2.6 million, or 13 per cent of the total population. Long-term health conditions are more common with increasing age. In 2005, nearly 100 per cent of older people reported at least one long-term health condition. The most commonly reported conditions were diseases of the eye, musculoskeletal conditions, diseases of the circulatory system, osteoarthritis, and respiratory conditions. Accidental falls are also a significant health problem with ageing. More than one in ten reported a very high level of psychological distress (ABS, 2006b).

In 2005, almost half of all older people (48 per cent) were classified as either overweight or obese, and around 8 per cent of older people were current smokers (ABS, 2006b). Over time, older people experience loss, not only of a partner, but often also incremental loss of independence through disability and other factors associated with ageing. A higher percentage of older Australians is socially isolated than for younger age groups.

Geographic characteristics and population health

People who live in rural and remote areas have limited access to health care services. They may need to travel long distances to visit a general practitioner, use preventive health services, and receive comprehensive treatments for their illnesses. Due to their work and declined economy in an agricultural sector, men who live in rural and remote areas have a high rate of psychological problems, including stress and psychosis (Fuller et al., 2002; Jirojwong et al., 2005). People in rural and remote areas also have poorer health than people in metropolitan and regional areas.

Following the migration of retired people to non-metropolitan areas in many states except Tasmania, there is a change in the demographic characteristics of people in regional, rural, and remote areas. An increased proportion of people aged 65 years and over, and more older women than older men, return to be close to family in non-metropolitan areas (Bell, 1995; Hugo, 2002). Since 2000, there has been a huge growth in the mining industry. A high proportion of mine workers travel to work on shift work on a fly-in fly-out basis, and this may be related to more family breakdown and children with behaviour problems (Gent, 2004).

Geography is also related to season, temperature, and humidity. People who live in tropical areas are at risk of exposure to more UV light and of having haemorrhagic fever and Ross River fever, with mosquitoes as a carrier. Children living in a tropical area and exposed to UV light are at risk of developing skin cancer when they reach adulthood (MacLennan et al., 1992, 1999).

Cultural characteristics and population health

Culture influences individuals' perception of health, behaviours to maintain health, response to a symptom of an illness, and types of care they seek (Kleinman, 1980; Huff & Kline, 1999). Australian migrants may have limited access to health care services. Migrants are healthier than the Australian-born population, due to self-selection and selection processes of the Australian government leading to 'healthy migrant effects' (Liamputtong Rice, 1999; Liamputtong et al., 2003). Despite relatively good health, migrants from Asian countries are less likely to exercise than Australian-born people. Female migrants are less likely to undergo cervical cancer screening or breast cancer screening (Kelaher et al., 1998; Jirojwong & Manderson, 1999, 2002; AIHW, 2003). More Lebanese-born men smoke than Australian-born men (Rissel et al., 1998). The longer migrants live in Australia, the higher the percentage that are overweight or obese. An adoption of new health behaviours, including food intake, by migrants is a good example of a relationship between the population's health and a community (Wahlqvist, 2002) (see Figure 1.1).

The effect of culture on health of the population is also evident among Australian Aboriginal people. Australian Aborigines are the most disadvantaged group, with a poor health status that is similar to people in many developing countries. The complexity of biological, cultural, social, and psychological issues, and a history of colonisation, have led to family breakdown, poor psychological health, high rates of alcohol and substance abuse, and high rates of chronic diseases and premature death. Chapter 4 discusses the health of Australian Aborigines specifically, and provides examples of effective health promotion programs. Chapter 12 discusses issues relating to the delivery of health promotion programs in Australian migrant populations.

In summary, the health of a population group is influenced by their social, physical, demographic, and cultural characteristics. These characteristics are also interrelated, and their complexity determines the health promotion programs that need to be provided to address a particular health issue. Active involvement of the population group is also required to ensure the success of the program. Therefore, it is important to gain knowledge relating to relationships between characteristics of a community and the delivery of a health program.

Characteristics of communities and their relationships with health promotion

We contend that at least three major components need to be considered when designing a health promotion intervention: the level of organisation that the intervention targets (individual, group, or society), the theory or framework to be applied in the intervention, and the characteristics of the target community. We discuss the first two components in detail in Chapter 2, but the need to consider the characteristics of a community is discussed below.

Health promotion interventions can target an individual or group, or act at society level. The interventions also can range from promoting health at a healthy stage to rehabilitating physical and psychological functions at an illness stage. In order to address a health issue in a particular group, their characteristics, categorised by social, physical, demographic, and cultural factors, need to be understood, as these will influence the type of health promotion message, mode of delivery, target groups, and the size of the target groups. The attractiveness, appropriate language, congruence, and presentation of the health promotion message all have to be suitable for the age group and the socio-economic status of the target group (Egger et al., 1999). For example, a mental health care team aimed to increase an awareness of mental health services among adolescent students needs to design the content, packaging of the message, and method of message delivery by getting direct input from the target group.

In order to reach target groups whose first language is not English, the message needs to be linguistically and culturally appropriate. For example, a breast cancer screening campaign targeting Chinese women in Sydney had a message focusing on preserving and promoting health and overall well-being in everyday life, rather than attempting to detect hidden disease by screening. The message was delivered via the Chinese-language radio station to which the majority of the women listened. It was also aired at the time when the women were at home (Kwok &

Sullivan, 2007). Pictorial messages with a story presentation are more acceptable to Australian Aboriginal people than using a text message. English literacy, culture, and beliefs are underlying reasons for using such a design (Vindigni et al., 2004; Hermeston, 2005).

At the organisation level, a health promotion intervention may be delivered at a workplace, a general practitioner clinic, or a hospital, according to the health issue and the occupation of the target group. Examples of health promotion interventions in a workplace are regular hand, arm and shoulder exercises in a workplace to reduce repetitive strain injuries among typists, and compulsory immunisation to protect against Q fever among workers in an abattoir (Department of Health and Ageing, 2003). A general practitioner clinic and a hospital are settings where a number of health promotion programs are expected to be delivered to people with particular diseases. These include an asthma management program and chronic disease self-management projects (NHMRC, 2007).

Current issues in population health and health promotion

During the early 1980s, the term 'health promotion' was increasingly used due to the perceived top-down approach of health education and disease prevention. In 1986, the Ottawa Charter on Health Promotion was adopted by the World Health Organization as a strategy to reduce the burden of chronic diseases (WHO, 1986). Social epidemiology studies have shown that social and economic factors at a community or population level are increasingly important to explain the health inequity of different population groups. There is a distinction between population health and individual health, and the relative influence of various factors on each.

It can be said that population health and health promotion are relatively new and have gained momentum in public health in the past four decades. It is important to acknowledge that no single widely accepted definition of population health exists. Kindig and Stoddart (2003: 381) call for debates of their proposed definition: 'Population health is the health of groups, families and communities. Populations may be defined as locality, biological criteria such as age, gender, social criteria such as socio-economic status or cultural criteria.'

There are a number of current issues in population health and health promotion (Abel et al., 2007; McQueen et al., 2007; Rootman et al., 2007). Some of these are:

➤ difficulties in measuring the effectiveness of health promotion interventions and programs targeted at a population due to long lead times to measure

outcomes and the complexity of factors determining health behaviours of the population
- the lack of a model to be used for operationalisation, which limits the ability to compare interventions across different settings and cultural contexts
- difficulties in translating research results, in particular findings from social epidemiology studies to health interventions, and
- the shift towards wellness for health interventions needing clearly defined outcomes and standardised measurement tools.

Conclusion

This chapter aimed to provide general information relating to communities, population health, and health promotion. We have discussed basic concepts of health, disease, and illness and have provided examples of illness and wellness measurements in order to understand better how health can be compared through time and across different settings. Some models of health and the context of the model's development are outlined. The evolution of the concept of population health, and its relationship with the characteristics of a community, have also been discussed, based on reviewed studies and discussions in the field. We have also described the importance of community characteristics to the design of a health promotion program, and included current issues relating to population health and health promotion. What we have done is to set the scene for this volume, and we hope that it has served as a basic framework for the chapters to come.

CRITICAL THINKING EXERCISES

1. You are required to talk to three people. The first is a person with long-term illness, the second is a healthy adolescent, and the third is a person from a non-English-speaking background. Ask each person:
   - How do they know that they are healthy?
   - What makes them healthy?
   - What was the last time they were sick? What was the sickness?
   - What did they do to get over the sickness?

2. Search the publications by the Australian Institute of Health and Welfare and the Australian Bureau of Statistics to compare the health status of the general Australian population and Aboriginal people. Use the following measurements:

> life expectancy
> self-assessed health status.

How can these differences in health status be explained by genetics and social institutions? Use Figure 1.1 as a guide for discussion.

FURTHER READING

Ashton, J. (ed.) (1992) *Healthy Cities*. Open University Press: Philadelphia.

Baum, F. (2008) *The New Public Health: An Australian Perspective*. Oxford University Press: Melbourne.

Beaglehole, R., & Bonita, R. (eds) (2004) *Public Health at the Crossroads: Achievements and Prospects.* Cambridge University Press: Cambridge.

Friedman, D.J., & Starfield, B. (2003) Editorial: Models of Population Health: Their Value for US Public Health Practice, Policy, and Research. *American Journal of Public Health*, 93(3): 366–9.

Germov, J. (ed.) (2005) *Second Opinion: An Introduction to Health Sociology.* Oxford University Press: Melbourne.

Moodie, R. (ed.) (2004) *Hands-on Health Promotion*. IP Communications: East Hawthorn.

WEBPAGE RESOURCES

Expert Patients Programme: www.expertpatients.co.uk/public/default.aspx. Provides information about a type of self-help group. A similar Australian program is the Chronic Disease Management program.

Health Promoting Hospital: www.euro.who.int/healthpromohosp. One of the World Health Organization programs that is likely to serve as a model in many developed and developing countries.

Healthy Cities: www.euro.who.int/healthy-cities. The site of the initial international health promotion program.

Social Determinants of Health: www.euro.who.int/document/e81384.pdf. Has summaries of research in developed and developing countries.

Population Health: www.health.nsw.gov.au/org_structure. An example of the development of population health programs at a state level in New South Wales.

The Australian Institute of Health and Welfare (AIHW): www.aihw.gov.au. Good source of federal government publications.

World Health Organization: www.who.int. A number of publications can be found at this website.

Sansnee Jirojwong & Pranee Liamputtong

2

Primary Health Care and Health Promotion

Sansnee Jirojwong &
Pranee Liamputtong

Objectives

After reading this chapter, readers will be able to:

➤ Explain the development of primary health care and health promotion in the context of changing health and illness patterns and the determinants of health at individual, society and community levels

➤ Understand concepts of health promotion models and theories and their use at different organisational levels

➤ Describe underlying reasons for the development of health promotion programs at global, national and local levels

➤ Analyse the use of models and theories in health promotion.

Key terms

communication
model
social integration
social network
theory

Introduction

In 1978, primary health care (PHC) was adopted by the World Health Organization as the major principle of health care delivery. 'Health for all by the year 2000' was announced as the aim to be achieved by many countries. Since then, PHC has been used as a philosophy of health services, and has served as the foundation of subsequent health developments including health promotion and population health (Ashton, 1992a; Hills & McQueen, 2007). In this chapter, we describe the development of PHC and health promotion over the past thirty years. We provide examples of health promotion in an organisation and among population groups. We also explain eight selected health promotion theories and models that are frequently applied in health practices and research projects.

Primary health care and its development in developed and developing countries

As a part of the increasing postwar scientific and technology developments, a number of antibiotics, steroids, and therapeutic innovations were invented and used for treatments. These medical technologies for curative services and specialist care led to increased health costs. In the late 1970s, leaders in medical and public health fields pointed to limited benefits of newly developed medical technologies, and curative and pharmaceutical services on individuals' health, and the inability to maintain the use of curative services (WHO, 1978: 37–8; Le Fanu, 1999: 242).

In 1978, an important joint meeting between the World Health Organization and UNICEF was held at Alma-Ata, in the Soviet Union. As a result, the Declaration of Alma-Ata, which adopted primary health care (PHC) as the principal mechanism of health care delivery, was formally passed. 'Health for all by the year 2000' was the aim of this declaration. The essential elements of the declaration were that health is seen as a fundamental human right (WHO, 1978). There is inequality in the health of people within a country and between countries. Social and economic development is required to reduce this health inequality. Individuals and communities need to be actively involved in the planning and implementation of health care, with self-reliance and self-determination essential to that involvement.

The declaration also emphasises health promotion and protection as essential health components which contribute to a better quality of life, and that these should use socially acceptable methods and technology at a cost that the community and country can afford. The main health problems can be addressed by the provision of health promotion, prevention, curative, and rehabilitation services.

Sansnee Jirojwong & Pranee Liamputtong

Governments have responsibility for the health of their population through the provision of adequate health and social measures. Health sectors and non-health sectors should work together in coordinated efforts. Political action and cooperation between countries are required to formulate partnerships and to ensure that health benefits are distributed to people in every country. Primary health care should be an integral part of the health care system, and the community's overall social and economic development should proceed in the spirit of social justice. Primary health care is also the first level of contact with the health system.

In the following sections, we describe various strategies used to adopt PHC by developing and developed countries. The main purpose is to outline the variations in translating a global health care philosophy into practical activities at national and local levels. Similar issues are also likely to be found when applying the Ottawa Charter of Health Promotion in different contexts and settings.

Primary health care in developing countries

The concept of PHC has been widely adopted in many developing countries, and various programs have been initiated using PHC as their philosophy. One example is the expansion of the scope of practices of health care personnel. Nurses, traditional birth attendants, and volunteer health workers have been educated and trained in order to provide curative, health promotion, and disease prevention services (Flahault & Roemer, 1986). They collect health surveillance data at a local community level. 'Low cost' health care services have also been developed. The use of traditional health care methods, including herbal medicines and acupuncture, has been encouraged or its effectiveness explored further. Maternal and child health services, including family planning, are delivered in rural communities and in densely populated metropolitan areas in cities (Flahault & Roemer, 1986; Mir, 1998).

Primary health care in developed countries

Compared to developing countries, application of PHC in developed countries has been relatively slower. A number of health care initiatives have been developed to improve the health of high-risk groups, including children and teenage mothers. These initiatives use the input and participation of the target groups or key stakeholders as a part of their planning, implementation, and evaluation (Gottschalk & Baker, 2004).

However, criticism of PHC includes the unrealistic aims and difficulties in translating it into health care policies. The fundamental changes in some countries have been minimal. Some health practitioners and planners perceive PHC as just for developing countries (Wass, 2000). This probably could be explained by the emphasis on 'developing countries' in the Alma-Ata Declaration (WHO, 1978). Wass (2000: 10–11) also indicates that there was confusion between PHC and primary medical care or primary care, primary nursing, community-based health care, and the Third World health care.

In Australia, a few initiatives have been developed that adopt PHC components. Efforts have been made to provide health promotion services and coordinated health care throughout the community health program. The program has had some success for various reasons, despite the lack of cohesion of various health care organisations (see detailed discussion in Duckett, 2007: 221–65). Other national initiatives, including the National Better Health Program, the National Public Health Partnership and the Australian Better Health Initiatives have been developed using the PHC philosophy and health promotion as a framework. An example is the Better Health Commission, developed in 1986 and aimed to reduce the impact of three health issues: injury, cardiovascular disease, and poor nutrition.

The fragmentation of Australian health services is a major barrier to the full adoption of PHC. The report by Malcolm (1994) stated that there was a need for a clear health strategic direction and coordination at the national level. The different roles of a national health promotion program and the national Health for All strategy also needed to be clarified.

Since 2006, the federal government, along with the states and territories, has agreed to strengthen the focus of the health care system on prevention, health promotion, and management of chronic diseases. The Australian Better Health Initiative has been developed to reduce the impact of chronic diseases. Broad components of PHC and health promotion have been applied. Five major approaches of the Australian Better Health Initiative are: promoting healthier life styles, supporting early detection of risk factors and chronic disease, supporting lifestyle and risk modification, encouraging active patient self-management of chronic conditions, and improving communication and coordination between services and the introduction of care coordinators (Department of Health and Ageing, 2006). The focus of these approaches is mainly at an individual level, while there is a need to address underlying risk factors at a community or population level (Turrell et al., 1999; Duckett, 2007).

The Ottawa Charter of Health Promotion

During the early 1980s, the term 'health promotion' was increasingly used by health promotion practitioners. Health promotion combines health education and specific interventions (Modeste & Tamayose, 2004: 680). Increased and recognisable roles of health promotion at the global level primarily originated at the PHC declaration and the introduction of the Ottawa Charter of Health Promotion (Ashton, 1992a: Hills & McQueen, 2007).

In 1986, the Ottawa Charter of Health Promotion was adopted at an international conference in Ottawa, Canada. Many sources, including the reports by Lalonde (1974), Department of Health and Social Security, United Kingdom (1976), and McKeown (1979) were used for the development of the charter. The charter clearly stated the prerequisites for health, including peace, a stable ecosystem, social justice and equity, and resources such as education and income (WHO, 1986). It highlighted the roles of organisations, systems, and communities, as well as individual behaviours and capacities, in creating choices and opportunities for better health. The Ottawa Charter's five health promotion strategies are building healthy public policy, creating supportive environments, strengthening community actions, developing personal skills, and reorientating health services.

Building healthy public policy

The policy should combine diverse and complementary approaches, including legislation, fiscal measures, and organisational change. It fosters greater equity and contributes to ensuring healthier goods and services, healthier public services, and cleaner, more enjoyable environments.

Creating supportive environments

Reciprocal maintenance of individuals, communities, and natural environment is needed to ensure the promotion of living and working conditions that are safe, stimulating, satisfying, and enjoyable. The protection of the natural and built environments and the conservation of natural resources must be addressed in a health promotion strategy.

Strengthening community actions

Community empowerment is needed throughout a health promotion process. Existing human and material resources in the community need to be developed with flexible systems so that self-help and social support can be enhanced.

Developing personal skills

Information, education for health, and enhancing life skills will help the development of personal and social skills. This development will assist people to exercise more control over their own health and environments. Health promotion should enable people to learn, and then prepare them to cope with chronic ill and injuries.

Reorientating health services

Health promotion is shared between individuals, and government and non-government sectors through collaborative efforts. The health sector must increasingly move beyond clinical and curative services in the direction of health promotion. Health services need to focus on the total needs of the individual as a whole person, and be sensitive to and respect their cultural needs. Reorientating health services also requires research and professional education and training.

Since the Ottawa Charter in 1986, a series of follow-up conferences has been organised, with a specific health promotion strategy being explored (Catford, 2007). For example, the 'building healthy public policy' strategy was further discussed in 1988 at the Second International Conference in Adelaide, Australia. The beneficial results of health promotion policies and practices on health and quality of life of people in developing countries was also emphasised at the Fifth Conference in Mexico. Significant changes in the world, and better understanding of the determinants of health, have also been considered as an additional context of health promotion. These changes include internet usage, knowledge about the human genome, climate change, terrorism, Third World debt, and globalisation. At the 2007 International Union for Health Promotion and Education (IUHPE) Conference in Canada, the social determinants of health were also explored in depth (see also Chapter 1).

Health promotion: International, national, and local levels

Health promotion was initially driven by many developed countries so that the primary health care philosophy and the aim of Health for All would be taken up (WHO, 1986: 1). Since Ottawa, health promotion has been widely integrated into health care policies in many developed and developing countries in order to improve the population's health (Kickbusch, 2007). Examples are Health21: The Health for All Policy Framework for the WHO European Region, and the USA's Healthy People 2010. They emphasise health promotion and disease prevention as important components of health care services to address the impact of chronic diseases in developed and developing countries (WHO European Region, 1999a, 1999b; Department of Health and Human Services, USA, 2005).

Health21 has specific targets to be achieved by 2020 in 51 countries in the European Union that range from highly developed socio-economically to poorly developed Eastern European countries. It has excellent examples of specific targets with a defined timeframe (WHO, 1999a: 6; 1999b: 177–202). Various health promotion initiatives, including the Health Promoting Hospital, have been developed to reach these specific targets. Other countries, including Australia, have gained knowledge from research results of these Health21 initiatives (Department of Human Services, 2002).

Australia has also been one of the leading countries in pioneering health promotion as an essential part of health care services. As mentioned above, a few national initiatives, including the National Better Health Program, the National Public Health Partnership, and the Australian Better Health Initiatives, have been developed using the PHC philosophy and health promotion as a framework. Duckett (2007) has analysed the policy developments of these health promotion initiatives. Compared with other initiatives, the Australian Better Health Initiatives has a holistic approach to addressing chronic diseases and focusing on the individual level. However, programs that focus on social and community levels are needed (see also Duckett, 2007: 207–20).

At the local government level, a National Public Health Partnership project explored the role of local government in public health regulation (National Public Health Partnership, 2002). The results show that there are substantial differences between the content and function of local government and public health legislation in each jurisdiction. However, there are some common functions shared by the majority of local governments, and these include the prevention and control of infectious disease, control of nuisances and offensive trades, food safety, and responding to emergency situations (National Public Health Partnership, 2002: 69). Several health promotion projects have been conducted and some demonstrate strong partnership between local governments, state governments, health services, non-health services, and volunteer organisations.

Health promotion: Healthy settings

The first major international health promotion program was the Healthy Cities program, which originated in 1986 (Ashton, 1992b: xiii). It was based on the principle that health is created by people within the settings of their everyday life (WHO, 1986: 3). Each setting should have physical and social environments contributing to the health and well-being of individuals and the communities in which they live, work, rest, and take their leisure. The framework of the Healthy Cities program for a public health policy is a group of executive decision-makers who take a strategic overview of health in the city. It aims to develop healthy urban communities through on-going changes in the environment and ecological systems (see also Ashton, 1992b; Goldstein, 1992). The program is perceived to be a 'field laboratory' for testing health promotion strategies at the local level, and has grown to include more than 800 cities (Tsouros, 1995; Harpham et al., 2001). In 1987, three locations in Australia—Canberra (ACT), Illawarra (New South Wales) and Noarlunga (South Australia)—served as pilot sites for the Healthy Cities program (Kaplan 1992: 57–58). Each location had its own strategies and activities and achieved different levels of success. These ranged from putting the public health on the political agenda, using volunteers and local organisations' collaborative efforts to clean up Lake Illawarra, and bringing conflicting groups together to discuss the issue of clean water for the southern suburbs of Adelaide.

The idea of the 'healthy setting' has developed substantially. At an international level, the Health Promoting Hospital project and Health Promoting Universities are other programs with their own networks and conferences to exchange information (WHO, 2007). The overall concept of Health Promoting Hospitals is broad and complex, and includes the reduction of hospital waste, provision of a healthy working environment for workers, and promoting health behaviours of patients (WHO, 2007). The underlying characteristics of each healthy setting also differ from one setting to another (see also Moodie & Hulme, 2004). Examples of Australian 'healthy settings' are Healthy Schools and the on-going Healthy Cities (Department of Health and Ageing, 2007; Alliance for Healthy Cities, 2007).

Health promotion: Healthy population groups

In this section, we focus on elderly people as an example of a population group targeted by health promotion programs. Elderly people are defined as people aged 65 years and older. The impact of their health and illness status is significant for several reasons. First, the percentage of this age group in the population is projected to increase from 13.0 per cent of total population (2.6 million) in 2004 to 20 per cent of total population (5.0 million) in 2024. Second, they will typically have one or more degenerative diseases, and these will require health care resources. The older people become, the greater the level of disease severity. Third, the proportion of elderly Australians from culturally and linguistically diverse (CALD) backgrounds will increase from 20 per cent of older Australians (518,100) in 2003 to 22.5 per cent of older Australians (939,800) in 2026. The CALD population ages more rapidly than other Australians as a consequence of migration patterns and the age at arrival of CALD migrants (AIHW, 2002, 2004a, 2004b, 2005, 2006), and they need health care services that are culturally and linguistically sensitive to their needs. Fourth, elderly people tend to have limited financial resources. A high proportion (80 per cent) receives an age pension or a Department of Veterans' Affairs pension (AIHW, 2005).

Ill health is not a criterion of ageing; however, certain diseases are more frequent in older people. Older people can have a high quality of life throughout their old age, as indicated by several studies among older Japanese (Tsuji et al., 1995). In Australia, the majority of older people (74.1 per cent) still live in a private residence. Less than half (44.7 per cent) require assistance from private and government organisations, and 21.5 per cent have severe or profound limitations to their ability to conduct their core daily activities (see AIHW, 2005). However, when they need carers, sometimes these carers are not well themselves (Cummins & Hughes, 2007).

Some of the aims of the current Australian Better Health Initiatives are to manage chronic diseases and to strengthen the focus of the health system on disease prevention and health promotion. A range of health promotion projects has received financial support to address the needs of elderly people. Two of these are the Self-Management of Chronic Diseases and Lifestyle Prescriptions programs, which aim to provide comprehensive health checks for older people to improve their quality of life (Department of Health and Ageing, 2006). Other wellness programs focusing on a social model of health developed at state and local government levels include the 60 and Better Program and the University of the Third Age (U3A), which help older people to develop social support and increase their skills and knowledge of current issues (Rockhampton–60 and Better Program, 2007; University of the Third Age, Adelaide, 2007).

Most of the Australian health promotion programs focus on the individual, with some attention paid to the spiritual and psychological aspects of health. The outcomes for this particular population group still need to be assessed. However, for older people from some cultural backgrounds, such as Spanish and Japanese, family members have significant roles in maintaining the health of their elders (Sheykhi, 2007). It will be a challenge to design health programs that target older people within the context of their family and community.

Health promotion: Theories and models

The complexity of human behaviour in relation to preventing a disease and promoting health can be demonstrated by the decreasing rate of smoking among the middle-aged while a high percentage of young girls are now taking up smoking (McDermott et al., 2002). The benefits of exercise are known to the general public, but the rate of obesity and numbers with a sedentary life style have increased (AIHW, 2006).

The process of taking up positive health behaviours or giving up a negative behaviour may not be the same as when both these actions are undertaken simultaneously. The complexity of the factors influencing health is also shown by the results of epidemiological studies (see also Chen et al., 1992; Marmot & Wilkinson 1999; Berkman & Kawachi, 2000). Reducing the risk of having a chronic disease may require changes in a range of behaviours. For example, weight reduction as measured by body mass index may not help reduce the risk of having cardiovascular disease or diabetes (Hodge et al., 2004).

A theoretical framework helps program developers and researchers to organise knowledge and interpret factors and events. It helps to describe the at-risk and intervention groups, and understand health-promoting behaviour and environmental conditions. It describes possible determinants of both risk and health behaviours, and identifies methods to promote changes in the determinants, behaviours, and environmental conditions (Bartholomew et al., 2006: 82). A theory and model is chosen in order to meet the objectives of the program. For example, the 'health belief model' aims for change in the individual, and the 'ecological model of health behaviour' aims for change at a community level. Theories and models can be categorised according to the level of organisation, including individual, interpersonal, organisation, and community levels (see Figure 2.1).

Theory: an integrated set of propositions that serves as an explanation for a phenomenon. It is introduced after a phenomenon has already revealed a systematic set of uniformities.

FIGURE 2.1 Health promotion approaches at different organisational levels

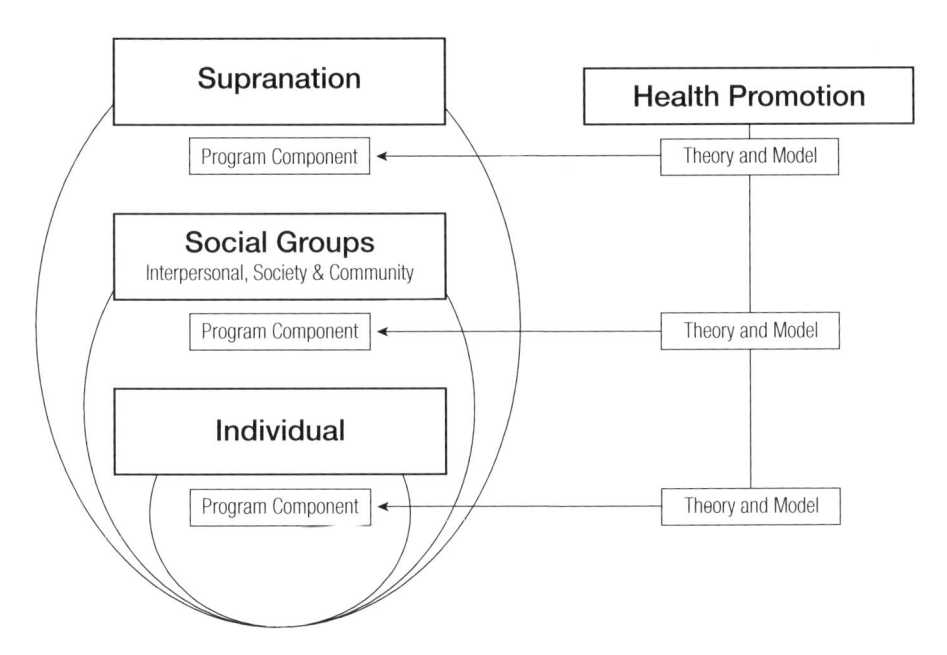

Source: Modified from Richard et al. (1996) and Germov (2005)

Model: a subclass of a theory, providing a plan for investigating or addressing a phenomenon. It does not attempt to explain processes, only to represent them. It also provides the vehicle for applying the theories.

There are more than forty models and theories used in health promotion. We describe eight models here as they are frequently used by researchers and practitioners. Some other models and theories are listed in Appendix 1. Combinations of different models are also used. An example is Pender's health promotion model (Pender, 1996).

Behaviour change theories: Individual level

Three models used to explain the behaviour changes at an individual level are briefly described in this section: the health belief model, the theory of reasoned action, and the transtheoretical model of change.

Health belief model (HBM)

This model is based on cognitive expectation (Rosenstock, 1974). Human behaviour depends mainly on the value that an individual places on a particular goal and on the individual's estimate of the likelihood that a given action will achieve that goal. People want to avoid illness or to get well, and to believe that a specific behaviour will prevent or reduce illness. The HBM comprises the major variables:

- perceived susceptibility: a person's subjective perception of the risk of contracting a particular condition or illness
- perceived severity: a person's feelings concerning the seriousness of contracting an illness
- perceived benefits: a person's beliefs regarding the effectiveness of various actions available to reduce the threat of a disease
- perceived barriers: potentially negative aspects of a particular health action
- self-efficacy: the conviction that one can successfully execute the behaviour required to produce the outcomes.

There are other modifying factors included in the model (Rosenstock, 1974). These include age, sex, personality, cue to action, and knowledge about the illness or health promotion behaviour.

Theory of reasoned action

The theory of reasoned action and the similar theory of planned behaviour are concerned with individual motivational factors as determinants of the likelihood of performing a specific behaviour. The theory of reasoned action is a highly specific theory outlining cognitive and attitudinal determinants of behaviour. Attitudes and subjective norms determine a person's intentions, which are predictive of behaviour. Attitudes are composed of two beliefs: to what extent the participant believes a certain behaviour will lead to a certain consequence, and whether or not the participant values the consequence. Social norms also are measured by using two constructs: the participant's perception of his or her referent group's desires, and the participant's predilection to conform to the referent group's desires (Montaño & Kasprzyk, 2002; Bartholomew et al., 2006).

Transtheoretical model (TTM) of change

The transtheoretical model of change has two major sets of constructs: stages of change, and process of change. In the stages of change, people are thought to move from having no motivation to change to internalising the new behaviour. Prochaska and colleagues (2002) list the stages as follows:

➤ precontemplation, in which people have no intention of changing their behaviour
➤ contemplation, in which people are thinking about changing the problem behaviour in the future
➤ preparation, in which people are planning to change the behaviour in the short term and are taking steps to get ready for the change
➤ action, in which people have recently changed the behaviour
➤ maintenance, in which people have performed the new behaviour for a required time frame.

People in the action and maintenance stages may lapse and then return to action, or relapse to contemplation or even precontemplation. The stages are consistent with predisposing, enabling and reinforcing factors in the PRECEDE model (Chapter 8) and represent a time course for examining when shifts in attitudes, intentions, and behaviours occur. Change may involve multiple techniques, methods, and interventions. Change processes include consciousness raising, self-reevaluation, improving self-efficacy and skills, relevancy, tailoring, and individualisation (Frankish et al., 1999: 58; Bartholomew et al., 2006: 113–15).

Behaviour change theories: Group level

When group interactions are a component of a health promotion program, appropriate behavioural change theories at this level need to be considered. Social relationships can affect individuals' health behaviours, decision-making, and health status. Two theories at a group level, the social networks and social support theory, and diffusion of innovation, are described in this section. Other theoretical frameworks, including community organisation and capacity building, are also useful when designing a health promotion to operate at a group level.

Sansnee Jirojwong & Pranee Liamputtong

Social networks and social support

Social integration: the existence of social ties.

Social network: the web of social relationships that surround individuals. The provision of social support is one of the important functions of social relationships.

A social network is an analytic framework for understanding relationships among members of social systems. Networks are classified as either personal or the whole network. The personal or egocentric network is based on the ties an individual has with other people, while the whole network allows the identification of cliques of individuals and the identification of roles, such as occupational positions, that extend across networks and act as boundary spanners.

Networks can be horizontal (peers) or vertical (hierarchy) and can provide a way to understand power relationships in organisations. A community can be understood as networks of networks in which the nodes of the larger network consist of smaller-scale networks. Individuals in the network provide social support, defined as aid and assistance exchanged through social relationships and interpersonal transactions (Heaney & Israel, 2002). Four main types of social support are emotional (affective), instrumental (tangible), information (cognitive), and appraisal supports. Different types of social networks are associated with specific types of social support.

Diffusion of innovation

An innovation is an idea, practice or product that is new to the adopter, which may be an individual or an organisation. For example, Self-Management of Chronic Disease or Health Promoting Hospital may be an innovation in an organisation. According to Bartholomew and colleagues (2006: 132), diffusion should be thought of as moving from awareness of an innovation, through a decision to adopt the innovation, to initial use and maintenance. From an organisational perspective, there are essentially three stages:

- adoption, which depends on knowledge of an innovation, awareness of an unmet need, and the decision that a certain innovation may meet the perceived need and will be given a trial
- implementation, or the use of innovation to a trial point
- sustainability, or the maintenance and institutionalisation of an innovation or its outcomes.

The adopters need to assess the innovation and their current 'products'. They evaluate the relative advantage of the innovation compared to what is being used and its compatibility with the intended users' current behaviour. Other aspects of the innovation being assessed are its complexity, potential results, impact on social relations, reversibility in case of discontinuation, communicability, required time, risk and uncertainty, required commitment, and ability to modify. The diffusion of innovation model can be combined with other theories targeted at an individual level.

Behaviour change theories: Population level

Social marketing and the ecological model of health behaviour are examples that guide health promotion at a community or population level.

Social marketing

Social marketing is the application of commercial marketing technologies to the analysis, planning, execution, and evaluation of programs designed to influence the voluntary behaviour of target audiences in order to improve their personal welfare and that of their society (Baibach et al., 2002: 438). Rothschild (1999) includes mutual fulfilment of self-interest through voluntary exchange. Social marketing defines success primarily in terms of benefits to members of the target market or to society as a whole. It could be compared to commercial marketing, which focuses on financial gain as the indicator of its success.

Baibach and others (2002) clearly indicate that education is often a component of marketing. The benefits of a recommended behaviour are attractive when the barriers are minor. The use of incentives and other benefits reinforces the desired behaviour, and direct benefits are an immediate reinforcement. Social marketing programs make every effort to identify and reduce barriers that interfere with the target members' ability to perform the desired behaviour. The use of law is another approach to behavioural influence. The elements of marketing are known as the four Ps—product, price, place, and promotion—and are also used by promoters. Product is the overall benefit, and the price is the reduction of the overall barriers of cost. Place is delivering the benefits and costs to the right place at the right time. Promotion is informing and persuading the consumers about the costs and benefits, and also involves communication or education.

Communication and media

Communication is defined as the production and exchange of information and meaning by use of signs and symbols (Finnegan & Viswanath, 2002: 361). It involves processes of encoding, transmission, reception or decoding, and synthesis of information and meaning. Some key components of communication are the sender, the content or message, the channel, the receiver, and the effect. The effect of communication on health behaviour at a micro level can be provided by an individual's social network through interpersonal communication. At a macro level, communication can be made through mass media. Kegler and colleagues

(2002: 368) comment that when both mass media and individualised media programs are used and these have an effects on a significant influential group, the changes in this group will become another important source of change for a larger section of the population.

Various steps are needed to communicate health information to a community. They include identifying the scope and sequence of the program, having a program theme, and selecting a channel and vehicle to deliver the information (Bartholomew et al., 2006: 380–438; see also Finnegan & Viswanath, 2002). For example, the theme 'Go for 2 Fruit and 5 vegetables' uses billboards and posters as vehicles, and display print as a communication channel. Computer-assisted interventions and computerised tailoring of interventions have also been increasingly used to target a selected population group.

Communication: the production and exchange of information and meaning by use of signs and symbols.

The ecological model of health behaviour

The development of the ecological model of health behaviour was based on studies by several researchers, including McLeroy and colleagues (1988), Bronfenbrenner (1979), and Sallis and Owen (2002). McLeroy and others proposed that health behaviour has five levels of influence: intrapersonal factors, interpersonal processes and primary groups, institutional factors, community factors, and public policy.

There are four assumptions:

- that health is influenced by multiple facets of the physical and social environments
- that environments are multidimensional and can be social, physical, actual, or perceived
- that human–environment interactions can be described at varying levels of aggregation: individuals, families, work, cultural organisations, communities, and whole populations
- that there is feedback across different levels of environments and aggregates of persons.

Although this has been accepted as a useful model to improve a population's health, there is a need to operationalise and apply the model more specifically to health behaviour change and to evaluate the effectiveness of multilevel interventions (Sallis & Owen, 2002).

There are also other theories and models used in health promotion, some of which help health promotion planners understand why a program is effective with the target population group. If it is not effective, reasons for such failure can be identified through a monitoring and evaluation process. This monitoring and evaluation process is crucial, and is discussed in Chapters 14 and 15. Chapter 8 discusses the PROCEDE–PROCEED model in detail as it is useful for planning a health program targeted at the population level.

Conclusion

In this chapter, we have thus far described the brief history of primary health care and health promotion at global, national, and local levels, and major concepts behind it. We have suggested that a range of health promotion programs have been developed in order to reduce the impact of chronic diseases. We have also suggested various theories and models that can be used to explain an individual's health behaviours, and other theories that have been developed to design a program while taking into account group interactions and the complexity of a population. We suggest that students and health practitioners need to select a theory or model appropriate to the health issue and the target group with which they are concerned.

CRITICAL THINKING EXERCISES

1. A number of health promotion programs have been developed to reduce health problems. List two of these programs and use them to answer the following questions:
   - Is there any media or advertisement used to increase the adoption of health behaviours among the target group? List three types of these media.
   - Is the message easily understood by its target audience? Explain your reasons.

2. In the recent years, immunisation against cervical cancer has been recommended to young women. However, there is resistance to this immunisation as some parents believe that it will lead to promiscuity. What health promotion theories can be used to reduce these beliefs?

FURTHER READING

Duckett, S.J. (2007) *The Australian Health Care System*. Oxford University Press: Melbourne.

Sansnee Jirojwong & Pranee Liamputtong

Moodie, R., Hulme, A. (eds) (2004) *Hands on Health Promotion*. IP Communications: East Hawthorn.

Promotion & Education (2007) Supplement 2.

WEBPAGE RESOURCES

Department of Health and Human Services (US): www.healthypeople.gov/. Sets out health outcomes and measurable outcomes to be achieved in 2010. The Healthy People 2020 program is currently being developed.

ABC Radio National websites: www.abc.net.au/rn. Current health and family issues are published on two good pages: the Health Report, and Life Matters. International researchers provide data on their work.

Expert Patients Programme, UK: www.expertpatients.nhs.uk. The UK Expert Patients Programme can be compared with the Self-Management of Chronic Diseases program undertaken by the Australian Department of Health and Ageing.

Department of Health and Ageing: www.health.gov.au/internet/wcms/Publishing.nsf/Content/pq-ncds. Focuses on health priorities and provides updated information relating to health services relevant to each health priority.

PART 2

Needs Assessment

Chapter 3	Health Needs Assessment of Communities and Populations	45
Chapter 4	Health of Indigenous Australians and Health Promotion	69
Chapter 5	Emerging Population Health Issues and Health Promotion	92
Chapter 6	Assessing the Needs of Health Professionals and Stakeholders	104

Health Needs Assessment of Communities and Populations

Pranee Liamputtong
& Sansnee Jirojwong

Objectives

After reading this chapter, readers will be able to:

➤ Describe what needs assessment is
➤ Provide a rationale for conducting needs assessment
➤ Describe the process of needs assessment
➤ Describe methods for needs assessment including both quantitative and qualitative methods
➤ Identify characteristics of the population for needs assessment, particularly disadvantaged and vulnerable groups as the target population
➤ Prioritise identified health needs of population.

Key terms

mixed method
needs assessment
qualitative methods
quantitative methods
vulnerable target group

Needs assessment in health: An introduction

Needs assessment: a systematic means for researchers to be able to identify the unmet health and health care needs of a target group, as well as to make changes to meet those unmet needs.

The focus of this chapter is on needs assessment in health. As such, it is crucial that we commence the chapter by discussing the definition of needs and needs assessment in community groups. Following Bradshaw's theory (1972, see also 1994), Payne (1999: 5) contends that there are four kinds of needs, including 'normative (as defined by professionals/experts): felt (wants, wishes, desires); expressed (felt need turned into action or vocalized: for example asking for pain relief, striking for more pay), and comparative need (inequalities)' (see also Petersen & Alexander, 2001). These distinctions, according to Payne, are valuable for the purposes of clarification, but they are insufficient for examining the health needs of communities. Perceived health needs or felt needs of people can be influenced not only by 'expert' definitions, but also by comparisons with the health statuses of other individuals and community groups. Therefore, health needs should be defined 'in terms of comparative standards or inequalities'. As such, Payne (1999: 6) suggests that need can be referred to 'felt or expressed need', which is 'responsive to the needs and preferences' of those who use health services, and so on.

What then is a needs assessment? Gilmore and colleagues (1989) define a needs assessment as a process that is employed to indicate the needs reported by an individual or a group. For individuals, they may carry out needs assessment to express their personal needs. Their needs, their importance, and practicality are reviewed, and steps to address them are taken. For groups, they may be represented by smaller sub-groups who carry out the needs assessment process with the groups. The reported needs from this representative group can then be adopted for planning purposes.

For Reviere and colleagues (1996: 6), a needs assessment is 'a systematic and ongoing process of providing usable and useful information about the needs of the target population—to those who can and will utilise it to make judgments about policy and program'. They also further explain that needs assessment needs to be 'population-specific, systematically focused, empirically based and outcome-oriented'. As such, needs assessment is a form of applied research that is more than data collection and analysis but includes the use of the findings from these processes.

Wright and colleagues (1998) define a health needs assessment as a new discourse adopted to explain the establishment and refinement of well-developed approaches to appreciating the needs of local communities. However, Wright and colleagues. (1998: 2) also contend that this discourse has now been referred to as 'an objective and valid method of tailoring health services, an evidence based approach to commissioning and planning health services'.

According to Wright and colleagues (1998), health care needs are those needs that can benefit from health care, such as illness prevention, health education, diagnosis and treatment, rehabilitation, and palliative care. Most health professionals perceive health needs in terms of the health care services that they can offer. Consumers, however, may consider other critical factors that would make them healthier, for instance having a decent job, money to pay for a bus to travel to the hospital or health centre, or a house in which to live. Health needs, as such, embody a wide range of social and environmental determinants of health. This wider definition of health needs permits health professionals to look beyond the medical model of health and health services to incorporate the wider influences on health. This is because health needs of a community or group will be constantly changing, and medical interventions alone may not provide the answer to all health needs.

Jonathan Bradshaw (1994: 50) suggests that the definition of health needs must be based on what we mean by health. According to the medical model, health is perceived as 'the absence of clinically ascertainable disease'. Within this context, needs are associated with the presence of disease that can be treated. In this model of health, the emphasis is on the treatment of specific conditions, the assessment of health needs using waiting-lists for treatment, the number of operations performed over a period of time, or patients treated per bed. Bradshaw (1994) alerts us to the alternative view of a social model of health recently defined by the World Health Organization (WHO, 1985). Health, accordingly, is 'the extent to which an individual or group is able, on the one hand, to realise aspiration and satisfy needs and on the other hand, to change or cope with the environment' (Bradshaw, 1994: 50). As such, health is perceived as resources for everyday life, not the objective of living. Health is a positive concept emphasising social and personal resources as well as physical capacities (WHO, 1986; see also Chapter 1 this volume).

This social model of health focuses on prevention, recovery, and rehabilitation (Bradshaw, 1994). The interaction between health and the social structure is the essence of this model. The impact of disadvantage and inequalities is emphasised. Need is not an absolute state, not just an untreated condition, an impairment or a disability, but also an absence of well-being or quality of life. Need is socially defined (Bradshaw, 1994: 50). Therefore, to fulfil the needs of people is to consider whether quality of life is promoted, not only whether the disease is treated. He argues that if the meeting of health needs is to be sufficient, health professionals should look into 'changes in the material conditions in which people live and the life-changes they have available to them' in order to pinpoint ill-health. Bradshaw (1994) strongly argues that we have to rely on other methods rather than the diagnostic skills of medical practitioners to assess individual health needs. The reports of personal experiences, subjective feelings and assessments of needs, to be precise the felt needs, are more important and reliable than medical assessments. Researchers and health professionals need to adopt a social definition of health when assessing health needs. We too argue that a wider range of issues, rather than simply the assessment of the prevalence of medical conditions, needs to be incorporated in our research. Thus, health needs assessment of community members is a crucial part of sensitive health care.

Health needs assessment, according to Wright and colleagues (1998: 6) is:

> A systematic method of identifying unmet health and health care needs of a population, and making changes to meet these unmet needs. It involves an epidemiological and qualitative approach to determining priorities, which incorporates clinical and cost effectiveness and patients' perspectives. This approach must balance clinical, ethical, and economic considerations of need, that is what should be done, what can be done, what can be afforded.

Why do we need to conduct a needs assessment?

Needs assessment provides a logical starting point for individual action and program development. It also acts as a continuing process for keeping activities on track (Gilmore et al., 1989). A needs assessment process helps health professionals in several ways. For instance, reported needs can be used to develop a health program, and target groups can take part in more meaningful and appropriate activities. The target groups can be more closely characterised, and health professionals can assess changes and trends over a period of time.

Needs assessment also enables health professionals to examine a number of factors that affect the health of the target groups and their ability to influence them positively. It is a crucial aspect of program planning, implementation and functioning as the starting point of program evaluation. Specifically, needs assessment, as suggested by Hodges and Videto (2005: 2–4), allows:

- the target groups to establish a sense of connection and ownership of the program
- identification of programming goals and objectives
- identification of barriers to and limitations of a program that health professionals attempt to implement
- collection of baseline data used for evaluation.

Through needs assessment, the health problems in a target group and gaps in the levels of the group's wellness can be pinpointed. Once health professionals have identified these, they can prioritise the problems and make decisions about which health needs should be developed to provide direction to program developers. Through this process, programming that is efficiently developed, implemented, and presented will result, and it will be more likely to be effective in reaching its goals and objectives (Hodges & Videto, 2005).

The needs assessment process aims to identify the health, educational, and resource needs of the target group (Hodges & Videto, 2005; see also Simons-Morton et al., 1995). Once this is identified, program planners can use the information to develop health education and health promotion programs that are designed to meets the needs of their target groups. A well-targeted program is more likely to be accepted by the group and be successful. This will save money and time. A program that is not accepted will have to be abandoned.

Wright and colleagues (1998: 6–7) propose that health needs assessment provides the opportunities for health promoters to:

➤ learn about the needs and priorities of their consumers and the local community group
➤ exhibit the areas of unmet needs and suggest a clear set of goals to work to meet these needs
➤ make decisions about how to use resources to improve the health of their local population in the most efficient and effective way
➤ influence the policy-making process, collaboration between agencies, or priorities development and research.

Most importantly, health needs assessment not only permits a method of measuring and enhancing equity in the provision and use of health services, but also addresses health inequalities in the target groups.

As a conclusion, all health needs assessment have three crucial aspects: health problems (need), resources, and outcomes (health gain) (Robinson & Elkan, 1996). Based on Bradshaw's theory (1994), meeting the health needs of local communities is a moral or ethical question. It is a question of what a society values, and what goals or outcomes we desire to bring about (Robinson & Elkan, 1996).

Needs assessment processes

Wright and colleagues (1998: 8) propose a framework of questions to ask when assessing health needs, as follows:

➤ What is the problem and its size?
➤ What are the current services available for people?
➤ What do local people want?

Pranee Liamputtong & Sansnee Jirojwong

➤ What are the most appropriate and effective solutions?
➤ What are the resource implications?
➤ What are the outcomes to evaluate change and the criteria to measure success?

The World Health Organization (WHO, 2000; cited in Hodges and Videto, 2005: 6) proposes a nine-step model for undertaking a needs assessment. The model provides valuable guidelines for health promoters and professionals to plan their needs assessment. These steps include the following:

1 Deciding when to carry out the needs assessment
2 Reviewing available data to assess what information is already available and what needs to be collected
3 Making decisions about appropriate data collection method(s)
4 Developing a concrete and realistic plan that incorporates approximate cost and time frames
5 Identifying and training the assessment team
6 Collecting data
7 Analysing data
8 Interpreting the analysis to pinpoint priority needs and intervention strategies and resources
9 Reporting the results of the needs assessment to all agencies and communities involved.

As an example and in practical terms, the New Zealand Ministry of Health sets out a guide for District Health Boards (DHBs) to undertake health-needs assessments of the New Zealand population. The needs assessment process incorporates data collection on the need and demand for health services of the population. These data are then analysed to examine future needs and the ability of health services to meet them. If needs are not being met, a process of evaluation of different options that feeds into the prioritisation process of the Ministry of Health should be carried out. Essentially, the evidence required for the Minister to make a decision is based on the health-needs assessments (Ministry of Health, 2000).

Strategies for needs assessment: What methods?

How will we obtain the information we require for needs assessment? There are several strategies that we may adopt to assess needs in the population with whom we work. Existing literature on needs assessment suggests that two approaches have been utilised: quantitative methods, and qualitative methods (see Reviere et al., 1996; Payne, 1999; Hodges & Videto, 2005). Payne (1999) points out that quantitative techniques are used to gain information that can be counted (for example, how many people use the local health care centre) and often necessitates the conduct of surveys. Qualitative methods are utilised to obtain in-depth information about people's perceptions, feelings, and experiences (Liamputtong & Ezzy, 2005). An example is how pregnant women make sense of their childbearing needs and experiences.

However, we feel that this distinction is not useful, as some of the quantitative methods can also be seen as qualitative, and vice versa. Good quality needs assessment should be based on the ways that we collect and organise the information appropriately (Hodges & Videto 2005). We need to consider which method would be best for the target group that we work with. We also argue that a mixed methodology is more appropriate for health needs assessment. Researchers also argue that, when possible, a needs assessment should contain both quantitative and qualitative data (see also Gilmore et al., 1989; Payne, 1999; Hodges & Videto, 2005). Several methods for health needs assessment are discussed in the following sections. Human needs differ, and continue to change (Gilmore et al., 1989). As such, no single method of assessing them will be appropriate and sufficient. A combination of quantitative and qualitative methods might be more efficient.

The choice of methods will determine the types of data that will be collected, and this will lead to what can legitimately be concluded about the findings (Berkowitz, 1996). Hence, the method or combination of methods we select to undertake a needs assessment is critically important. Methodologically, Berkowitz suggests there is no reason for us to restrict our data collection method to only qualitative or only quantitative approaches. Rather, the strength of a research design can be enhanced by careful and artful combination of both methods.

Whatever method is adopted for a needs assessment, Hodges and Videto (2005: 133) contend, 'the big picture' should be considered. There are several forms of data collection, and some are more suited to certain people/groups, environments, and situations than others. The best ways to obtain the needed information for a particular needs assessment should be considered by the person in charge. The following are suggestions from Hodges and Videto (2005: 133) for the production of a quality needs assessment:

➤ When choosing data collection methods, several factors including age, gender, education and literacy levels, first language, accessibility, information needed, and resources should be considered.
➤ Use triangulation whenever possible; that is obtaining data in more than one way and from more than one source.
➤ The process should be identified and essential approvals must be obtained as early as possible.
➤ Ensure the protocol and manual is written and procedures and instruments should be pilot-tested.

Quantitative methods: research methods that rely on standardised research tools such as surveys and are used to gain information that can be counted.

Qualitative methods: research methods employed when researchers wish to understand the health needs of their target group. Qualitative methods are employed to obtain in-depth information about people's perceptions, feelings, and experiences, and do not rely on numbers.

Mixed method: the use of both quantitative and qualitative methods in needs assessment.

- ➤ Data collectors must be appropriately trained.
- ➤ A data analysis plan must be developed prior to data collection.
- ➤ If requiring help with the needs assessment or evaluation process, this should be established early.
- ➤ As there are many ways to collect data, consider all options in order to identify the best ways to suit a particular circumstance.

The use of existing data

This method of using existing data, sometime referred to as 'document review', gathers relevant existing information about the local community, their health status, the health services they use, and gaps in services. This information can be obtained from existing records and reports, which can be found in hospitals, health departments, health care centres, clinics, and also in libraries. The following records and reports are of value in assessing the health needs of local communities (Ministry of Public Works and Government Services Canada, 2000: 8):

- ➤ data from facilities such as hospitals, nursing homes, medical clinics, and government records on numbers of population for the whole community
- ➤ reports from earlier needs assessments which were undertaken for health, environment, social services, and crime prevention
- ➤ periodic reports or special reports of data on use of health services by different population groups to examine rates and causes of injuries, illnesses, death, disabilities, use of antenatal care, pregnancy outcomes, and use of substance-abuse services or prescription drugs
- ➤ reports about particular health services or programs.

Existing data such as records and reports are easily accessible. They tend not to be dependent on access or ethical constraints. As they can be obtained quickly, the needs assessment can be done quickly. Hence, the results become known early for further actions to be taken (Liamputtong & Ezzy, 2005). However, the use of existing data has its own limitations. The issue of accuracy is at the core of the controversy. How can we be sure that the existing data are accurate in the first place? How can we make sense of information that other researchers have collected and with which we have not had any involvement? According to Kellehear (1993), if researchers have doubts about the accuracy of the existing data, they need to combine this method with other research methods. This is in line with the triangulation approach. The combination of research methods allows researchers to validate the results they obtain from the use of existing data. If the results appear to support each other, then the existing data should be sufficiently reliable.

Survey and questionnaire method

The sample survey, according to Berkowitz (1996), is primarily the method of choice in quantitative data collection for needs assessment. Typically, the survey method utilises a standardised and structured survey instrument to gather primary data from a probability sample of participants. Surveys and questionnaires, Hodges and Videto (2005) suggest, produce data through written responses to a standard set of questions. Depending on the nature of the questions, the data collected can be quantitative or qualitative. However, surveys and questionnaires tend to produce quantitative data because they have more closed questions and answers than open-ended questions. The questions asked in survey research are often highly standardised, and all the participants will be asked the same questions and in the same order. All the questions are written down in a standardised form (questionnaire), even though they will be asked by an interviewer (Payne, 1999).

It is quick and easy to administer surveys and questionnaires. They can be sent to many people at once. The answers can be done by means of paper and pencil, on the telephone, through the mail, and also electronically through email or web pages (Berkowitz, 1996; Hodges & Videto, 2005; Liamputtong, 2007). In needs assessment surveys, however, surveys will often be undertaken face-to-face. Survey interviews conducted face-to-face allow the researchers to establish a closer relationship with the participants. Thus, people are less likely to refuse to participate than in other methods. Face-to-face surveys are also more useful when a survey contains some open-ended questions, as the researcher can prompt by simply asking 'Anything else?' (Payne, 1999: 75).

Typically, self-completion questionnaire surveys are cheaper and quicker than face-to-face survey interviews. Researchers need to provide reply-paid envelopes for the survey to be returned, or organise to have them collected. Self-completion questionnaires tend to have lower response rates than face-to-face surveys. As participants fill in the forms themselves, researchers need to be more cautious about the instructions, the wording of the questions, the range of topics, and types of questions included in the survey. Self-completing questionnaires can be problematic for certain groups of people. For example, those who are physically disabled or have problems understanding the questions due to language barriers or learning difficulties may not be able to complete a questionnaire themselves (Payne, 1999). A self-completing questionnaire is best used with some interest-based groups who are able to comprehend the questions posed, or if the questionnaire is to be treated as part of a larger study (Payne, 1999).

Sample surveys have their limitations. A simple assumption that people can be asked to state their needs and are able to articulate about them is too dangerous.

People's recognitions of their own needs are essentially impacted by social, cultural, political, and historical contexts (Berkowitz, 1996). Their roles and power in society also influence their needs. People may not be able to recognise and identify their own needs. Berkowitz (1996: 33) argues, 'it is essential to recognize that all perceptions of need have a subjective element'. A standardised tool such as surveys and questionnaires may not be appropriate in health needs assessment.

In any needs assessment using the survey method, Hodges and Videto (2005) suggest that, if possible, researchers may adapt and utilise existing surveys that previous researchers have developed and tested to see if they work with the target group (see also Thompson & McClintock, 1998; Payne, 1999). There may be surveys and questionnaires which were developed or used to measure a similar concept or to examine needs from a similar target group. However, researchers need to consider people's characteristics, such as age, gender, literacy level, language, and culture, which may have an impact on the ability of the target group to really comprehend the questions asked. It is essential to pilot-test the adopted surveys with the target group. This should determine if the survey is appropriate for use with the target population, and if it can be completed within the set timeframe.

Delphi method

The Delphi technique is valuable for pinpointing problems and identifying priorities within a group (Hodges & Videto, 2005; see also Delbecq et al., 1975; Duffield, 1993; Ziglio, 1996; Jackson et al., 1998). The aim of the Delphi method is to provide a reliable tool to explore ideas creatively or produce suitable data for making decisions (Ziglio, 1996). The method relies on a structural process for collecting and distilling knowledge from a number of experts by using a series of questionnaires interspersed with controlled opinion feedback. The Delphi method is an activity in group communication among a panel of geographically dispersed experts (Ziglio, 1996). The technique allows the experts to communicate or interact systematically with a complex problem or task. The Delphi method, Ziglio claimed (1996: 3), is 'creative or informed decision-making'.

The methodological procedures adopted in the Delphi method focus on eliciting and orchestrating a large amount of information which has not yet been formalised as concrete evidence in order to reach 'informed judgment and decision-making' (Ziglio, 1996: 6). The results of a Delphi research project can be used to enhance traditional face-to-face meetings. For example, a supplementary group communication process obtained through the Delphi method can increase the efficiency of face-to-face meetings. When time and cost constraints make frequent face-to-face meetings difficult to organise, the Delphi method can be adopted. This method is particularly useful when the heterogeneity of the participants must be preserved. It also assures anonymity in order to avoid the domination of the communication process by a particular profession, vested interest, or strong personality (Ziglio, 1996).

In public health, Ziglio (1996) concludes, the Delphi method is a valuable tool to improve data collection, generate ideas, explore future plans, and make informed decisions. The method is an essential tool for decision-makers who are facing uncertainty about how to explore the nature of a specific public health problem, assess its magnitude, and evaluate different means of addressing it. Appropriate applications of the Delphi method can offer results that policy makers can use to make their decisions when accurate information is not readily available.

The Delphi method is composed of a series of questionnaires distributed to a group of pre-selected experts. These questionnaires are designed to gather and establish responses from individual experts. This allows them to refine their opinions while the group's work on the assigned task continues. The questions may be either broad and open-ended or specific and closed. These responses are then returned for analysis. The next set of questionnaires is constructed and sent to the same experts. Subsequent questionnaires summarise previous responses and articulate new questions related to the decision being sought. This process continues until a consensus is achieved (Hodges & Videto, 2005). Ziglio (1996: 9) summarises the method as follows:

> In most applications, the first questionnaire (Q1) poses the problem in broad terms and invites answers and comments. The replies to Q1 are summarised and used to construct a second questionnaire (Q2). Q2 represents the result of Q1 and gives the respondents an opportunity to re-evaluate their original answers in the light of comprehensive feedback on the responses of the whole group. During this interactive process, which can be repeated as many times as are judged appropriate in the circumstances, issues can be clarified, areas of agreement and disagreement can be identified, and an understanding of the priorities can be developed.

Observation

Observation, according to Payne (1999: 90, original emphasis), is a research tool perceived as '*systematic looking and listening*'. As a research tool, observation is '*active looking* and listening: seeing, noticing, hearing and *recording*'. Observation, according to Hodges and Videto (2005: 121), is a method for 'seeing and hearing events, situations, and behavior'. It is frequently employed to assess people's behaviours, but it may also be utilised to measure some environmental factors and assess quality of life (WHO, 2000). Individuals or groups of people are observed so that their behaviour and skills can be evaluated. People's daily life can also be assessed by an observational method. Observation, Payne (1999: 91) contends, is not strictly a qualitative method, as it may involve 'complex sampling, counting and coding procedures'.

The observation method allows researchers to observe people's behaviours, skills, and conditions, rather than relying on their self-reports. It also provides an opportunity for researchers to document people's interests in the 'real world'. Thus, it provides an opportunity to improve researchers' interpretations and to prioritise or assess people's needs. A large amount of information about a community or target group can be gained by undertaking observational studies. This is especially so when observations are used with other methods as part of a mixed-method approach. The weakness of this method includes the possibility of the researcher making incorrect observations and interpretations. Those who are being observed may react to the presence of the researcher, and bias may occur (Hodges & Videto, 2005). Also, it is not the best method to use if a researcher wishes to examine people's opinions and attitudes, or to determine past and future events (Payne, 1999).

Observation here refers to the researcher recording what is seen and heard without taking part in any activities, unlike the participant observation used in ethnography (Liamputtong & Ezzy, 2005). A non-participant observation may include observations of small group activities, which is often referred to as 'the community walk' or 'casing the joint' (Payne, 1999: 92–3). Those being studied are told about the research, hence the observation is overt. Observation can also be covert. Overt observation may pose the risk of error and bias being introduced by the research process. It is likely that the people observed may act differently because they know that they are being observed. On the other hand, covert observation is perceived by many researchers as unethical because it breaches the principle of informed consent. There are others who would suggest that research is ethical as long as it does not cause any harm to the participants and when no one is identifiable in any writing stemming from the research. This type of observation tends to be labelled as unobtrusive rather than covert (Payne, 1999).

A good example of non-participant observation in community needs assessment is perhaps 'the community walk' (Payne, 1999: 93; see also Murray & Graham, 1995). Often, this form of observation is carried out as a preliminary or exploratory stage. The researchers 'case the joint' to become familiar with the physical environments and to examine how these environments affect the community's social life. However, the community walk can be employed as part of a mixed-method approach so that a greater depth of information can be added to a survey or other type of needs assessment method (Payne, 1999). Nevertheless, as Payne (1999) argues, in community health needs assessments, researchers are more likely to participate in community life in some ways, for example as a community member, a patient, or a health professional. Therefore, participant observation is often used.

In-depth interviewing method

The method of in-depth interviewing is most commonly adopted by qualitative researchers. This method assumes that people have particular and important knowledge about the social world that is obtainable through verbal messages. The in-depth interviewing method aims to obtain detailed information from the perspective of a particular person and on a selected topic. In-depth interviewing allows researchers to access complex knowledge from an insider 'without the preconceived biases inherent in using existing structured instruments that may contain items irrelevant to local populations' (Schoenberg et al., 2005: 92). This method, they maintain, allows the participants to express their views freely and at the same time permits researchers to focus on the research topic.

The in-depth interviewing method, according to Johnson (2002), usually refers to a fact-to-face and one-on-one interaction between a participant and a researcher. This method is especially of value for 'accessing subjugated voices and getting at subjugated knowledge' (Hesse-Biber & Leavy, 2005: 123). It is a valuable method for collecting information about health needs assessment from vulnerable and marginalised people. The method is particularly preferred among researchers who wish their participants to speak about their needs in greater depth (Nicholson & Burr, 2003; Hesse-Biber & Leavy, 2005; Liamputtong & Ezzy, 2005). As the method 'seeks "deep" information and understanding' (Johnson, 2002: 106), it permits researchers to make sense of the multiple meanings and interpretations of a specific action, occasion, location, or cultural practice. The method is, therefore, conducive to needs assessment of community groups in any setting.

Within the in-depth interviewing method, key informant interviews are frequently adopted (Hodges & Videto, 2005). Key informants are individuals living in the community who possess knowledge or have access to information about the community group, or professional people who are working with the community group (WHO, 2000). These key informants are able to provide information about the community group the researchers are working with. Key informant interviews may assist researchers in identifying potentially controversial issues. They also can provide guidance on how to address issues in a way that may be more acceptable to local people.

Focus group interview

A focus group interview is a qualitative method 'with the primary aim of describing and understanding perceptions, interpretations, and beliefs of a select population to gain understanding of a particular issue from the perspective of the group's participants' (Khan & Manderson, 1992: 57). A focus group interview usually involves about six to ten people who come from similar social and cultural backgrounds, or who have similar experiences or concerns. They come together to discuss a particular issue, with the assistance of a moderator, in a specific setting where participants feel comfortable enough to interact in a dynamic discussion for at least one to two hours (Krueger & Casey, 2000; Liamputtong & Ezzy, 2005; Barbour, 2007; Colucci, 2007).

The focus group interviewing method is a group discussion that relies heavily on the interaction between participants. It is successful only when the participants are able to talk to each other, rather than individually answering the moderator's questions. Interaction is a unique feature of the focus group interview. Indeed, this characteristic differentiates the method from the individual in-depth interview. It is based on the idea that group processes assist people to explore and clarify their points of view. Such processes tend to be less accessible in an individual interview. As Morgan (1988: 12) suggests, the focus group makes 'explicit use of the group interaction to produce data and insights that would be less accessible without the interaction found in a group'. Recent writers on focus groups have termed this 'the group effect'.

In needs assessment, a focus group interview is a useful research tool when the researcher does not have deep knowledge about the participants or local community. Focus groups 'represent a remarkably flexible research tool in that they can be adapted to obtain information about almost any topic in a wide array of settings and from very different types of individuals' (Stewart & Shamdasani, 1990: 140).

When a researcher wishes to explore people's knowledge and experiences, focus groups are particularly useful. They can be employed to examine not only what people think, but also how and why they think the way they do (Kitzinger, 1995). This is especially essential when the researcher needs to explore the perspective and experience of people whose social and cultural backgrounds differ from theirs, or when there is little information about the group of people under investigation (Liamputtong, 2007).

Focus groups have been used to 'give a voice' to marginalised groups such as the poor, minority ethnic groups, women, or those affected by HIV/AIDS. This enables researchers, policy makers and others to 'listen' to people who may have little chance to express an opinion about their health and needs (Kitzinger, 1994, 1995; Madriz, 1998; Winslow, et al. 2002; Umaña-Taylor & Bámaca, 2004). In early HIV/AIDS research, Joseph and others (1984) employed focus groups as a means to understand the lived experiences of gay and bisexual men. These were perceived as at-risk groups, but their health behaviours and needs were not well understood by the researchers and the wider public.

In health needs assessment, focus groups are invaluable. Focus groups are commonly utilised in the exploratory studies in health issues and health needs assessment, or in the assessment of the acceptance of new health service programs. Focus groups are often employed in health education and promotion, particularly as part of the process of program planning (Goldman & Schmalz, 2001).

In needs assessment, it is wise to undertake a number of focus groups that consist of representatives of different sub-groups in the local community. This way, information gathered will be sufficient for making decision in health promotion programs developed for the community. For example, as part of a needs assessment for planning a Queensland Rural Chronic Disease Initiative, the project team carried out focus group interviews with several interest groups, including senior citizens and male farmers from four rural Queensland communities (Jirojwong et al., 2005).

Nominal group technique

The nominal group technique is very similar to the Delphi method. Like the Delphi method, the nominal group technique is employed for 'aggregating group judgement and for distilling information on highly complex problems characterised by uncertainty' (Ziglio, 1996: 12). The nominal group technique is a process that brings experts together. It combines non-verbal and verbal stages using a highly structured communication procedure (Ziglio, 1996).

According to Ziglio (1996: 12), the nominal group technique is composed of three phases: independent idea generation, structured feedback, and independent mathematical judgment. The structure of a group meeting applying the nominal group technique is summarised below.

1. Individual participants generate their ideas in writing in silence.
2. Group members provide their opinion in a round-robin feedback tradition on a flip chart.
3. Each recorded idea is discussed for clarification and evaluation.
4. Priority ideas are voted on individually, and the group decision is derived through rating or rank-ordering.
5. The final vote is carried out and the outcome of the meeting is set.

Through the nominal group technique, a group can be formed to make decisions about complex issues, and this permits all needs and ideas to be heard and taken into consideration (Jackson et al., 1998; Hodges & Videto, 2005). Selected participants are chosen on the basis of their knowledge of the issue under consideration. Usually, five to seven people are involved in this process (Gilmore & Campbell, 1996). The moderator commences the research by inviting all participants to provide one area of response to the question or problem being considered, for instance, which of the health issues that older people are facing is in most urgent need of attention in this community? Each participant provides his or her own responses. When all responses are identified, they are listed for all members to consider. Each participant in the group is then invited to rank the top three to five items from the compiled list (Jackson et al., 1998). The votes are counted by the moderator. Issues of agreement and disagreement are then identified and discussed. The group continues its discussion after considering the initial listing of items. The votes are then reviewed to examine clear priorities. If these are identified, the initial items are eliminated from the process. The group repeats the ranking and discussion with the remaining items. When all members agree on the priority list, the process is finalised (Hodges & Videto, 2005).

The nominal group technique offers both quantitative and qualitative data (Gilmore et al., 1989: 61). While quantitative data provides results 'in the sense of voted-upon priorities', qualitative data provides 'a descriptive discussion of the problem'. The qualitative data is often generated from the group discussion, which is the main characteristic of the nominal group technique, as the group members tend to refer to their critical circumstances of personal experiences, a subjective form of evidence. A combination of qualitative and quantitative data greatly enhances appropriate professional responses to the needs of their consumers.

Rapid appraisal method

The rapid appraisal method has become popular in health needs assessment. According to Payne (1999: 29–30), the rapid appraisal method is essentially a mixed-method approach; it is based on what Denzin (1970) refers to as 'data triangulation' (see also Beebe, 2001). For a number of years, the method has been commonly employed in social research. Examples are projects by the United Kingdom Institute of Community Studies in the East End during the 1950s and 1960s, and public-health related studies (see Manderson, 1998; Pelto et al., 1998; Stimson et al., 1999; Fitch et al., 2002; Needle et al., 2003; Sanderowitz et al., 2003).

The techniques used in this method are not new, but they offer a framework to guide a health needs assessment. The method can identify the broad areas on which researchers can focus. The rapid appraisal method draws on both qualitative and quantitative research techniques, but qualitative techniques tend to be employed more (Beebe, 2001). The method is used when information is needed quickly and when conventional research methods cannot be undertaken because of resource and time constraints (Fitch et al., 2002). The main weakness of this method is its heavy reliance on key informants to provide detailed information. However, when used with a survey and other research methods, the rapid appraisal method can offer the basis for a thorough health needs assessment of a local community (Payne, 1999).

In the field of rural development in developing countries, methodologies that permit not only rapid but also reliable and cheap profiling of community characteristics and resources have become popular (Scrimshaw & Gleason, 1992; Ong & Humphris, 1994; Pelto et al., 1998; Beebe, 2001; Needle et al., 2003). The rapid appraisal method is one of most popular methods. It includes several different techniques, but has its common framework as follows:

- Researchers are working in the 'field'.
- Its focus is on learning directly from local people.
- It is a semi-structured, multidisciplinary approach that allows more flexibility and new ideas to be developed.
- The ultimate aim is to produce 'timely insights, hypotheses or "best bets" rather than final truths or fixed recommendations'.
- In comparison with other conventional methods, it has a greater speed (Ong & Humphris, 1994: 64).

The rapid appraisal method attempts to elicit information that can aid resource allocation and that encourages and supports community participation (Ong & Humphris 1994: 65). The method aims to reach two goals: continuity (a commitment to a community), and action (delivering tangible results). Assessment of the needs of a community is a complex task. Researchers need to develop alternative methods to use alongside the orthodox or conventional approaches if the totality of need is to be understood. This method, as Ong and Humphris (1994: 80) suggest, 'has the potential for being developed into a tool that involves communities directly and fundamentally in defining health needs and health gains, and thus in the process of decision-making'.

Community-based methods

There are other community-based methods adopted to assess the needs of a local population. Here, we describe two methods that we believe are valuable.

Windshield tours

Windshield tours, according to Hodges and Videto (2005), are an effective means to assess the needs of the target group or community. The tours can also function as part of an evaluation. Often, windshield tours are undertaken by professionals, with the help of trained community members. The tours involve researchers walking, driving, or cycling through the chosen area at different times during the day and on different days in order to observe and record general impressions of the area, such as types and conditions of housing, the maintenance of buildings and grounds, and the amount and types of social interactions and observable health-related behavior (Eng & Blanchard, 1990; Sharpe et al., 2000). Observations and impressions can be recorded as written notes of key observations, but the use of audiotape recorders, maps, videotapes, and laptop computers may also be utilised.

Pranee Liamputtong & Sansnee Jirojwong

Photovoice method

The photovoice method is employed in needs assessment to explore the needs of people in order to 'promote dialogue, encourage action, and inform polity' (Wang & Burris, 1994: 172). Essentially, photovoice is 'an innovative participatory action research (PAR) method based on health promotion principles and the theoretical literature on education for critical consciousness, feminist theory and non-traditional approach to documentary photography' (Wang 1999: 185; Brooks et al. in press). The photovoice method allows people to record and reflect the concerns and needs of their community via taking photographs. It also promotes critical discussion through dialogue about important issues from the photographs they have taken. Their concerns may reach policy makers through public forums and the display of their photographs. By using a camera to record their concerns and needs, individuals who rarely have contact with those who make decisions over their lives can make their voices heard.

Characteristics of the population for needs assessment

Disadvantaged and vulnerable groups as the target population

Quest and Marco (2003: 1297) contend that some population groups face particular social vulnerability. These groups include children, unemployed people, homeless people, drug-addicted people, sex workers, refugees, and ethnic and religious minority groups. These groups are often referred to as people with 'social vulnerability' (Liamputtong, 2007). When involved in their needs assessment, these groups of people need special care from the researchers. According to Wright and colleagues (1998), these people are difficult to access in health needs assessment, and hence they deserve special attention.

The reasons for their invisibility are many, and may include their marginality, lack of opportunity to voice their concerns, fear of their identity being disrespected, stigma attached to their social conditions, heavy responsibilities, language barriers, and scepticism about being involved in research (Liamputtong, 2007). Women from ethnic backgrounds and low socio-economic backgrounds are less willing or able to participate in research due to their heavy responsibilities and their well-founded scepticism about the value of their input (Liamputtong, 2007). Some vulnerable people may face pressing socio-economic needs that limit their participation in research (Anderson & Hatton, 2000). Birman (2005: 197) suggests that most

Vulnerable target group: a group of people who face particular social vulnerability. These include children, unemployed people, homeless people, drug-addicted people, sex workers, refugees, and ethnic and religious minority groups.

so-called 'illegal' immigrants do not wish to be identified and, hence, will avoid participation in any research, especially if the research may reveal their identity to authorities. Refugees may 'feel vulnerable' in taking part in any research as a result of their past experiences of dealing with authorities (Liamputtong Rice 1995; Birman 2005; Schweitzer & Steel, in press). These people are 'distrustful of non-members, do whatever they can to avoid revealing their identities, and are likely to refuse to cooperate with outsiders or to give unreliable answers to questions about themselves and their networks' (Benoit et al., 2005: 264).

It is also crucial that the characteristics of the participants, such as developmental levels, reading abilities, and social and cultural factors, must be taken into account when choosing data collection methods (Hodges & Videto, 2005). Self-administered surveys and questionnaires, for example, will not be suitable for young children, illiterate people, and those with reading difficulties. Questionnaires that contain only English will often be problematic for many people from non-English-speaking and refugee backgrounds. Individual and face-to-face interviews may be less acceptable culturally if the interviewers are strangers or of a different gender to the participants.

One contentious issue involved in needs assessment is the issue of the power imbalance between the participant and the researcher (Payne, 1999). These power imbalances stem from either real or perceived differences in social or professional status, including culture, gender, age, and social class. It is important that researchers recognise these differences. They must attempt to minimise these sensitivities, which can be done by adopting an appropriate research design. In health needs assessments, researchers are more likely to encounter these power imbalances when carrying out research within an ethnically mixed community. In such cases, it is crucial to involve representatives from all ethnic groups in the local community in the development and design of the research.

Prioritising identified health needs of a population

In prioritising health needs of community groups, there are several questions that need to be considered (Hodges & Videto, 2005: 34):

- How do the target community and the stakeholders perceive health needs?
- Are the data they provide similar or different from the other data which have been collected in the community?
- Do particular groups of people have disproportionate rates of health problems?
- What resources can be drawn on to address a problem?
- Is the community able to address the problem?
- What difficulty may arise if the problem is not addressed?

Pranee Liamputtong & Sansnee Jirojwong

It is imperative that the agencies and stakeholders involved participate in the selection of priorities in the health needs of community group (Hodges & Videto, 2005: 33–34). This can be done through a 'coalition structure', such as community forums or any other open communication method. Another way of setting priorities is by establishing working groups or ad hoc committees. Frequently, a group process, such as a nominal group technique (see above) is employed. Recently, community-based participatory research, which is becoming popular in health promotion and education, is utilised in setting priorities. The methodology takes the stance that community members must engage equally with researchers in all stages of the needs-assessment process as well as the decision-making process (Minkler & Wallerstein, 2003). As such, community members are able to make their voices heard in setting priorities for their own health needs (Liamputtong & Ezzy, 2005; Liamputtong, 2007). The involvement of local communities in promoting their own health, and their active participation in setting priorities and allocating sresources was a focus of the World Health Organization Health for All 2000 (WHO, 1985).

Jordan and colleagues (1996: 65) suggest innovative and interesting methods for setting priorities: citizens' juries and user-consultation panels. In the citizens' juries method, participants are chosen to represent the public or local viewpoint. Citizen juries sit for a set period of time, and they are provided with information to assist them to make decisions. Jurors are able to ask questions or to discuss relevant issues while experts provide the evidence (see also Lenaghan et al., 1996).

User-consultation panels consist of several people from local communities who are selected to represent the local people. Members are rotated to ensure that a wide range of opinion is expressed and heard. Issues for consideration are set beforehand, and members are provided with essential and relevant information so that informed discussion can take place. The consultative panels meeting is usually facilitated by a moderator (see Bowie et al., 1995).

CASE STUDY

1. Health needs assessment—St Ives, Sydney

Assessment of health needs in St Ives was carried out by Piper and Krolik (1991). Like all other communities in Australia, St Ives deals with the many health needs (both physical and social) of its local people as well as the changing physical environment in which the community exists. The population in St Ives has increased dramatically. The composition of the population has also changed; for example, there has been an increase in the number of older people (over 60 years of age). Hence, the existing health services within the community need to be redirected. It is also important that the community itself should be informed of and have access to health services that are provided within both the local area and its surrounding settings. It is, therefore, essential for service planners and providers to be aware of the needs of the local community.

It was felt that the issues that local people see as important in their community should be determined. The identification of these important issues would permit service providers and the community to work towards strategies to address these important issues. The Ku-ring-gai Hospital organised a health needs assessment of the community in 1991. A mixed-method approach was adopted, comprising a survey and focus-group interviews. The target groups included residents of St Ives, health professionals, and business people working in the St Ives area. A total of 520 residents, male and female, were recruited randomly from the electoral roll and telephone directory. Only 131 returned the survey. Fourteen focus-group interviews (94 participants) were undertaken with residents of St Ives. Seventeen health professionals and fifty-three business persons returned the questionnaires.

The study showed that several issues were important for people living in St Ives, and these issues were shared by most participants across the three groups. These included: stress, medical conditions, accidents and injuries, loneliness, lack of facilities and activities, boredom, isolation, public transport, traffic safety, and access to information. The results of this health needs assessment, it was claimed, provided relevant information to service providers for the planning and redirection of services, facilities, and activities in St Ives.

2. Reproductive and sexual health initiative— The Photovoice Project and Indigenous Australians

A photovoice method of research was employed by Marie Stopes International Australia (2005) in innovative research with young Indigenous people in rural Victoria, Australia. In their research on developing reproductive and sexual health initiatives for Indigenous communities, Marie Stopes International formed a partnership with local Indigenous communities in Mildura, Shepparton and Warrnambool. It aimed to allow Indigenous

Pranee Liamputtong & Sansnee Jirojwong

communities to identify, control and develop their own health solutions and build capacity for Aboriginal self-determination and community control. It had to be culturally sensitive to the needs of Indigenous communities.

One important aspect of their development was to empower, motivate, and inspire young Indigenous people to have more control over their sexual health through the photovoice project. A six-day workshop was organised. The first and second days focused on information regarding written consent, a briefing about photovoice, and photographic and ethical training. These young people spent the third day taking photographs and had them developed overnight. On the fourth day, the photos were selected by the young people for discussion. Their discussions were documented. These photos were then enlarged and framed by the participants. On the fifth day, the framed photos were transported to Mildura Art Gallery. The participants categorised the themes of the photos and then exhibited them. On the sixth day, an opening of the local community exhibition was organised with a traditional welcome from Indigenous communities.

This photovoice project provided powerful insights into the sexual health issues important to young Indigenous people in Victorian rural communities. The outcomes of this project enabled Marie Stopes International and the Victorian Aboriginal Community Controlled Health Organisation (VACCHO) to design sexual health initiatives that were culturally appropriate to the specific needs of Indigenous young people, and to identify important issues for discussion with decision-makers, community leaders, government departments, and donors.

Conclusion

In this chapter, we discussed essential issues relating to health needs assessment in target populations. It is claimed that needs assessment is an essential step in planning any health promotion and programs, as the target community can be involved in the process. This way, the programs developed will be more sensitive to the needs of the local community. There are many methods that researchers may adopt in their needs assessment endeavours, including both quantitative and qualitative approaches. As we have suggested in this chapter, a mixed-method approach, and a combination of conventional and innovative methods, may be more appropriate in assessing health needs. We hope that this chapter has provided some useful examples for readers to follow if embarking on a needs assessment project. We wish to leave the chapter with the following quote, as we believe it captures the essence of this chapter very well.

> Conducting a community health needs assessment is a little like finding your way at a service station. Many of us travel; at some point in our travels, almost every one of us has looked around and asked ourselves where we are ... If you are just starting out, it gives you a starting point. If you are along the way, it helps you evaluate your progress and measure your distance from your ultimate goal. If you have reached your goal, an assessment will show you other routes (Bosworth, 1999: 13).

CRITICAL THINKING EXERCISES

1. You are a health promoter and are asked to assess the health needs of Aboriginal women in the Western Desert area. How would you go about the needs assessment process in order to obtain information that is relevant and sensitive to the local women?

2. In order to assess the health needs of homeless young people in inner Melbourne, what method(s) of needs assessment do you believe is best adopted, and what makes you select such method(s)? Discuss.

FURTHER READING

Adler, M., & Ziglio, E. (eds) (1996) *Gazing into the Oracle: The Delphi Method and its Application to Social Policy and Public Health*. Jessica Kingsley: London.

Atlas, B., & Molloy, R. (2005) *Photo Voice*. Paper presented at the Melbourne Interest Group in International Health, the University of Melbourne, Melbourne, 9 August.

Beebe, J. (2001) *Rapid Assessment Process: An Introduction*. AltaMira Press: Walnut Creek.

Hodges, B.C., & Videto, D.M. (2005) *Assessment and Planning in Health Programs*. Jones and Bartlett Publishers: Boston.

Liamputtong, P., & Ezzy, D. (2005) *Qualitative Research Methods*, 2nd edn. Oxford University Press: Melbourne.

Liamputtong, P. (2007) *Researching the Vulnerable: A Guide to Sensitive Research Methods*. Sage Publications: London.

Payne, J. (1999) *Researching Health Needs*. Sage Publications: London.

Piper, D., & Krolik, P. (1991) *A Needs Assessment: St Ives Sydney*. Health Promotion Unit, Ku-ring-gai Hospital and Community Health: Hornsby.

Southern Community Health Research Unit (1991) *Planning Healthy Communities: A Guide to Doing Community Needs Assessment*. Flinders Medical Centre: Bedford Park.

Wang, C.C., Morrel-Samuels, S., & Hutchison, P. (2004) Flint Photovoice: Community Building among Youth, Adults, and Policy Makers. *American Journal of Public Health* 94(6): 911–13.

WEBPAGE RESOURCES

Community Health Needs Assessment Tool Kit: courses.essex.ac.uk/hs/hs915/Mid%20Hampshire%20PCT%20HNA%20Toolkit.pdf. This tool kit provides a step-by-step guide for conducting a needs assessment, and includes several methodologies that researchers can adopt in their assessment of the health needs of their target groups.

Health Needs Assessment for New Zealand: www.moh.govt.nz/moh.nsf/pagesmh/1327?Open. This website provides a full review of health needs assessment for New Zealand.

Orange County Needs Assessment: Partnership for Health: http://www.ochna.org/publications/index.htm. The Orange County Health Needs Assessment (OCHNA) performs a survey of health needs every three years for the people of Orange County and the hospitals and organisations that serve them.

Centre for Research on Minority Health: www.mdanderson.org/departments/CRMH/. The first phase of the Asian–American Health Needs Assessment project, conducted by the first-ever comprehensive telephone survey to assess the health issues of Chinese and Vietnamese populations in Houston and surrounding areas.

Photovoice: Social Change through Photography: www.photovoice.com. This website provides details and case study examples of 'Photovoice', a participatory tool designed to bring about social change through photography and social action.

4

Health of Indigenous Australians and Health Promotion

Janya McCalman, Komla Tsey, Teresa Gibson & Bradley Baird

Objectives

After reading this chapter, readers will be able to:

- Provide a definition for Indigenous health promotion
- Analyse whether there should be other cultural health promotion concepts or ways of knowing about health which can be different from the Ottawa Charter for Health Promotion
- Understand approaches that make health promotion projects successful in an Indigenous population
- Identify the main challenges of Indigenous health promotion programs
- Explore learning opportunities for the future of Indigenous health promotion.

Key terms

Aboriginal health
equity in health
Indigenous Australians

Disclaimer

We would like to acknowledge that different views are held by different Aboriginal people and groups. The following content does not claim to represent the situation or opinion of all Aboriginal people.

Introduction

Equity in health: reducing or eliminating health differences that result from factors that are considered to be both avoidable and unfair.

In 1995, the National Health and Medical Research Council (NH&MRC) completed a comprehensive review and analysis of past and current Australian health promotion initiatives. They concluded that there had been progress towards an effective health promotion workforce and infrastructure. But there was still a strong focus on the prevention of disease and reduction in individual behavioural risk factors, rather than the physical, socio-economic and environmental determinants of health and their implications for equity and social justice. The review acknowledged that programs did endeavour to take account of marginalised groups such as Indigenous people, but the effort fell short of expectations that national effort should be focused on improving health and reducing inequalities in access and outcomes (NH&MRC, 1997).

Indigenous Australians: people of Aboriginal or Torres Strait Islander descent who identify as Aboriginal or Torres Strait Islander and are accepted as such by the community with which they are associated (AIHW, 2003).

Since the early 1990s, there has been international and national recognition that many years of policy and intervention effort have not delivered desired health outcomes to disadvantaged peoples. Indeed, in Australia, in some important respects the circumstances of Indigenous people appear to have either deteriorated or regressed (Gary Banks, quoted in Steering Committee for the Review of Government Service Provision, 2005: i) or health inequity has increased. In the Northern Territory, for example, Indigenous all-cause mortality rates declined overall and for all age groups over a long period (1967–2000). Declines in Indigenous mortality, however, 'did not keep pace with the relative decline for the total Australian population' (Wilson et al., 2007). This has led to an evolution of health promotion away from simple mono-causal models focused on behavioural risk factors towards a greater emphasis on the broader social and economic determinants of health, with an ultimate goal of improving health outcomes, particularly for disadvantaged populations.

Indigenous health promotion is important because there are huge health inequalities within Australia. Despite Australia's world-class health system, the life expectancy of Indigenous people is estimated to be around 17 years lower than that for the total Australian population. The difference in life expectancy between Indigenous people and other citizens in North America and New Zealand has been reduced to around seven years, showing that concerted action can make a difference (Steering Committee for the Review of Government Service Provision, 2007). In a wealthy country, this inequality is avoidable, amenable to reduction, and is an issue of social justice.

In the context of Indigenous health, the goal of health promotion programs may include individual health gain, community health gain, equity and/or cultural appropriateness (NH&MRC, 1997; Ivers, 2003; Davis et al., 2004; McLennan & Khavarpour, 2004). Indigenous health promotion practitioners call for a health promotion practice that is well-resourced, consistent, and based on sustained long-term strategies that address the underlying determinants of health. It needs to be respectful and appropriate, and take into account culture, diversity within the population, socio-economic circumstances, languages and dialects, geographic location, and the consequences of colonisation (including the social, economic, and physical living conditions of Indigenous people).

Before we continue our discussion in this chapter, we wish to acknowledge that there are different views held by different Indigenous groups. Hence, what we express in this chapter may not reflect the views of all Indigenous people.

Historical context of Indigenous Australians' health

Australian Aboriginal and Torres Strait Islander cultures go back at least 50,000 years and some argue closer to 65,000 years. They are the oldest living cultures in the world—their ability to survive being closely related to their capacity to adapt and change over time. There were about 600 different clan groups or 'nations' around the continent when Europeans arrived, many with distinctive cultures and beliefs. All were semi-nomadic hunters and gatherers, with each clan having its own 'traditional lands', defined by geographic boundaries such as rivers, lakes, and mountains. Land is fundamental to the well-being of Aboriginal people, sustaining and sustained by people and culture, and is the core of all spirituality. Aborigines and Torres Strait Islanders identify themselves through their land areas, their relationship to others, and their language and stories—which may be expressed through ceremony, the arts, family, religion, and sports (Australian Government Culture and Recreation Portal, 2007a).

Australia's history of European settlement since 1788 was characterised by the dispossession of over 400 million hectares of land, massacres of unarmed Aboriginal people, and the decimation of the Indigenous population through introduced illnesses, poverty, and exclusion from health care (Mitchell, 2007).

Aboriginal health: not just the physical well-being of an individual but also the social, emotional and cultural well-being of the whole community in which each individual is able to achieve the full potential as a human being, thereby bringing about the total well-being of the community. It is a whole-of-life view and includes the cyclical concept of life-death-life (National Aboriginal Health Strategy Working Party, 1989).

Janya McCalman, Komla Tsey, Teresa Gibson & Bradley Baird

Between 1790 and 1890, Aboriginal clans realised that their land, resources, and the order of their life were becoming seriously disrupted and undertook a series of campaigns of resistance against the British colonisers (Australian Government Culture and Recreation Portal, 2007b).

By the late 1890s, Aboriginal resistance had been effectively broken and the land taken. State governments believed Aboriginal people to be 'doomed to extinction', and enacted legislation to 'protect' the welfare of the survivors through isolation and segregation. Reserves or missions were established, and state governments increased their efforts to remove Aboriginal people to reserves. All Aborigines and 'half-castes' became wards of the state, and were subjected to repressive regulations, taboos on marriage between Indigenous and non-Indigenous people, compulsory medical examinations, and imprisonment without trial (Kelly & Lenthall, 1997). Since the demise of Indigenous Australians was seen as inevitable, little concern about their health status was expressed by non-Indigenous Australians (Saggers & Gray, 2007). Between 1910 and 1970, thousands of Indigenous Australians were forcibly removed by the state from their families as children and raised in government institutions and foster homes (Human Rights and Equal Opportunity Commission, 2006).

In 1937, a national meeting of state and federal governments was held to develop the first common national approach towards Aborigines. The resulting policy of assimilation differentiated 'full bloods', who were to remain segregated on reserves and expected to die out, from 'half castes', who were to be educated to white standards for employment which would not 'bring them into economic or social conflict with the white community i.e. domestic labourers'. In 1965, at a federal conference, the goal of 'assimilation' was modified to voluntary 'integration', and in 1972, this was again modified to self-determination and self-management (Kelly & Lenthall, 1997). The Indigenous population began to increase over the first half of the twentieth century, and, unable to ignore their poor health and living conditions, governments responded primarily by funding biomedical interventions.

Since the late 1960s, as a result of passive welfare and rise of substance abuse epidemics in Indigenous communities, there has been what Pearson (2006) describes as a collapse of social norms concerning responsibility, respect, authority, obligations, and behaviour. He depicts Aboriginal communities where the majority of people may personally hold positive values and behaviour, but have adopted a neutral or non-judgmental norm which is permissive of the deviant values and behaviours of sub-groups (Pearson, 2006). Substance use and different forms of antisocial behaviours seem to be a way of life for many Indigenous youth. Some suffer from depression, which later leads to suicide. Winch (1999: 22) indicates that these issues are broader as Indigenous parents and children attempt to succeed in modern Australia. Children experience on-going pressure in the classroom and their social environments. They also have to learn to change or adopt Western culture or risk being dropped out of the wider society. There are consequences for school participation rates and expectations of educational success on these groups (Winch, 1999).

Despite activism from the nineteenth century onwards by Indigenous and non-Indigenous people to improve health standards and support Indigenous empowerment (Mitchell, 2007), until recently Indigenous people have had little control over their lives or capacity to address their own health issues. It was not until the 1970s that Aboriginal and Torres Strait Islander health workers began to form a professional group, and the first Aboriginal community-controlled health service was established in 1971 in Redfern, Sydney. As the limited impact of biomedical approaches became evident, some researchers began to emphasise the importance on health of environmental and social conditions, colonial history, and dispossession (Saggers & Gray, 2007).

The first network of Australian Indigenous health promotion practitioners was formed as recently as 1995. It is based at Sydney University, and aims to improve the health of Indigenous Australians through education and professional development, mobilisation of relevant resources, and advocacy. In 2006, it initiated a process towards developing a model for Indigenous health promotion (Australian Indigenous Health Promotion Network, 2006). Though recent, the Indigenous health field has grown rapidly and there are now more than 130 community-controlled health services throughout Australia. They aim to ensure that primary health care services are delivered in a holistic, comprehensive, and culturally appropriate way to the community (which controls it through a locally elected Board of Management), and often have a strong health promotion focus (National Aboriginal Community Controlled Health Organisation, 2006).

The diversity of Indigenous Australians

The latest Australian Bureau of Statistics (ABS, 2007) preliminary count estimates the Indigenous population at just over 517,000, or 2.5 per cent of the total population. Of Australia's Indigenous people, 90 per cent identify as being Aboriginal, 6 per cent Torres Strait Islander, and 4 per cent as being of both Aboriginal and Torres Strait Islander origin. New South Wales (148,200) and Queensland (146,400) had the largest Indigenous populations, followed by Western Australia (77,900) and the Northern Territory (66,600). However, the Northern Territory had the highest proportion of Indigenous people among its population (32 per cent), and Victoria

Janya McCalman, Komla Tsey, Teresa Gibson & Bradley Baird

the lowest (0.6 per cent). As expected, most Torres Strait Islander people live in Queensland (ABS, 2007).

Higher levels of fertility and mortality than the non-Indigenous population mean that the Indigenous population is much younger, with a median age of 21 years compared to 36 years for the non-Indigenous population (see Figure 4.1). Only about 3 out of 100 Indigenous people are aged 65 years or over, compared with 10 out of 100 non-Indigenous people (ABS & AIHW, 2005).

FIGURE 4.1   Population pyramid of Indigenous and non-Indigenous populations—2001

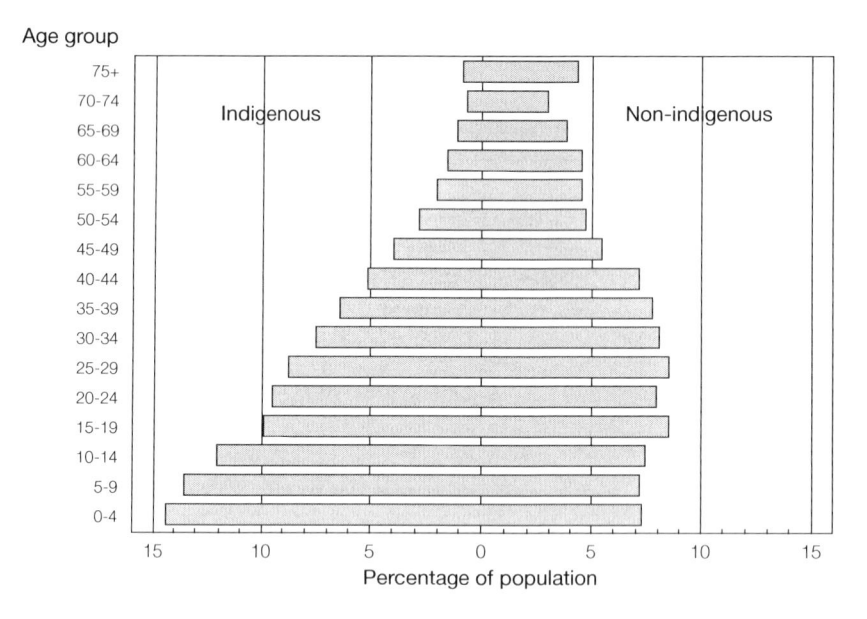

Source: Australian Bureau of Statistics (2001) *Census of Population and Housing*, cited in Australian Bureau of Statistics & Australian Institute of Health and Welfare (2005)

Slightly more than one-half of the Indigenous population now lives in 'major cities' or 'inner regional' areas (compared with almost nine-tenths of the non-Indigenous population). But the Indigenous population is much more widely dispersed across Australia than is the non-Indigenous population, with about one-quarter of Indigenous people (compared to 2 per cent of non-Indigenous people) living in areas classified as 'remote' or 'very remote' in relation to having 'very little or very restricted access to goods and services and opportunities for social interaction' (ABS & AIHW, 2003: 17).

The importance of cultural ties and connection to homelands or traditional country is illustrated in Figure 4.2 by a recent Australian Institute of Health and Welfare survey of Aboriginal and Torres Strait Islander health (ABS & AIHW,

2005). Some Aboriginal people have returned to homelands communities, and although they are struggling to maintain their traditional ways in the face of the ever-increasing pressures of modernisation, a recent government report found that small remote Indigenous communities have healthier environments than larger towns and also have stronger economic possibilities (Office of Indigenous Policy Coordination, 2007).

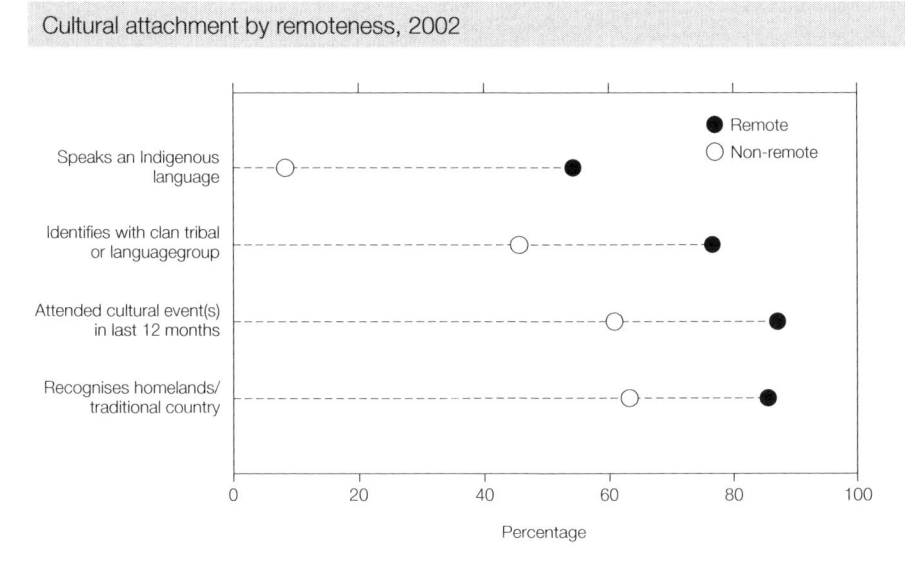

Cultural attachment by remoteness, 2002 — FIGURE 4.2

Source: Australian Bureau of Statistics, *2002 National Aboriginal and Torres Strait Islander Social Survey*, cited in Australian Bureau of Statistics & Australian Institute of Health and Welfare, 2005

Ties to family, clan and tribal groups are also strong despite the removal of family members through the 'stolen generation'. The extent and impact of this policy was revealed through a national survey in 2004, in which 40 per cent of Indigenous people aged 15 years or over reported that they or one of their relatives had been removed from their natural family (Human Rights and Equal Opportunity Commission, 2006).

Indigenous Australians and their health indicators

Australia's overall good health is not shared by all Australians. There are substantial, avoidable, and systematic health inequalities that cannot be explained by individual make-up or behaviour. Headline indicators for overcoming Indigenous disadvantage include:

- life expectancy—59 years for Indigenous men (compared to 77 years for all Australian men) and 65 years for women (compared to 82 years) (Steering Committee for the Review of Government Service Provision, 2007)
- mortality—age-standardised death rates from all causes combined were more than three times as high for Indigenous people as those for non-Indigenous people 2001–05 (2043.7 per 100,000 compared with 621.7 per 100,000) (Steering Committee for the Review of Government Service Provision, 2007). The major contributor to premature mortality in Indigenous Australians was non-communicable diseases in adults. These include cardiovascular disease, cancers, endocrine, nutritional and metabolic diseases (including diabetes), external causes (violence), respiratory disorders, and digestive diseases (Australian Indigenous Health*InfoNet*, 2007)
- serious illness being treated in hospitals—Indigenous people experience more illness at more acute levels. and later hospital presentations (Steering Committee for the Review of Government Service Provision, 2007)
- school retention—in 2006, Indigenous students were half as likely as non-Indigenous students to continue to Year 12 (Steering Committee for the Review of Government Service Provision, 2007)
- labour force participation—in 2004–05, after adjusting for age differences, the labour force participation rate for Indigenous people (58.5 per cent) was about three-quarters of that for non-Indigenous people (78.1 per cent). The unemployment rate for Indigenous people (12.9 per cent) was about three times the rate for non-Indigenous people (4.4 per cent) (Steering Committee for the Review of Government Service Provision, 2007)
- household and individual income—for the period 2004–05, median gross weekly household income for Indigenous people was $340, compared with $618 for non-Indigenous households. In 2004–05, over half of Indigenous people (51.6 per cent) received most of their individual income from government pensions and allowances, followed by salaries and wages (33.9 per cent) and CDEP (Community Development Employment Projects) (10.1 per cent) (Steering Committee for the Review of Government Service Provision, 2007)
- home ownership—in 2002, 27 per cent of Indigenous people nationally lived in homes that someone in their household owned or was purchasing, compared with 74 per cent of non-Indigenous people (Steering Committee for the Review of Government Service Provision, 2007).

In general, health data currently under-represents the health experience of Aboriginal communities and, unfortunately, health status may be worse than the figures indicate (Collaborative Centre for Aboriginal Health Promotion, 2006).

The Human Rights and Equal Opportunity Commission (HREOC, 1997) predicts that, in Australia, the level of inequality is likely to worsen substantially over the next decade due to the faster growth rate of the Indigenous population.

So far in this chapter, we have tried to portray the historical, demographic and socio-economic context within which health promotion initiatives are being implemented. These are important because they shape Indigenous people's expectations, relationships, willingness to encompass health promotion messages, and capacities, and hence the effectiveness of health promotion interventions. The remainder of this chapter is based on data from two major sources. The first source was a group of North Queensland Indigenous graduates of Sydney University's Graduate Diploma in Indigenous Health Promotion, who provide a direct voice of their reflection of their work in communities. The second is a literature review using various databases on Indigenous health promotion. Evaluations of more than thirty Indigenous health promotion interventions were retrieved and analysed.

What do Indigenous health promotion practitioners say?

This section describes the reflections of Indigenous health promotion practitioners, two of whom co-authored this chapter. The discussion was guided by the objectives cited at the start of this chapter. Although both Indigenous and non-Indigenous health promotion practitioners participated, we quote only the insights of the Indigenous practitioners here.

Consistent with the Aboriginal definition of health, Indigenous health promotion practitioners defined health promotion as 'part of raising up the spirit'. 'When you have got no culture you get people who have got nothing. We have got to meet the need of our people and their need is that their spirit is crying out—for our way again, you know? Our land.'

From their experience of implementing interventions in their communities, the group reflected that programs work well when they have strong emotional, spiritual, and cultural underpinnings. Addressing emotional resistance to change as a result of shame, grief, feelings of inadequacy or low self-esteem, and the promotion of spiritual forgiveness and reconciliation, can be important. Building on cultural attachment, identity, and the restoration of cultural values can also work well. 'We start dancing and this time it was a different dance, you know. Not like a puppet on a string no more. We dancing in our spirit now, you know. Oh man!'

Janya McCalman, Komla Tsey, Teresa Gibson & Bradley Baird

Small groups can provide support for personal and community-level empowerment. 'Being part of a group … gives them a stronger voice to speak out and I have seen people take action, take control. But there needs to be that ongoing support within the family construct, within the community construct.'

Reflecting on personal stories can also be a powerful way of reinforcing oral traditions and promoting messages of health and wellness. 'Passing on the skills and knowledge to your siblings or to your cousins or so on. It's a natural process. The story telling'.

The main challenges for health promotion interventions arise from the frustration and sense of hopelessness engendered by the long struggle for equality and equity in Australian society, and the lack of acknowledgment by mainstream Australia of past and present injustices.

> This country here, we have not acknowledged what is wrong—how they have treated Aboriginal people … And that is the thing that I believe breaks Aboriginal people down, they give up. It's funny but I feel very strong about that. White Australia don't realise how hard it is for Indigenous people. There is a lot of us want to move up the chain, and want to own a house and want to have a car and want to be able to have materialistic things. But when you keep getting kicked and kicked and kicked you just give up. So that is the struggle I guess. I wish people would—step in our shoes for one day and you will see what it is like to be an Aboriginal person.

and

> As a people we have been fighting for change and it is not ten years, it is not twenty years, it has been a hundred years and a lot of that stuff still exists today, we are still fighting and fighting and fighting. And sometimes I think in myself is there hope. Are we still going to be living in a system that is very racist. That is how I feel. Is it going to improve for our children. Our children here.

The health promotion practitioners felt that ongoing 'strength and courage' was critical to the future of health promotion. 'That is the challenge—it is that getting up and keeping fighting, and looking for new ways to combat the things that make us sick. To build a fighting spirit and not give up.'

Thus, from the point of view of this group of Indigenous health promotion practitioners, effective health promotion needs to be underpinned by strong emotional, spiritual, and cultural understandings; an acknowledgment of past injustice, and will-power to address current inequities. Above all, it needs strength, courage, and hope to make things better.

What does the literature say?

This section was developed from a review of more than thirty papers and reports that described Indigenous health promotion evaluations, and a scan of the mainstream and Indigenous health promotion literature concerning theory, methods, and evaluation.

What is Indigenous health promotion?

By combining the Ottawa Charter for Health Promotion's definition of 'health promotion', and the National Aboriginal Health Strategy Working Party's definition of 'health', Indigenous health promotion can be defined as the 'process of enabling Indigenous people to increase control over, and to improve, not just the physical wellbeing of the individual, but the social, emotional and cultural wellbeing of the whole community in which each individual is able to achieve their full potential as a human being, thereby bringing about the total wellbeing of their community' (WHO, 1986; National Aboriginal Health Strategy Working Party, 1989: x).

What this means in practice was discussed by 65 Indigenous and non-Indigenous health professionals at an Australian Indigenous Health Promotion Network workshop at the Sixteenth National Health Promotion Conference in Alice Springs in 2006 (Australian Indigenous Health Promotion Network, 2006). Participants concluded that there were fine distinctions between mainstream health promotion, as expressed in the Ottawa Charter, and Indigenous health promotion. The essential elements of an Australian Indigenous health promotion model were identified as community ownership, empowerment, consultation, and partnerships. Participants did not elaborate specifically on what these meant for health promotion practice in general, but described how they related to the Ottawa Charter action areas as follows (Australian Indigenous Health Promotion Network, 2006):

- Building healthy Indigenous public policy: means active involvement and consultation with Indigenous health professionals and communities that is flexible, equitable, accessible and responsive to Indigenous culture. Ongoing effective partnerships should enable community ownership of the policies that will impact on their health.
- Strengthening Indigenous community action: means Indigenous people taking ownership and control over what happens in their communities, and making empowered and informed decisions. Indigenous health professionals can engage and consult communities in culturally appropriate ways, form

partnerships, build community capacity to ensure they are empowered to make their own decisions, show respect and support, and ultimately bridge the gap between health professionals and the community.
- Creating supportive environments for Indigenous people: means environments that are safe and sustainable for Indigenous people by supporting and encouraging workers and communities, such as developing youth skills, leadership qualities, building on existing strengths of family and kin, and providing workforce development opportunities.
- Developing Indigenous people's personal skills: means improving literacy and health literacy and having an understanding of the health system, medical terminology and available resources.
- Reorientating health services to be more appropriate for Indigenous people: means becoming more appropriate and respectful of Indigenous people by strengthening community control and developing Indigenous models of access and care, strengthening the Indigenous health workforce, communicating with communities, integrating service delivery, collaborating between disciplines and measuring outcomes in Indigenous terms.

What is working well?

It can be difficult to determine the effectiveness of varying health promotion approaches. It is costly to measure complex interventions, often with multiple components and intended outcomes, goals of long-term social change, diverse target groups, mixed evaluation designs, and different contexts, intervention designs and implementation, and it can be both pragmatically and ethically challenging (Jackson & Waters, 2005). However, four recurrent and interrelated themes were selected from our review of the Australian and international literature as being fundamental to effective Indigenous health promotion policy and interventions. These were the need to reduce socio-economic health inequalities by:

1. addressing both the material conditions for good health and capability, responsibility, spiritual and psychological needs
2. increasing Indigenous people's control over life circumstances and meaningful participation in decision-making
3. addressing the 'causes of the causes' of health through long-term strategies at multiple levels, and
4. engaging with expressions of Indigenous culture to convey health messages.

On this first point, Marmot (2005) suggests that remedying the gradient in health and improving the health of disadvantaged people can be built on two intertwining pillars: the material conditions for good health, and addressing capability and spiritual or psychological needs through control of life circumstances or empowerment. In the first category come availability of healthy food, opportunities for exercise, and crime-free neighbourhoods. The second pillar is empowerment at the individual level or at the level of the community, to reduce chronic stress and secure resources for health (Marmot, 2005). In the Australian Indigenous context, Pearson (2006) emphasises that capabilities need to go hand-in-hand with responsibility because of the relative breakdown of social norms in communities.

On the second point, it is critical to the health of people that they have control over their lives and meaningful participation in decision-making. The inability to control one's life (self-determination) is closely related to higher rates of morbidity and mortality (Marmot, 2005). Indigenous community leaders and health professionals have called for more innovative and empowering interventions that enhance people's capacity to take greater control and responsibility for their own situation (Oldenburg et al., 2000; Pearson, 2000). Empowerment has been defined as a process by which people, organisations and communities gain mastery over their affairs (Wallerstein, 2006).

Drawing on the findings of a multi-strategic health promotion project conducted within the Indigenous urban communities of Brisbane, Logan and Ipswich in 2001–03, Brough and others (2004) argue that a community-strengths approach that starts with a valuing of existing capacity can result in a positive, empowering focus on cultural identity, sense of community, knowledge and skills, political activism, extended family, organisational involvement, volunteerism, and community networks. Community strength can be defined as the extent to which people provide personal support for one another, engage in wider networks, and access the resources of organisations. In contrast, the conventional starting point for planning health promotion—a needs analysis—focuses attention on community deficits such as unhealthy behaviours, poor nutrition, lack of exercise, alcohol and substance use, loss of culture, crime and incarceration, educational disadvantage, poverty, unemployment, and poor housing, and naturally leads to tunnel vision concerned only with changing unhealthy behaviours (Brough et al., 2004).

Figure 4.3 illustrates that for Indigenous people, family members and friends are by far the most important sources of support in times of crisis, and health services played a relatively minor role (ABS & AIHW, 2005). Strengthening family and community support networks can therefore lead more effectively into value-adding activities compared with 'grand' new projects (Brough et al., 2004).

The third key theme from the literature describes the importance of addressing the social and economic determinants of health or the 'causes of the causes' (Rose, 1992). Mortality rates for most major causes of death, ill-health (both physiological

> **FIGURE 4.3** Selected sources of support in time of crisis by remoteness area—2002

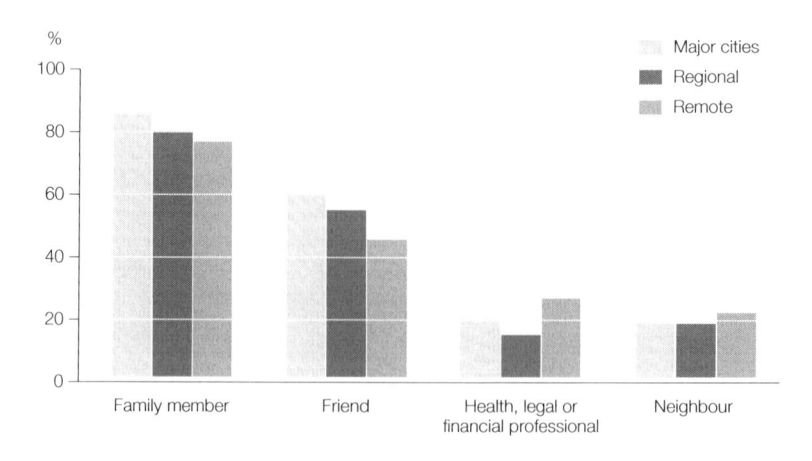

Source: Australian Bureau of Statistics, *2002 National Aboriginal and Torres Strait Islander Social Survey*, cited in Australian Bureau of Statistics & Australian Institute of Health and Welfare, 2005

and psychosocial), and use of health care services are all directly related to socio-economic status (Turrell et al., 1999). But Marmot attributes the poor health of Indigenous Australians not only to their social and economic exclusion, but also to their relative deprivation within Australia in relation to broader social functioning and meeting human needs.

The critical risk factors for adult non-communicable diseases include overweight, smoking, alcohol, and poor diet. However, Marmot (2005: 1102) questions whether it would be helpful to go into a deprived Australian Aboriginal population and point out that they should really take better care of themselves—'that their smoking and obesity are killing them; and if they must drink, please do so in moderation'. Attempts to focus solely on a key message about a specific problematic behaviour, such as smoking, alcohol, dietary habits, physical activity, immunisation, or health screening, are potentially important, but often do little to engage with the interests and priorities of community members, or the upstream chain of events leading to their occurrence.

The health promotion literature suggests that addressing the 'causes of the causes' of health requires multi-level approaches that intervene simultaneously at different levels of people's lives—individual/family, organisation/group, and community/structural levels (Wallerstein, 1992). There are examples of well-designed and evaluated long-term multi-level health programs in Indigenous Australian settings. One is the Yaba Bimbie Men's Group, developed in 1998 to address dysfunctional social norms in the north Queensland community of

Yarrabah by making clear distinctions between responsible and non-responsible behaviour for men. At an individual level, men's group strategies have increased the strength, confidence, and capacity of its members. Men have developed a greater sense of direction, enhanced awareness of themselves and their needs, and a greater willingness to seek help when needed (Tsey et al., 2004a, 2004b). There is evidence that Yarrabah men are taking a partnership approach to parenting, sharing house work, taking a stand against violence and abuse, and embracing meaningful work. Although issues such as men's alcohol misuse, drug use, violence, and gambling are still clearly manifest, there are also indications of community-level changes in Yarrabah. The number of suicides has fallen from three to four suicides each year in 1997 to two in 2006. The men's group has also developed an enhanced capacity to bring in additional resources to address a range of priority issues. These have spawned sub-projects to address family violence; prevention of crime by young people, and professional development of cultural dance troupe members (Tsey et al., 2004a, 2004b).

Attempts to address the fundamental inequalities and broader determinants of Indigenous health through changing macroeconomic and social policy, improving living and working conditions in disadvantaged areas through community development programs, changing unhealthy behaviours and/or reforming health care, and redistributing resources (Turrell et al., 1999) require long-term approaches and coordinated intersectoral collaboration. There are multiple stakeholders in Aboriginal health, including state and federal government departments, Indigenous community-controlled services, universities, research centres and related bodies, other national or local community-based organisations, and affected community members.

Finally, the literature provides examples of health promotion interventions that are not only culturally appropriate, but effectively engage with traditional expressions of Indigenous culture to convey health messages. This practice involves much more than 'Indigenising' mainstream health programs. An example is a health initiative developed collaboratively by health professionals and Aboriginal people from West Kimberley communities. The focus on learning was derived from the cultural context of the local people, and involved the development of two health booklets and a video using traditional art and language. The use of traditional art provided a means for linking spiritual and cultural life with preventive health messages about how to look after yourself and women's business. The messages were defined by community members, particularly Elders. The resources led to modest changes towards health-enhancing behaviours, improved health awareness, spiritual, emotional and cultural benefits, and greater control of health promotion by local people (Davis et al., 2004).

Janya McCalman, Komla Tsey, Teresa Gibson & Bradley Baird

What is difficult?

The key challenges for health promotion practice in Indigenous settings cited in the literature were:

1. top-down approaches focused on single issues will not be effective unless related issues are also addressed
2. bottom-up approaches can be slow, resource intensive, and require new ways of working, and
3. evaluation is critical but can pose political, pragmatic, resourcing, and ethical challenges.

Traditional public health approaches that emphasise expert knowledge, advanced detailed planning, and separation of research from intervention may not be appropriate in Aboriginal communities (Potvin et al., 2003). If not carefully designed, health promotion programs can exacerbate inequalities and hence have unintended negative health effects. The ATSI Social Justice Commissioner expressed concern that top-down initiatives such as Shared Responsibility Agreements could become less about capacity building than about punitive or coercive funding models in pursuit of behaviour change (Human Rights and Equal Opportunity Commission, 2006).

Despite new thinking about health promotion approaches, mono-causal models focused on behavioural risk factors were still a part of government-led policy and interventions in early 2008. The vigorous involvement of the Australian government in addressing issues of child abuse in Aboriginal communities in the Northern Territory (Ring & Wenitong, 2007) provides a good example. Ring and Wenitong (2007) describe the intervention as an attempt to confront a real and acute problem of child sexual abuse, using a legalistic and 'tough love' policy approach. But like any health issue, they argue, the abuse of children cannot be dealt with effectively as a separate issue without also finding sustainable solutions to the related health, social, education, and economic issues—and it will not occur without the full engagement of Aboriginal communities. Attempts to confront this emergency will immediately come up against longstanding problems, including the welfare system, exposure to alcohol and pornography, environmental and housing issues; deficiencies in mental and other health services, in the law enforcement system, and in social services; and the manifest weaknesses of the criminal justice system. There are also problems related to workforce, training, and accommodation for staff working in Aboriginal communities. Most importantly, there is also the lack of self-esteem, the need for cultural strengthening, and the paucity of meaningful activities for individuals and communities (Ring & Wenitong 2007).

On the other hand, working from the 'bottom up' can be slow and resource intensive. Laverack and Labonte (2000) estimate that community empowerment typically takes at least seven years to generate significant social and policy change. Funding sources are generally short term and often inadequate, so it is difficult to sustain such work. The review by Gray and colleagues (2000), which evaluated alcohol misuse interventions among Aboriginal Australians, for example, found that the impact of most interventions appears limited, but, in part, this may have been due to inadequate resourcing and program support.

Supporting Indigenous Australians to take their 'rightful place' (Tsey et al., 2002) implies support for Indigenous political, economic, and personal self-determination, as well as reconciliation, and cultural recovery (including connection with country). This often means that the health promotion practitioner's role is not as 'expert' but as a facilitator or support person, and that the political and ethical context to the work can be challenging. Campbell and colleagues (2007) cited deeply embedded power inequalities within health services, together with reluctance by some non-Aboriginal clinic staff to share control of health decisions with Aboriginal participants. As Professor Sue Kildea said of nursing in remote Northern Territory communities, 'this can be hard because it's not how we were taught to work' (Anonymous, 2006). Her examples of working in culturally appropriate ways included working with elders to ensure adequate nutrition for young pregnant women rather than providing direct individual dietary advice, and liaising with local council to fix or maintain a local water supply rather than dispense antibiotics to a child with gastroenteritis.

Evaluation of programs can also be challenging. Our literature search found acknowledgment of a range of limitations to evaluation designs. These include the pilot/feasibility or exploratory nature of the study, small and non-representative sample sizes, lack of Indigenous involvement at the design stage of the study, inability to clarify the exact component activities within the overall program that are responsible for any measured effect, practical difficulties caused by lack of evaluation experience, lack of technical or cultural appropriateness of evaluations, under-resourcing of evaluation, lack of measurement of specific health gain, and self-selection of participants or intervention communities (Gray et al., 1998; Johnston et al., 1998; Gray et al., 2000; Shannon et al., 2001; Ivers, 2003; Poelina et al., 2004; Hurst & Nader, 2006). Since health outcomes are a function of both health promotion interventions and a range of other factors, it can also be difficult to attribute precise effects to individual interventions and determinants (Swerissen et al., 2001).

Evaluation can also drain a community's resources. The evaluation of a peer support and skills training program for school students in a remote West Australian community, for example, provided some indications of limited positive changes in knowledge and behaviour. But the evaluation was compromised by methodological difficulties stemming from the program staff's lack of evaluation expertise and lack of support for them. The project received grants of $17,300 but implementation of the program cost an additional $32,000 in donations of community time and resources (Gray et al., 2000).

Intervention or evaluation research can support community programs by providing evidence of how to create change, produce change as it occurs, and improve health outcomes. The NH&MRC's Aboriginal and Torres Strait Islander Research Agenda Working Group (NH&MRC, 2002) prioritised intervention research for these reasons. However, a review of Indigenous health publications across three timeframes between 1987 and 2003 found that 78 per cent of recent Australian studies were purely descriptive, and the proportion of intervention studies was not increasing. Presumed reasons for the lack of intervention research publications were the need for a substantial budget if evaluating multi-strategic whole community interventions, potential design, pragmatic, cost, and ethical issues, difficulty of publishing interventions studies that produce a negative result, the political and pragmatic challenges associated with identifying and engaging Indigenous people and communities to collaborate in health interventions, and the predominance of 'researcher-driven' versus 'strategic' or 'development and evaluation' health research (Sanson-Fisher et al., 2006). A further concern is the apparent lack of reference in evaluation studies to ethical guidelines for Aboriginal and Torres Strait Islander people (Mikhailovich et al., 2007).

Learnings for the future

It can be difficult to know where to start to address the disadvantage of Indigenous Australians. Local people may not specify a health problem that fits neatly with mainstream health service agendas, but working with the issue/s that local people have energy for is likely to be an effective starting point for addressing their health needs, building partnerships, and creating ripple effects towards other subsequent issues (Campbell et al., 2007).

Based on several previous Indigenous health initiatives, a Consensus Statement on Principles for Better Practice in Aboriginal Health Promotion was developed in 2002 by a national consultation workshop hosted by NSW Health (NSW Health, 2002). These nine points reflect guidelines for ethical research practice and provide a checklist of best practice principles. According to these guidelines, health initiatives should:

1. acknowledge Aboriginal cultural influences and the historical, social, and cultural context of communities
2. be based on available evidence
3. build the capacities of the community, government, service systems, organisations, and the workforce, ensuring equitable resource allocation (flexible purchaser–provider arrangements), cultural security, and respect in the workplace
4. ensure ongoing community involvement and consultation
5. practically apply Aboriginal self-determination principles in all Aboriginal health promotion planning
6. adhere to the holistic definition of health and acknowledge that primary health care in Aboriginal communities incorporates Aboriginal health promotion
7. establish effective partnerships to address many of the determinants of health
8. aim to be sustainable and transferable, and
9. demonstrate transparency of operations and accountability.

Conclusion

Since the 1930s, when Australians realised that the 'doomed race' would *not* inevitably die out, government-led Indigenous policy experiments have 'lurched erratically between rather pessimistic realism to over-optimistic hope' (Manne, 2007). Although the health improvement of other global Indigenous populations has shown that concerted action can make a difference, in Australia there has been a lack of progress or even deterioration in some health indicators (Steering Committee for the Review of Government Service Provision, 2007). Hence, the dominant image of Indigenous Australia portrayed by health statistics and the media remains that of a traumatised people beset by chronic and debilitating disease, incompetent governance systems, alcoholism, violence, unemployment, boredom, and appalling education outcomes.

The issue has not been about whether there is a need to act, but about the way in which action should be taken. It has become evident that biomedical approaches and simple mono-causal models focused on behavioural risk factors (which have been largely driven by the non-Indigenous community and lacked full Indigenous partnership) have not delivered desired health outcomes, nor reduced inequalities in access and outcomes (NH&MRC, 1995). Disempowerment of Aboriginal people is a significant factor in the complex set of problems, and measures that lead to further disempowerment have, at best, doubtful prospects (Ring & Wenitong 2007).

Janya McCalman, Komla Tsey, Teresa Gibson & Bradley Baird

In responding to health crises, it is important not to throw the baby out with the bathwater. The foundation has already been laid for the emergence of Indigenous health professionals with distinctive world views and understandings of what works in Indigenous health promotion. Although Indigenous health promotion is still a new profession, there is a clear emphasis on the underlying social and economic determinants of health, recognition that Indigenous ill health must be understood in the context of a history of dispossession, and that substantial, avoidable, and systematic health inequalities in Australia cannot be explained simply by individual make-up or behaviour. Indigenous health promotion practice also reflects a holistic view of 'raising up the spirit', incorporating not only individual well-being, but also the social, emotional, and cultural well-being of the whole community. It needs to be respectful and appropriate, and to take into account the material conditions for good health, and capability, responsibility, and spiritual and psychological needs (Marmot, 2006; Pearson, 2006). At the 16th National Health Promotion Conference in Alice Springs in 2006, the essential elements of an Australian Indigenous health promotion were identified as community ownership, empowerment, consultation, and partnerships (Australian Indigenous Health Promotion Network, 2006).

Indigenous communities, like all human societies, mainly consist of people trying as best as they can to go about the daily business of living a meaningful life. Equally important is that no matter how desperate the situation might look to the outsider, communities often have pockets of exceptional strength, resilience, creativity, and innovation. Health promotion processes can work to harness and support those strengths from within. Creating environments where people feel safe to interact and share experience, and to learn from and support one another, is critical to developing personal and community empowerment. Processes that enhance discussion between people who bring different experiences and knowledge provide opportunities for broadening understanding, reinforcing potential connections, minimising divisions, and building confidence to plan and work together. Rather than 'fixing up' problems, the solution lies in taking action *with* Aboriginal people.

Acknowledgment

The authors would like to acknowledge the contribution of Dr Susan Vlack and Dennis Warta for their assistance with the early stages of this chapter.

CRITICAL THINKING EXERCISES

1. Why is understanding the history of Indigenous health relevant to studying contemporary health promotion approaches?

2. Choose a paper in a peer-reviewed journal that describes an Australian Indigenous health promotion intervention, and analyse it critically against the nine-point checklist of the Consensus Statement on Principles for Better Practice in Aboriginal Health Promotion (above). Does the intervention described in the paper meet the best practice principles?

3. What are some of the critical social determinants of Indigenous Australian health and well-being from the point of view of Indigenous health promotion workers? How do they operate at the level of the individual and the community?

4. What do 'healthy public policy', 'supportive environments', 'community action', 'personal knowledge and skills', and 'reorienting health services' mean to Aboriginal and Torres Strait Islander people? How can their implementation be improved?

FURTHER READING

Carson, B., Dunbar, T., Chenhall, R., & Bailie, R. (eds) (2007) *Social Determinants of Indigenous Health*. Allen & Unwin: Sydney.

Couzos, S., & Murray, R. (2007) *Aboriginal Primary Health Care: An Evidence-based Approach*, 3rd edn. Oxford University Press: Melbourne.

McLennan, V., & Khavarpour, F. (2004) Culturally Appropriate Health Promotion: Its Meaning and Application in Aboriginal Communities. *Health Promotion Journal of Australia*, 15(3): 237–9.

Mikhailovich, K., Morrison, P., & Arabena, K. (2007) Evaluating Australian Indigenous Community Health Promotion Initiatives: A Selective Review. *Rural and Remote Health* 7: 746 (available online at www.rrh.org.au/publishedarticles/article_print_746.pdf).

National Health and Medical Research Council (NH&MRC) (1997) Promoting the Health of Aboriginal and Torres Strait Islander Communities: Case Studies and Principles of Good Practice. National Health and Medical Research Council: Canberra.

Janya McCalman, Komla Tsey, Teresa Gibson & Bradley Baird

National Health and Medical Research Council (NH&MRC) (2003) *Values and Ethics: Guidelines for Ethical Conduct in Aboriginal and Torres Strait Islander Health Research*. National Health and Medical Research Council: Canberra.

Sanson-Fisher, R., Campbell, E., Perkins, J., Blunden, S., & Davis, B. (2006) Indigenous Health Research: A Critical Review of Outputs Over Time. *Medical Journal of Australia*, 184(10): 502–5.

Tsey, K., Travers, H., Gibson, T., Whiteside, M., Cadet-James, Y., Haswell- Elkins, M., McCalman, J. & Wilson, A. (2005) The Role of Empowerment through Life Skills Development in Building Comprehensive Primary Health Care Systems in Indigenous Australia. *Australian Journal of Primary Care*, 11(2): 16–25.

Wallerstein, N. (1992) Powerlessness, Empowerment and Health: Implications for Health Promotion Programs. *American Journal of Health Promotion*, 6(3), 197–205.

WEBPAGE RESOURCES

Auseinet: www.auseinet.com/atsi/index.php. This website provides a guide to information that focuses on Aboriginal and Torres Strait Islander mental health and related issues.

Australian Department of Health and Ageing's Indigenous Health Site: www.health.gov.au/internet/main/publishing.nsf/Content/Aboriginal+and+Torres+Strait+Islander+Health-1lp. This is the Australian Department of Health and Ageing's Indigenous health site. DoHA takes a whole-of-government approach to improving Indigenous health. This site contains Aboriginal and Torres Strait Islander health information from mainstream areas of the Department of Health and Ageing as well as from the Office of Aboriginal and Torres Strait Islander Health (OATSIH).

Australian Health Promotion Association: www.healthpromotion.org.au/index.php. The mission of the Australian Health Promotion Association is to provide knowledge, resources and perspectives needed to improve health promotion research and practice.

Australian Indigenous Health*InfoNet*: www.healthinfonet.ecu.edu.au. The Australian Indigenous Health*InfoNet* is an innovative web resource that makes knowledge and information on Indigenous health easily accessible to inform practice and policy. It provides quality, up-to-date knowledge and information about many aspects of Indigenous health, and supports 'yarning places' (electronic networks) that encourage information-sharing and collaboration among people working in health and related sectors.

Australian Indigenous Health Promotion Network: www.indigenoushealth.med.usyd.edu.au/. The Australian Indigenous Health Promotion Network (AIHPN) provides access to the latest information in Indigenous health, including employment, skills and educational development opportunities, conferences, and publications.

Cooperative Research Centre for Aboriginal Health: www.crcah.org.au. This website from the Cooperative Research Centre for Aboriginal Health provides details of their programs and a useful newsletter.

National Aboriginal Community Controlled Health Organisation: www.naccho.org.au. This website describes the purpose and programs of the National Aboriginal Community Controlled Health Organisation, a peak organisation for Australia's 130 community-controlled health organisations.

Reconciliation Australia: www.reconciliation.org.au. Reconciliation Australia was established in 2000 by the former Council for Aboriginal Reconciliation. It is an independent, not-for-profit organisation which aims to build relationships for change between Indigenous and non-Indigenous Australians.

World Health Organization: www.who.int/healthpromotion/conferences/previous/ottawa/en/index1.html. This website of the World Health Organization (1986) provides information about the Ottawa Charter for Health Promotion.

Janya McCalman, Komla Tsey, Teresa Gibson & Bradley Baird

5

Emerging Population Health Issues and Health Promotion

Diane Goldsworthy,
Sansnee Jirojwong
& Pranee Liamputtong

Objectives

After reading this chapter, readers will be able to:

- Identify and discuss the emerging population health issues in the early twenty-first century with a focus on health promotion strategies for optimal health for travel
- Discuss the evidence for causal links between ecological change and its impact on human health and how life styles can be adjusted to maximise health status
- Critically analyse how social and lifestyle changes may impact on the overall health status of an individual and their society.

Key terms

displaced persons
ecosystem
global burden of disease
zoonotic diseases

Introduction

Since the late 1990s, the concept of the world as a 'global village' has increasingly embedded in the human psyche. Global trade, economies, investment, communication, and travel have been precursors to improved quality of life. Further, as more countries begin to industrialise, patterns of disease and illness reflect the new societal and demographic structures arising from such industrialisation and the changes in people's life styles. This has led to global ecological changes at an unprecedented rate. The importance of the relationship between health, the environment, and quality of life has become a global rather than a local concern.

The relationship between humans and the environment is complex. Gross disturbance of the balance between the maintenance of the environment and its exploitation inevitably has consequences for human health and, ultimately, life. Population growth makes demands on the environment for habitation, resources, and food. Health provision inequities emerge as people struggle to maintain health independence within increasingly unbalanced ecosystems. The aim of 'Health for All by the Year 2000' (WHO, 1978) was an attempt to reduce some of the disparities in health between prosperous and less developed countries, although its success has been limited (Hall & Taylor, 2003).

People in developing countries are coping with infectious diseases related to poverty, housing, inadequate nutrition, and lack of health care. This can be compared to people in Westernised industrial countries, who have the diseases related to their affluent life styles, including cardiovascular disease and cancers, as well as the re-emergence of some of the older infectious diseases once thought to be eradicated, such as measles.

Ecosystem: the integrated natural life-support system for humans and all other life forms. Environmental damage beyond the ability of the planet's ecosystems to recover results in climate change, natural disasters, and altered disease patterns.

Travel, health issues, and health promotion

Before the twentieth century, travel tended to be undertaken mainly by affluent members of society without passports or visas (Lloyd, 2003). In the current global village, travel is faster, cheaper, more available, acceptable, and more common. More people are travelling more frequently at home and overseas, by air, land, and sea, for trade, business, or pleasure (Kawachi & Wamala, 2007). In 2006, there were more than two million international travellers on the move at any one time, with more than 800 million international journeys completed (WHO, 2007a).

However, travel brings health risks. Transmission of infections through aircraft ventilation systems is a potential risk to health, particularly relevant to the spread of severe acute respiratory syndrome (SARS) (Olsen et al., 2003) and influenza (Moser et al., 1979). The World Health Organization also acknowledges avian influenza, measles, and meningococcal disease as pathogens potentially transmissible during long flights (WHO, 2007a). Long-haul air travel, more than eight hours, and being seated for a long period, may result in stress, jet lag, and deep vein thrombosis (WHO, 2007a). Individuals travelling from developed countries to developing countries may be exposed to diseases attributable to poor hygiene, unclean water, poor sanitation, and inadequate health care services (Hollingsworth et al., 2007). Those who travel by rail and road have similar problems, especially where the journey is long and immobility is unavoidable (Select Committee of Sciences and Technology, 2000). The guidelines for travellers (WHO, 2007a) warn about factors predisposing to health problems in long journeys. These include extended travel periods, a history of or tendency to deep vein thrombosis or prolonged clotting time, dehydration, and malignancy. Whatever the reason for travel, for some people, health behaviours can be problematic. Changes in diet, alcohol intake, dehydration, forgetting to take prescribed medications, pre-existing conditions, and any unprotected sexual activity may have health consequences.

Health promotion strategies for successful travel and the prevention of associated illness are provided by travel clinics, government departments, websites, and airlines. Planning for maintaining optimal health should begin as soon as a journey is decided upon, taking into consideration the uniqueness and environment of the target destination. To assist with planning, there are a number of websites with travel and health advice and guidance for travellers at international (WHO, 2007a), national (Department of Foreign Affairs & Trade, 2007), and local levels (see also Queensland Health, 2007).

Travelling is a complex process that requires knowledge and preparation, although the experienced traveller may organise his or her own travel through internet bookings (Travel Information Association, 2006). However, the question may be asked: 'What is the link between internet travel bookings and health?' The answer is simply that the responsibility for any associated health implications has been passed to the individual involved. The World Health Organization (2007a) clearly states that 'it is the traveller's responsibility to ask for information, to understand the risks involved, and to take the necessary precautions for the journey'. This seems unreasonable because of the complexity of organising travel, the increasing number of official government advisories and warnings, and the need for travellers to meet formal requirements of assorted governmental bodies. It is also assumed that the travellers have access to websites to search for information about travel and travel health. However, this is unlikely to be true in many cases.

If the traveller is to be 'travel-health wise', education must be available at all stages of travel planning, and presented via a range of vehicles and communication channels (see also Chapter 2). Travellers also need to know *what it is they don't know!* In other words, the responsibility is a joint one, and educating the 'traveller' is as much an obligation for society and the community as it is for the individual. Therefore, there need to be policies and strategies to promote awareness of potential health issues involved in travelling. Equally, health organisations and governments must encourage *positive* action aimed at maintaining personal health when travelling, rather than simply using the convenience of the internet and traditional media sources to abdicate their own responsibilities for health education and promotion (Macdowall et al., 2006). Failure to do so will result in some people continuing to travel without protecting themselves from possible injury and disease. Importantly, such travellers may also bring disease home, as evidenced by the severe acute respiratory syndrome pandemic of 2003.

While travel is a chosen option for many people, there are others for whom travel may be necessary and unavoidable to save their life. These people include refugees, who may have little preparation for their travel.

Population mobility and health

Many people in poor and economically deprived countries have moved to wealthier ones in search of a better life, security, and freedom from persecution. Although mass migration is not new, the speed and size of the phenomenon have significant effects on both home and host countries, and on the health of their populations. There have been demographic change, social change, and, importantly, changes in health and personal status. Some people move through choice, while others are forced to leave their home countries. According to the United Nations High Commission for refugees, in 2006 there were approximately 9.2 million refugees, one million asylum seekers, and 25 million displaced persons (UNHCR, 2006). The victims of 'forced migration' may be escaping from conflict, famine and political instability, persecution, poverty, and environmental disasters. Many are susceptible to disease because of the lack of basic sanitation, lack of clean water supplies, inadequate nutrition, and poor health care services. Not only do refugees have to cope with the trauma of forced migration, but they and their children also face uncertainty and the added insecurity of living in camps or detention centres. Health problems may be physical or, particularly in the case of children, both physical and psychological problems. Even the Global Commission on International Migration does not accord sufficient importance to migrant health when addressing migration issues (MacPherson et al., 2007). MacPherson and colleagues (2007) are also critical of the failure of host countries to provide basic health promotion services. An example of proactive measures was taken by the United States in 1997, when migrants who underwent health assessments on

Displaced persons: people forced to leave their homes because of conflict, natural disasters, or trauma. Internally displaced persons remain within their regional or national boundaries; externally displaced persons (refugees) move across national and international boundaries.

arrival were subsequently treated for malaria and helminthes infestations (Miller et al., 2000).

Not all people who experience conflict and trauma will have poorer physical health status as a result (Ugalde et al., 2000). However, Ugalde and colleagues warn that the less visible manifestations of war, such as psychological and psychosocial problems, may be missed, with consequently increased rates of disability of adjusted life years (DALY), a long-term health effect. Nevertheless, the health of refugees and other displaced persons remains a cause for concern as they attempt to cope with poor emotional and mental health, threats to their physical health, insecurity, and the trauma of dislocation from their homes (Allotey & Zwi, 2007).

Emerging and re-emerging infectious diseases

Wherever there is a group of people, there is a potential for pathogens to cause disease and ill health. Infectious disease has always co-existed with humans. In 2003, sudden acute respiratory syndrome (SARS) spread from Guangdong province in China to Hanoi, Hong Kong, Singapore, and Toronto in Canada, and this spread was facilitated by air travel. Within six months, there were 8000 cases of SARS reported, with 921 deaths (Schnur, 2006). The World Health Organization has developed guidelines and a surveillance system to coordinate international effort to reduce future occurrences (WHO, 2007b).

Although there has been a reduction in the overall mortality from infectious diseases, people in many poor countries still die from preventable diseases (Parashar et al., 2006). In developed countries, the economic impact of infectious diseases is also an issue. For example, in the USA, the financial cost of adolescent pertussis is estimated to reach US$3.2 billion by 2010 if preventative action is not taken (Purdy et al., 2004). There is also the economic and social cost of HIV/AIDS and the re-emerging diseases of syphilis, gonorrhoea, and chlamydia.

Zoonotic diseases: diseases caused by infectious agents that can be transmitted between, or are shared by, animals and humans.

Inappropriate farming practices lead to the emergence of new zoonotic diseases and threaten to increase the burden of disease, with subsequent economic, social, and community effects. Examples are SARS, avian influenza, and bovine spongiform encephalopathy (BSE), also known as mad-cow disease. King (2007) warns that demand-driven agriculture and the methods of producing livestock for human consumption contribute to the increase of infectious disease. Therefore, public health infrastructure and strategies for maintaining good animal health are needed to ensure safe crop and animal production. Failure to do this will see the evolution of new infectious zoonotic pathogens and a rapid spread of current zoonotic microbes. Indeed, air travel and globalisation of trade, and political and social exchanges, provide opportunities for accidental, opportunistic, and deliberate sharing of pathogens.

Society and health

In their paper to the Sixth Global Conference on Health Promotion in Bangkok in 2005, McMichael and Butler (2005: 2) warn us that:

> There are emerging risks to health from demographic shifts, large-scale environmental changes, the cultural and behavioural changes accompanying national development, and an economic system that emphasises the material over other elements of well-being.

The risks identified by McMichael and Butler (2005) were infectious diseases—both new and re-emerging ones. To these could be added inadequate public health resources, and civil and political conflict. The relationship between the environment, globalisation, health, and population mobility has been known for some time. The interest in this health issue is apparently motivated by the emergence of new infectious diseases together with the reappearance of old ones, as previously discussed. But infectious disease is, as indicated by McMichael and Butler, only part of the picture. Movement of people, agricultural, industrial, technological, and economic changes, and the rising population, are all contributors to change in today's societal structure and its subsequent relationship to health. Differences in cultures, societal mores, behaviour patterns, and religious beliefs impact on communities and their health status. The increase in world population is accompanied by an increase between the 'haves and have-nots', together with gross disparities in health status. As some developing countries moved towards industrialisation and affluence, their leading causes of illness and morbidity, such as cardiovascular disease, obesity, diabetes, and cancer, began to reflect those of the industrialised West.

Sub-Saharan Africa, Ethiopia, parts of Afghanistan, and Bangladesh are still very much agrarian-based societies where, for many, survival is still at subsistence level. The situation of some developing nations is further exacerbated by the drain on already scarce resources as a result of the migration of medical practitioners from sub-Saharan Africa to more affluent countries, especially the United States. These Sub-Saharan countries are further disadvantaged economically since they incur the initial cost of educating the medical practitioners (Hagopian et al., 2004).

Entrenched and long-standing government corruption found in some countries can be difficult to eradicate. In turn, social injustice, economic disadvantage, and

Global burden of disease: the gap between current health and an ideal health status in which individuals live a normal life span free of illness and disease. Populations of impoverished countries carry a greater burden of disease than wealthy countries.

religious fundamentalism, have been instrumental factors in bioterrorism, a new health issue. Infectious biological and chemical agents have the potential to become the weapons of choice for groups seeking to fulfil their political or other agendas. Biological attacks using anthrax, botulism, smallpox, plague, cholera, and viral haemorrhagic fever have the potential to cause high mortality and morbidity rates in communities where population immunity is low or non-existent (Radosavljevic & Jakovljevic, 2007). The World Health Organization (2005) warns that preparedness and a rapid coordinated response following an attack is essential to contain infection spread and minimise mortality and morbidity. Following the SARS outbreak, strategies and management processes have been developed to deal promptly with pandemics and epidemics and bioterrorism attacks. These incorporate the International Health Regulations (IHR, 2005a), designed for surveillance and response to any global health or epidemic threat.

In short, should there be a deliberate or natural biological epidemic, a chemical or radiological disaster, a collaborative, coordinated global response activates to deal with it. The IHR became effective worldwide as of 15 June 2007, their adoption binding on all WHO member states and other governments and organisations with which the World Health Organization collaborates (WHO, 2005). In addition, the

FIGURE 5.1 Flowchart of the World Health Organization's alert and verification activities

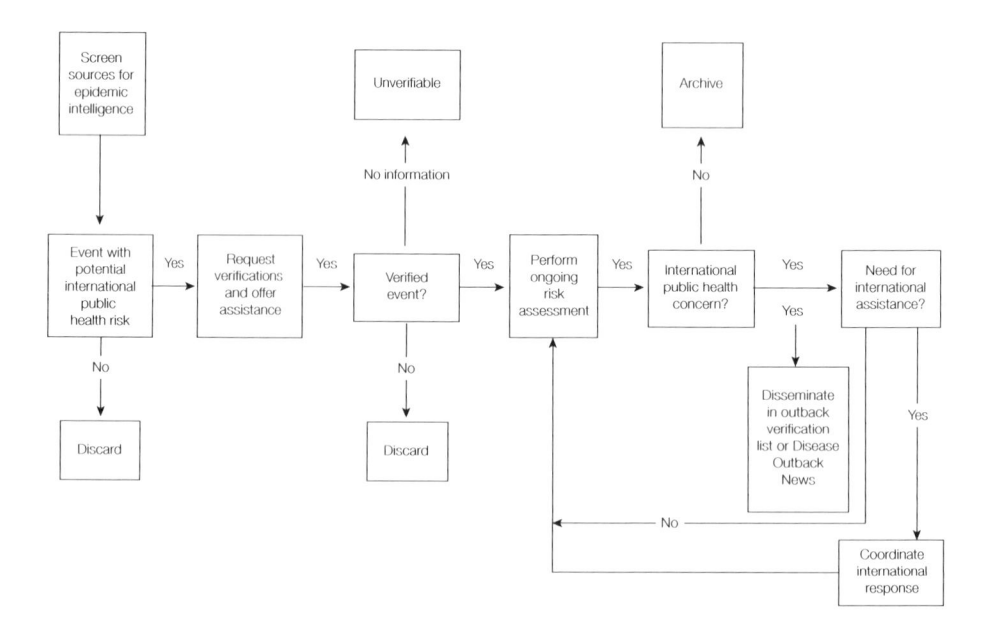

Adapted from World Health Organization (2006)

establishment of the Global Outbreak Alert and Response Network (GOARN), and a public health mapping program, together with computerised global information systems, enable the World Health Organization to maintain surveillance and monitoring when an infectious disease outbreak occurs (O'Neill & Meert, 2007). As soon as an international public health threat is identified, a process of assessment begins (Figure 5.1).

Environment and health

You are reading a travel brochure. The place advertised seems a paradise: clear blue skies, fresh clean streams and rivers, lush green surroundings, seas teeming with fish, a multitude of flora and fauna, warm days and cool evenings with occasional rainfall, and friendly locals. 'Perfect', you think to yourself, 'fresh air and exercise. I shall get some fishing in too.'

As you land at your destination, something seems not quite right. The clear blue skies are dark and cloudy with bits of matter floating in them. On landing, you set off exploring the surroundings. The fresh, clean stream you looked for is dirty with scum and debris floating on top with a few dead fish on the surface. Disappointed, you set off for the beach. 'I'll fish there,' you think. Going to the beach, you have to cross a field. When crossing the field, you notice the lush green grass is brown and dead; only weeds are growing. There aren't any trees or animals either, except a few penned cattle watching a man walking to them with some feed. 'Am I on the right path to the beach?' you ask. 'Yes,' is the reply, 'but watch out for the guerrillas, they've been seen in the area.' 'Guerrillas?' you ask, 'I thought this was a peaceful place.' 'Well, it was before the insurgents decided they wanted the land,' was the response. You see the sea in the distance and smile at the thought of some good fishing. But when you arrive, there is a notice on the beach: 'No fishing. No fish.' Disappointed, you walk back to the man, who is still with the cattle. 'What happened to the fish?' you ask. 'Fish?' replies the man, then laughs, 'There hasn't been any fish here for decades. The sea was all fished out years ago. There's nothing in the sea now, not even coral. That died when the sea temperature rose with climate change.' You think about this for a minute, then look around. 'It's very quiet. Aren't there any children here?' 'No,' says the man quietly, 'my two little boys died three years ago. The livestock died in the drought, because there wasn't any pasture for them. The children became undernourished because we didn't have enough food for them either. They caught a new bug that gave them diarrhoea and were dead in four days. My wife was drowned in the cyclones that came last year; she was caught in the field in a flash flood and got swept away. There is only me now, and these old

Diane Goldsworthy, Sansnee Jirojwong & Pranee Liamputtong

beasts I saved, and I won't live for much longer. The pollution from the factories in the town down the road has damaged my lungs, and poisoned what few crops I have.' The man moves towards the cattle, the conversation is finished.

You turn and walk away, wondering how all this happened. Taking the travel brochure out of your pocket you read it again. There, at the bottom, in very small writing is a date. You look at it again. The brochure was printed 150 years ago! You prepare to leave, thinking sadly about your dream of a good holiday.

Humans' relationship with their environment has always been one of dependence, where food, clothing, and shelter, the basic human needs for survival, have been provided by the environment itself. Where we live also influences how we live, and governs decision-making, social activities, belief structures, and, consequently, our state of health (Baum, 1999; Prüss-Űstűn & Corvalán, 2006). Safeguarding and maintaining a healthy environment is vital for optimum individual and population health. The US National Environmental Health Association describes this perfectly (Newton, per.com.):

> Environmental health and protection refers to protection against environmental factors that may adversely impact human health or the ecological balances essential to long-term human health and environmental quality, whether in the natural or man-made environment.

However, our ecosystem is under stress; the processes of global warming and climate change are well under way. It is unlikely they can now be stopped. The continuing degradation of the environment, pollution of the atmosphere, and contamination of seas and waterways ultimately manifest themselves in natural disasters, agricultural dysfunction, and ill health. These occurrences are responsible for approximately 24 per cent of the global disease burden and 23 per cent of all deaths (Prüss-Űstűn & Corvalán, 2006). The magnitude of the problems needs urgent action to address the environmental health problems. Yet, the health issues today result from many decades of environmental degradation and pollution, and continue to affect human health.

Climate change is not the only factor that determines the outcomes of health. Climate change is the product of human interference with the ecosystem through industrial development, industrial waste, pollution of water sources, atmospheric pollution, agricultural practices, land clearing, and use of pesticides and fertilisers. Agent Orange, a chemical defoliant used in Vietnam between 1962 and 1971, is now associated with a number of diseases in Vietnam veterans, including prostate cancer, with spina bifida and acute myelogenous leukaemia now appearing in their children (Frumkin, 2003). It is also blamed for serious health problems, including cancers, among the Vietnamese (Kramárová et al., 1998). A chemical widely used to control mosquitoes, DDT, is another example of a synthetic environmental contaminant (EPA, 1972).

In agrarian and livestock industries, workers can be exposed to allergens (Goldsworthy, 2005), pesticides, fungicides, insecticides, anti-helminthes, and herbicides, the multiplicity of chemicals potentially causing major health problems (Whyatt et al., 2002; Bertolote et al., 2006). Climate change may exacerbate this situation, where disease-causing organisms and allergenic flora may trigger illness in areas previously not conducive to their growth and survival. The impact of climate change has relevance for measuring health—the determinants of health status—and the resulting effect—health status. Figure 5.2 illustrates the pathways through which environmental change may result in a very different profile of the burden of disease, as climatic conditions change.

Should temperature changes occur as has been suggested, the outcome would be longer and hotter heat waves. Heat-related illness would affect elderly people, those with pre-existing cardiac and respiratory conditions, people in low socio-

FIGURE 5.2 Effects of climate change on health through the changes to environment and associated impacts on infectious diseases, food production, and communities

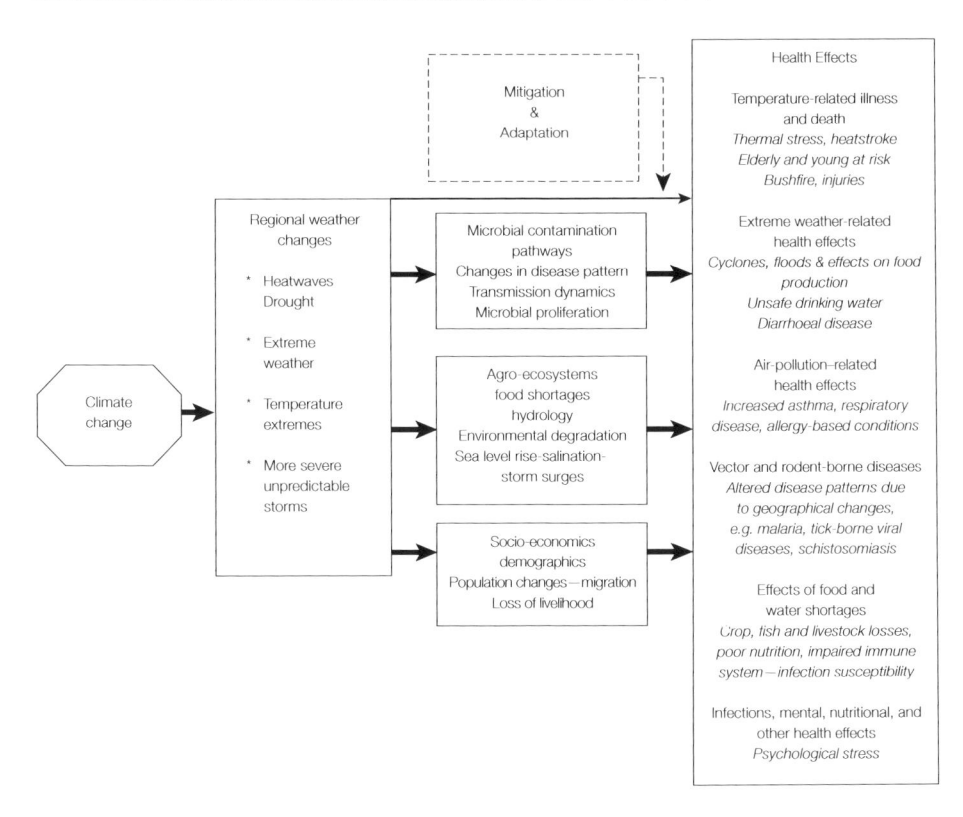

Source: Adapted from Paz et al. (2000: 368)

economic groups and young children. Meanwhile, studies need to be undertaken to identify whether increased temperature and ozone depletion is related to skin cancer, cataracts, non-Hodgkin's lymphoma, immuno-suppression, and genetic mutation (McMichael et al., 2006). Food shortages leading to malnutrition may occur as loss of habitat, agricultural land, and occupation will force people to seek other places to settle. Poor economic and social conditions in poor countries predispose to disease and may also lead to migration. Changes in life styles, housing construction, clothing, strong community cohesion, health promotion strategies and well developed public health infrastructures may assist in mitigating the effects of climate change (McCarthy et al., 2001). Human flexibility and planning will mean some adaptation, some accommodation of the population to the changing conditions (Corvalán et al., 2005).

Conclusion

Globalisation, population growth, and poor resources management are related to emerging health problems. These include zoonotic diseases and travel-related illnesses. Global warming and the depletion of the ozone layer may have results comparable to a large-scale natural disaster. Integrated and international collaborative efforts are required in order to monitor these environmental and health changes.

CRITICAL THINKING EXERCISES

1. You are intending to travel to Ethiopia as a volunteer health worker in a refugee camp. You have never travelled overseas before but are aware that you need to ensure you maintain optimum health during the 36-hour journey. Using the internet as an information source, identify how you would:
   (a) maintain adequate hydration and exercise levels during the flight
   (b) prepare yourself for the change in diet and any possible health issues on your arrival in Ethiopia.

2. Environmental issues including climate change have been debated for more than a decade. Discuss the impacts of growth of mining industries on health of two population groups: (i) Australian Aboriginal people who live in rural and remote areas, and (ii) miners and their families. After the closure of these mines, discuss immediate and long-term potential effects on both population groups.

FURTHER READING

Corvalán, C., Hales, S., & McMichael, M. (2005) *Ecosystems and Human Well-being: Health Synthesis: A Report of the Millenium Ecosystem Assessment*. World Health Organization: Geneva.

Kawachi, I., & Wamala, S. (2007) *Globalization and Health*. Oxford University Press: New York.

Prüss-Űstűn, A., & Corvalán, C. (2006) *Preventing Disease through Healthy Environments*. World Health Organization: Geneva.

World Health Organization (2004) *World Report on Knowledge for Better Health: Strengthening Health Systems*. World Health Organization: Geneva.

WEBPAGE RESOURCES

World Health Organization (WHO): www.who.int. A number of publications providing travel guidelines can be found at this website.

Smart Traveller, Australian Government: www.smartraveller.gov.au/tips/travelwell.html. Useful travel guidelines from the Australian government.

Queensland Health: access.health.qld.gov.au/hid/HealthConsumerInformation/TravelHealth/index.asp Health advice and guidance page from Queensland Health.

Airsafe: www.airsafe.com/index.html. An American website giving comprehensive information for people who are planning to fly.

Environmental Health: journal.aieh.org.au. An Australian environmental health journal site.

Environmental journal: www.ehjournal.net. An online journal for those who wish to explore environmental health more widely.

Global health: www.globalhealth.org. A web site for international health issues.

Centers for Disease Control: wwwn.cdc.gov/travel/default.aspx. The American government's site for advice on disease control and travellers' health. It has almost everything from destination advice to vaccination requirements.

Diane Goldsworthy, Sansnee Jirojwong & Pranee Liamputtong

6

Assessing the Needs of Health Professionals and Stakeholders

Omar Ha-Redeye

Objectives

By the end of this chapter, readers will be able to:

- Explain why there is a shortage of public health professionals in most industrialised nations
- Understand the different routes of entry into public health
- Reflect on the challenges of determining core competencies for public health
- Describe techniques for building community collaboration using Participatory Learning Action
- Use an appropriate ethical decision-making tool to help establish priorities between different needs.

Key terms

amenability
attributed influentials
deontologicalism
economic dominants
essential public health services
gap analysis
key informants
KSAs

Likert scale
MAPP
participatory learning action (PLA)
prescribed influentials
prevalence
SWOT analysis
utilitarianism

Introduction: Identifying health professionals and stakeholders

Australian researchers reviewing census figures in 2006 from the Australian Bureau of Statistics discovered that the existing shortage of health care workers in rural areas was expected to become worse. This has confirmed previous findings in countries with similar demographics (Schofield et al., 2006). The Association of State and Territorial Health Officials conducted a series of surveys across the USA between 2002 and 2005, which suggested that the reasons for this shortage included:

- an ageing public health workforce
- a shrinking labour pool
- workers taking advantage of their eligibility for retirement
- existing shortages in clinical and professional fields
- high turnover rates.

The baby boom population, which is expected to reach retirement age within the coming decades, also increases the need for health and public health services. Competition between health fields also means that public health will lose potential workers to clinical and administrative positions. These challenges are part of the reason why many claim that, although medicine is getting better in most industrialised nations, health care is getting worse (Barrett et al., 2004).

Human resource needs within nations are not geographically uniform either. The poorer status of health of individuals in rural and remote communities is clearly an issue as well. This disparity could be attributed in part to the decreased availability of health professionals in these areas (Hays et al., 1998). Most health care systems continue to be largely dependent on practitioners who are not from rural settings or experienced in a specialised rural curriculum (Dunabin & Levitt, 2003).

Many propose meeting human resources needs by importing foreign-trained professionals. However, the shuffling of health workers into different positions causes an even more serious complication within developing nations. The exodus of professionals from developing nations to industrialised nations has often left the source countries in desperate public health situations (Pang et al., 2002). Countries such as the Philippines are under immense strain to meet the needs of their own population as locally trained public health professionals seek to meet the needs of populations abroad (Bayron, 2006).

Regions with some of the worst public health issues have the smallest number of public health officials per capita. Six hundred medical graduates from South Africa are registered in New Zealand, costing the African nation, already struggling with HIV/AIDS, over $37 million (Bundred & Levitt, 2000). Meeting the public health needs of one region ideally should not be done at the expense of another.

Omar Ha-Redeye

Balancing the needs of competing populations, and finding the health workers to do so, may be the defining challenge of the twenty-first century. Another part of the challenge is that the public health workforce is comprised of individuals from many different academic and professional backgrounds. Some argue that the educational backgrounds and training routes for entry into public health make it the most diverse profession (Kennedy & Moore, 2001). The different types of careers found within a public health system include animal control officers, disaster relief workers, doctors, environmental engineers, epidemiologists, food scientists, pharmacists, health care administrators, health economists, industrial hygienists, laboratory technicians, librarians, mental health workers, nurses. nutritionists, politicians, sanitarians, social workers, statisticians, substance-abuse counsellors, and teachers (Telleen & Simpson, 2006).

The breadth of professional experiences brought into public health not only makes identifying appropriate health professionals tricky, but complicates the establishing of a common set of skills or body of knowledge needed to work in the field.

Assessing the needs of health professionals and stakeholders

Educators in public health have struggled to formulate an agreed set of competencies that can be used in the assessment of public health professionals. However, only 5–10 per cent of some public health professionals have formal education in public health (Kennedy & Moore, 2001). It is important to realise then that the most of the training and education of the public health workforce is likely to occur on the job, and is therefore also a responsibility of administrators in the field.

A number of different classification systems have been developed to organise core competencies needed in public health. One of the more validated systems is the CDC's National Public Health Performance Standards Program (NPHPSP) (Department of Health and Human Services, US, 1997). Ten different essential public health services have been identified by the NPHPSP:

1. Monitor health status to identify and solve community health problems.
2. Diagnose and investigate health problems and health hazards in the community.
3. Inform, educate, and empower people about health issues.
4. Mobilise community partnerships and take action to identify and solve health problems.

5. Develop policies and plans that support individual and community health efforts.
6. Enforce laws and regulations that protect health and ensure safety.
7. Link people to needed personal health services and assure the provision of health care when otherwise unavailable.
8. Assure a competent public and personal health care workforce.
9. Evaluate effectiveness, accessibility, and quality of personal and population-based health services.
10. Research for new insights and innovative solutions to health problems.

Essential public health services: ten core processes used in public health to promote health and prevent disease.

A public health workforce can be developed around these essential services through a four-part process (Potter et al., 2003):

- identifying a strategic need to improve a service by assessing effectiveness, accessibility, and quality
- identifying the analytical, communications, or cultural domains needed for training
- prioritising among competencies within a domain, and
- designing a curriculum for high-priority competencies.

MAPP: Mobilising Action through Planning and Partnership, a process developed by the CDC for planning in public health.

Identification of needed services can be accomplished through the Mobilizing Action through Planning and Partnership (MAPP) process developed by the CDC and the National Association of County and City Health Officials (Corso et al., 2000). The MAPP model and relevant tools are available online for use by practitioners (National Association of County & City Health Officials, 2008). Each competency can be further refined to assess knowledge, skills, and aptitudes, or KSAs (Reischl & Buss, 2005).

KSAs: knowledge, skills, attitudes; although knowledge and skills are separated from actual performance, they are important steps towards building competence.

Another important tool is the Public Health Workforce Questionnaire (PHWQ), which reflects the ten essential health services and a subset of core and new competencies. Respondents score three questions for each essential service on a five-point Likert scale (Chauvin et al., 2001):

- how necessary the knowledge or skill is to providing the essential service
- the personal level of confidence and self-efficacy of the knowledge or skill, and
- the perceived need for formal professional development or training in the specific knowledge or skill.

Likert scale: a graphic scale intended to quantify level of agreement or disagreement with a question or issue, typically numbered 3, 5, or 7.

A pre-test/post-test questionnaire developed by the Tulsa County Health Department has also been used in the literature (Brand et al., 2006). Once training areas or skill needs are identified through competency mapping as described above, a gap analysis can be conducted to meet these needs in order to create an appropriate training program (Calhoun et al., 2005).

Gap analysis: an assessment identifying differences between a current state of public health delivery and an optimal desired level.

Omar Ha-Redeye

Impact: a short-term measurable change in areas such as knowledge, attitudes, and behaviour.

Process objectives: a short-term assessment of the level of professional practice.

Outcome: a long-term change of health status of an individual, group, or population that can be directly attributed to a public health intervention; outcomes in MAPP are long-term measurable changes in areas such as mortality, morbidity, and disability.

Brand and colleagues (2006) described a four-stage process for evaluating public health training programs. The first stage is to identify their own abilities and skills. The second stage is that participants specify their learning objectives. The three types of objectives found in the MAPP process are outcomes, impact, and process. Outcomes are long-term measurable objects of interest, such as mortality, morbidity, and disability. Impact objectives are short-term measurable areas of interest, such as knowledge, attitudes, and behaviour. Process objectives are also short-term, and assess the level of professional practice through audits, peer reviews, accreditation, certification, or administrative surveillance. Projected timetables, production, distribution, utilisation of products, and financial audits can all be used to measure process objectives.

The third stage is to develop a scenario that can be used for evaluating the public health program. This scenario embeds the desired learning objectives in the response plan. In the fourth stage, sessions to assess, train, and evaluate are performed.

Although many of these techniques are useful in finding areas of deficiency among a workforce, a public health educator or administrator must still ensure these lessons are incorporated during in-services and course content. The Competency to Curriculum Toolkit (Center for Health Policy Columbia University School of Nursing & Association of Teachers of Preventive Medicine, 2004) describes some important steps needed to move from competencies to curricula:

- specifying the audience
- developing learning objectives
- assessing the time availability of the learner
- determining how and when learning will be measured
- determining expected outcomes
- determining content and availability
- matching teaching methods to the audience
- developing curriculum, and
- evaluating the learner after the materials have been presented.

Disadvantaged and vulnerable groups as stakeholders

Key informants: important individuals or organisations that provide valuable data, information, and context towards a public health assessment.

Key informants, whom I will discuss below, provide administrators with an invaluable starting point to conduct a needs assessment of health professionals, especially when participating in focused surveys. However, it is important to remember that their perspectives represent only elite segments of a community.

Conducting population-based surveys or creating in-depth plans requires highly comprehensive evaluations with input from the general population. The MAPP process promotes community collaboration through public health agencies and communities working towards common goals. Interaction with local leaders and the use of broader situational and problem analyses are needed to develop comprehensive social insights.

The MAPP process was developed in part from theory based in participatory learning action (PLA). PLA is a highly effective approach to obtaining broad input that uses a variety of established skills and methods such as facilitation, focus group discussions, social (wealth, well-being) maps, institutional diagrams, seasonality diagrams (pictorial representations of changes in such things as crops, labour availablity, and herd sizes associated with different times of the year), preference ranking, and matrices. PLA stems from the philosophy that elites should not control and direct the development of health promotion programs, and that marginalised populations with poorer health states know best how to address their problems (Dessel et al., 2006).

Participatory learning action (PLA): a collaborative approach towards collecting information in ways convenient and useful to the target population, characterised by engagement in a non-directive manner.

An equal emphasis on attitudes and behaviours is necessary to enhance the capacity of grass-roots groups. The ideal result is to provide underserviced groups with proven strategies for change by planning, controlling, and implementing strategies for themselves (Dessel et al., 2006). However, one of the challenges of PLA is they often do not address the systemic inequities that frequently result in disparity of health status (Castelloe et al., 2002).

While PLA is methodologically and analytically simple, it provides complex contextual understandings. The varied approaches it uses include secondary data review, direct observations, semi-structured interviews, analytical games, diagramming, stories, portraits, and workshops. PLA can also include symbolic representations to engage illiterate populations (Kuruvilla & Joseph, 1999). Techniques for PLA should be adaptable and appropriate for the respective population. The level of interaction with key informants and the larger community requires practitioners with strong communication skills, and the cultural context of a situation within a rural community often dictates the appropriateness of different communication styles. Differences in cultural contexts often present the greatest communication barriers between different groups (Dutton, 1998). Health care teams should therefore be designed to promote cultural competency for effective performance.

Managing competing interest groups

In conducting any appraisal or evaluation of existing health care personnel, it is imperative to engage local leadership and other prominent individuals who act

Omar Ha-Redeye

Prescribed influentials: people formally designated to positions of authority, such as mayors, sheriffs, chiefs.

Attributed influentials: people in informal leadership positions, such as religious leaders and health care professionals.

Economic dominants: people of wealth within a community.

as conduits. Targeting different leadership groups provides information about the specific population studied, allows public health interventions to be customised within a community, and confirms findings using different sources. Social planning using a top-down approach requires experienced community members who can influence community-wide behaviours and identify pathways for and barriers to community change. These individuals, often termed key informants, are of three types: economic dominants, prescribed influentials, and attributed influentials (Ayler et al., 1999).

Economic dominants are people of high financial position within the community, often businesspeople and industrialists. They typically have a shared interest in public health issues because their respective communities provide labour and customer bases for their operations. Businesses larger than a couple of dozen employees are typically more cooperative, as they are more likely to have public health initiatives for their employees. Industries with high turnover, such as seasonal and some retailers, may be omitted, given the lack of expertise that any individuals in positions for limited durations may have. Identifying these businesses in rural areas is usually less complex as they are typically fewer in number than in large urban areas, and they may be closely associated with natural resources in the area, such as mining or forestry. Business databases, focused news feeds, and consultancy resources are usually abundant in most industrialised and semi-industrialised nations, and can be useful tools of identification. One disadvantage with this approach is that respondents to written enquiries can easily be in positions of a secretarial nature and not in positions to influence the community.

Prescribed influentials are anyone formally designated to positions of authority, who can sanction or influence the effectiveness of public health programs. These are usually elected individuals in civic leadership positions who have a strong desire to align themselves publicly with any positive public health initiative for political gain. Rosters containing the name and contacts of these individuals are usually readily available in any stable democratic nation, and are often found detailed at the provincial, state, or territorial level. Examples include mayors, county commissioners, deputy directors, public administrators, sheriffs, or, in some cases, a village chief.

The final type of key informants is attributed influentials. These are leaders in informal leadership positions, often part of grass-roots or local community agencies. They are involved in community decision-making but do not necessarily hold official titles that clearly distinguish their identities, and can therefore be elusive and difficult to identify. Religious, cultural, and social leaders often play these types of roles, but existing health care professionals can also be useful. When dealing with small rural populations, it might be important to limit selection to those with larger or broader influence if large sample sizes will be required for a meaningful analysis of the program's effects on specific groups (Robinson et al., 2003).

Prioritising identified needs

Deciding between competing needs for resource allocation can be a challenge for any public health professional involved in planning. Some guidelines that have been established to assist in this process include determining the following (Wakefield & Wilson, 1986; Victorian Government Health Information, 2006):

- prevalence
- severity of the problem, from major debilitation to minor inconvenience
- selectivity of effects towards disadvantaged or unique populations
- amenability to intervention

However, these elements are typically not sufficient alone for dealing with more complex situations in which competing needs are equal in any combination of these five factors alone, and an ethical decision-making model can be useful to navigate the philosophical approach towards competing needs.

Health care professionals need cultural competence to understand value systems, customs, self-identification, and stereotypes that populations face. Many patients also expect greater sensitivity to complementary and alternative medicine and spirituality (Napoles-Springer et al., 2005). These factors are essential to retaining the individualised approach that distinct populations may need. Focusing on the patient in healthcare can be traced back to the Hippocratic Oath; however, paternalistic practices historically dominated most of health care, and it was assumed physicians knew best (Pellegrino, 1994). Today's benchmark for quality in healthcare is an emphasis on client-centred care (Nelligan et al., 2002), which has been linked to better outcomes for rural patients (Loveridge, 2006).

The cultural competence a health team develops will greatly assist its members in identifying relevant issues and concerns in advance, and meeting them where possible in the provision of care. Nevertheless, meeting every need and want of patient populations puts a strain on resources and procedures, the elements that client-centered focuses originally intended to challenge. These factors could respectively be characterised as a utilitarian ethos of maximising the common good, and a deontological ethos of doing the right thing. Rural areas may be more susceptible to medical dominance because human resource shortages place higher emphases and value on creating conditions favourable to professionals at the expense of other important issues. A balance between these competing needs

Amenability: how successful a public health intervention will be.

Prevalence: a measurement of how widespread a condition or disease is among a population.

Deontologicalism: an ethical approach that seeks a set action irrespective of consequences, most often used in law and legislation; ends do not justify the means.

Utilitarianism: an ethical approach commonly utilised in public health that seeks maximum benefit for the greatest number of people; the needs of the many outweigh the needs of the few.

Omar Ha-Redeye

should be established in the decision-making process to ensure that all perspectives are adequately considered. A bioethical tool can be used to assess the needs of competing interest groups and also prioritise identified needs (see Figure 6.1).

FIGURE 6.1 Bioethical model for decision-making

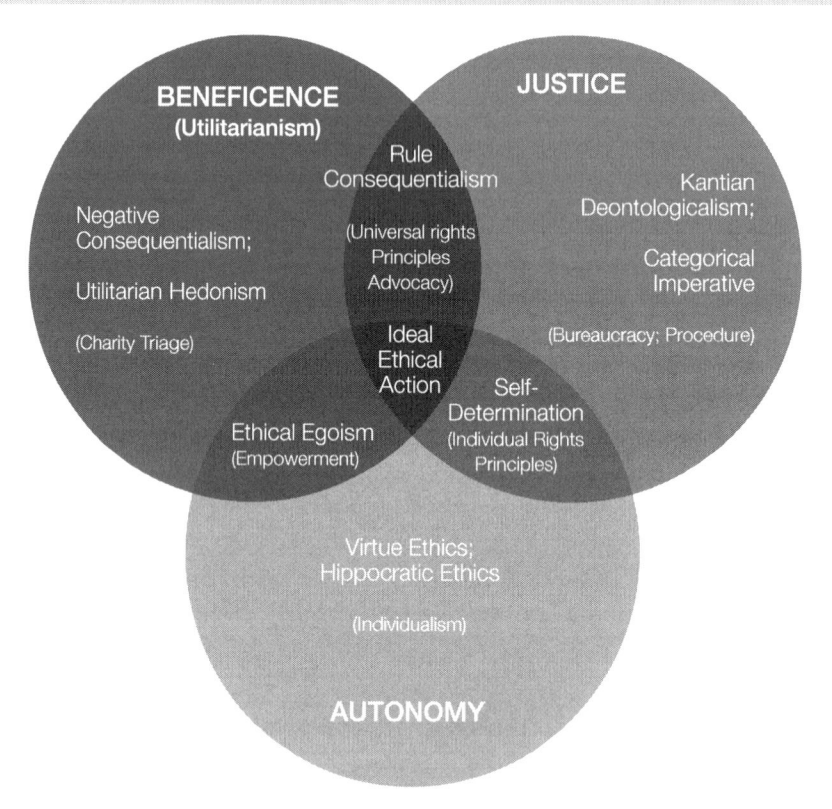

Venn diagram showing three overlapping circles:

- **BENEFICENCE (Utilitarianism)**: Negative Consequentialism; Utilitarian Hedonism (Charity Triage)
- **JUSTICE**: Kantian Deontologicalism; Categorical Imperative (Bureaucracy; Procedure)
- **AUTONOMY**: Virtue Ethics; Hippocratic Ethics (Individualism)

Overlaps:
- Beneficence ∩ Justice: Rule Consequentialism (Universal rights Principles Advocacy)
- Beneficence ∩ Autonomy: Ethical Egoism (Empowerment)
- Justice ∩ Autonomy: Self-Determination (Individual Rights Principles)
- Centre: Ideal Ethical Action

This bioethical model can be used for training, planning, and debriefing of public health programs (Ha-Redeye, 2006). A thematic approach for training could easily mirror the Action-Centred Leadership program used by the British Navy, involving task achievement, team building, and individual development (Adair, 2005). Problem-based scenarios can be used in outdoor training or classroom formats (Slack et al., 2002). Human resource limitations and the focus of public health interventions can be evaluated under beneficent distribution of resources, and examined under a key informant and PLA framework. Procedural concerns, such as organisational strategy and use of outdoor training to assist with the stages of team development, can be reviewed under justice principles with outdoor training using the bioethical model. Autonomy can be maintained through cultural competency development of individual team members as I have described above.

TABLE 6.1 Bioethical analysis guidelines

Bioethics principles	Ethical theories	Summary	Characteristics	Shortcomings	Examples
Beneficence	Negative consequentialism; utilitarian hedonism	Minimise bad consequences; maximise common good at any expense	Triage; charity	Impersonal view of life; may perpetuate injustices; undermines informed consent and joint decision-making	Emergency room
Justice	Kantian deontologicalism; categorical	Set action for all situations; decisions based on duty and rights of others	Bureaucracy; procedure	Inflexible, inefficient; red tape can render ineffective for practical purposes	Procedure wait times
Autonomy	Virtue ethics; Hippocratic ethics	Right character, not right action; protect from harm and promote welfare of single patient	Individualism	Can undermine group cohesiveness; may ignore choices of patients with different needs; impractical in mass casualty situations	Risks in alternative medicine
Beneficence; justice	Rule consequentialism	Rules of justice based on the results they create	Universal rights principles; advocacy	Susceptible to paternalistic tendencies; ignores cultural relativism	Most of historical healthcare
Beneficence; autonomy	Ethical egoism	Actions should be based on the results they create	Empowerment	Overlooks effects of actions on others; application of universal justice	Abortion; two-tiered system
Justice; autonomy	Self-determination	Everyone has entitlement to his or her own action	Individual rights principles	Individual entitlements can often conflict; eludes a standard definition of beneficent action	Assisted suicide
Beneficence; justice; autonomy	?	Ideal ethical action	All of the above	?	?

Omar Ha-Redeye

SWOT analysis: Strengths and Weaknesses (internal to organisation), Opportunities and Threats (external to organisation), plotted to assess strategic positioning.

Emerging trends in rural public health service delivery suggest a more localised service in the future with providers acting relatively independently of centralised services (Berkowitz, 2004). Providers can map their care plans and the rationale for decisions using the bioethical model in a manner similar to a Strengths, Weaknesses, Opportunities and Threats (SWOT) Analysis or an environmental scan as used by business in marketing. The shortcomings of each approach are considered so that a medium between all can be achieved (Table 6.1). Not only can this help provide justification for decisions, but can also be useful in conveying strategic elements to others on the healthcare team.

Decision-mapping can also be used for debriefing during and after deployment, which has been shown to be useful for health care workers, especially in high stress situations (Ellis & Kelly, 2005; Maggie et al., 2005). Culture shock often occurs when urban health workers move to rural areas, and this shock can last up to a year (Zapf, 1993). Framing emotions and rationalising situations can help in the process of making sense of situations in order to cope and adapt to the change (Dougherty & Drumheller, 2006). An ethical framework in particular can guide health care workers through dilemmas, and avoid the creation of moral distress (Kälvemark et al., 2004). Human rights issues, often otherwise neglected, can be emphasised and encouraged when an ethical framework is used.

CASE STUDY

1. MPHPs in the state of Victoria

Delivery of public health in Australia varies from state to state. The framework for delivery in Victoria is unique from other states in that it is largely mandated by law.

Legislation governing public health planning in Victoria includes the *Victorian Health Act 1958* and *General Amendment 1988*, the *Local Government Act 1989*, and the *Planning and Environment Act 1987*.

These laws mandate the creation of local government councils, each developing a municipal public health plan (MPHP), which has been operational for two decades. MPHPs are developed, with local agencies, to integrate national and state laws, identify priorities, and engage stakeholders. Internal multidisciplinary committees or advisory groups are often integrated into decision-making and management support.

A high level of participation by stakeholders is expected by the Environments for Health framework, aspiring to consultation with the community to identify problems and make key decisions. Planners are reminded to consider all of the following sectors when identifying stakeholders:

- national, state and local governments
- regional organisations
- private sector
- non-government organisations and community leaders
- potential users.

Each MPHP is directed to identify and assess potential and existing public health dangers and outline a program and strategy to address them in order to minimise the threat and achieve maximum well-being. An evaluation component of programs and strategies is also required.

A review, both of MPHPs in Victoria and of the *Health Act* nationally, has produced a number of findings. Most participants agree that the mandatory framework has improved the public health system in Victoria. However, due to differing interpretation of the legislation, the levels of formalised planning vary across the 79 local governments. Some have expressed a concern that there is an uneven balance between planning and operations, so that in some jurisdictions priorities are rarely turned into outcomes.

This last concern is related to one of the largest challenges faced by MPHPs—tensions over conflicting needs. Even if a priority is identified in the planning process, there is no guarantee that resources would be allocated to address the problem. Concrete examples cited in Victoria include low-cost housing, illicit drugs, and vaccinations.

Although housing has been consistently identified in public health literature as a socio-economic determinant of health, one municipality determined that their definition of public health (one shared by most) did not include the provision of housing, much to the dismay of some residents (Bagley et al., 2007).

A series of public deaths from the use of illicit drugs in another area of Victoria resulted in significant media coverage that translated into funding specifically targeted to reducing drug use. This occurred, and likely at the expense of other programs, even though the issue had not been identified as serious in the planning process.

But the opposite can occur as well. The Australian government at one point decided that all children up to 20 years should be provided with immunisation against meningococcal disease. The number of people requesting immunisation in some parts of Victoria tripled, but there were neither staff nor funding to provide the service. Funding of services consistently appears to be the limiting factor for most MPHP planning processes.

Recommendations for improving MPHPs include greater consultation during legislative changes, with scope and specifics of plans to be made more explicit. Reduced legislative ambiguity should foster a clearer mutual understanding of planning responsibilities among stakeholders. Although the support of leadership in the local community is indispensable, planning for workforce capacity and greater integration between agencies is also needed for the proper and effective engagement of all stakeholders (WHO, 1999; Victorian Government Health Information, 2006; Bagley et al., 2007).

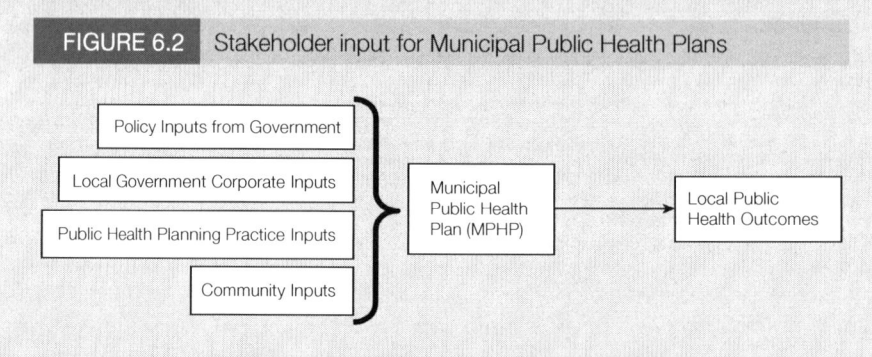

FIGURE 6.2 Stakeholder input for Municipal Public Health Plans

Policy Inputs from Government
Local Government Corporate Inputs
Public Health Planning Practice Inputs
Community Inputs
→ Municipal Public Health Plan (MPHP) → Local Public Health Outcomes

Source: adapted from: Victorian Government Health Information (2006)

2. Turf wars in rural Australia

Background

Victoria is Australia's smallest mainland state. Victoria is also the second most populous state in the nation and the most urbanised.

Although 70 per cent of the population lives in Melbourne, 18 per cent live in regional and remote areas, and only 12 per cent are scattered in rural areas. The sparse rural population is served by 69 rural public hospitals. These hospitals face a critical shortage of physicians, and struggle to provide adequate service.

This shortage of human resources has limited the ability of administrators to exert the importance of public health considerations in light of needs of individual physicians.

Tensions within the hospitals

Administrators had expressed fears of 'rocking the boat' because physicians previously employed had abandoned their facility when bureaucratic pressure was applied by senior management.

Physicians constantly threatened to withdraw services whenever new changes were implemented. The relationship between the two was so poor that some characterised it as animosity.

Some physicians even made demands for financial incentives in order to have their services retained.

Challenges to dominance

Challenges to medical dominance in Victoria and abroad are attributed to three major trends: 'McDonaldisation', deprofessionalisation, and proletarianisation.

'McDonaldisation' is a reference to the fast-food type of corporately owned managed care in public health, based on rules and regulations, where physician autonomy is severely limited.

Deprofessionalisation refers to a narrowing of the gap between physicians and the public, as demands for participatory care and patient knowledge increase. Deprofessionalisation is also caused by medical fraud and negligence leading to public scepticism and interest in alternative therapies.

The last challenge, proletarianisation, is a weakening of medicine's political position based on a number of trends, including the emergence nurse practitioners and other advanced care professionals in allied health that increasing infringe on physicians' scope of practice. Bureaucratisation and salaried physicians also add to the trend of proletarianisation.

Conclusion

Demographic changes in industrialised countries and population movements signal major shortages in the public health workforce in the coming years. Part of the existing challenge is to identify skill sets necessary to work in public health, largely arising from the diverse professional backgrounds of those who enter the field. A number of core competencies have been developed that can be used as a basis for training and evaluation.

Another important consideration in the planning process is the participation of stakeholders. Disadvantaged and vulnerable populations can be consulted directly using a variety of techniques. Economic, political, and community leaders should also be engaged to obtain insight and solicit support.

However, input from so many different groups and perspectives can result in conflicting calls for intervention. Consideration of how to allocate human resources should include prevalence, severity, selectivity, and amenability of a problem. More complex situations should use a bioethical model that takes into account utilitarian and deontological perspectives, while still maintaining the unique distinctiveness of the situation and autonomy of the population wherever possible.

CRITICAL THINKING EXERCISES

Case study 2 outlines some of the issues involving stakeholders in the provision of hospital-based health services in rural Victoria.

1. How does the influence of geography affect the medical dominance of physicians in Victoria?

2. How do the competing interests of the physicians, administrators, and the public play out?
   (a) What are the advantages and disadvantages of each of the challenges to medical dominance?
   (b) Where would each interest and challenge be plotted on a bioethical map?

3. (a) Which of these interests do you most relate to?
   (b) Are these affected by your values and beliefs, or professional background and experiences?
   (c) Have you considered the perspectives of other entities or organisations?
   (d) How would your perspectives change, if at all, if you represented a different party of those involved?

FURTHER READING

Duckett, S.J. (2007) *The Australian Health Care System*. Oxford University Press: Melbourne.

Wakefield, M.A., & Wilson, D.H. (1986) Community Organisation for Health Promotion. *Community Health Studies*, 10(4): 444–51.

WEBPAGE RESOURCES

Competency to Curriculum Toolkit: Developing Curricula for Public Health Workers: http://www.nursing.columbia.edu/chphsr/pdf/toolkit.pdf Developed by the Centers for Disease Control and Prevention (CDC), the toolkit is an aid to developing a competent public health workforce in all the essential public health services.

National Association of County & City Health Officials (NACCHO) *Mobilizing for Action through Planning and Partnerships (MAPP)* www.naccho.org/topics/infrastructure/MAPP.cfm The MAPP website provides access to the MAPP tool and related resources, including further publications and case studies.

Centers for Disease Control and Prevention (CDC) *National Public Health Performance Standards Program (NPHPSP)*. Department of Health and Human Services. www.cdc.gov/od/ocphp/nphpsp/ The NHPS site provides information and resources on assessment instruments used by the Centers for Disease Control and Prevention (CDC).

Centers for Disease Control and Prevention (2002) *Bioterrorism & Emergency Readiness. Competencies for All Public Health Workers*. Columbia University School of Nursing Center for Health Policy. www.cumc.columbia.edu/dept/nursing/chphsr/pdf/btcomps.pdf This guide by the Centers for Disease Control and Prevention provides core competencies for public health workers in bioterrorism and emergency readiness scenarios.

Council on Linkages between Academia and Public Health Practice. *Competencies for Providing Essential Public Health Services*. www.trainingfinder.org/competencies/list_ephs.htm The Council was originally responsible for developing the core competencies for the CDC, and provides real examples of how they have been used by other agencies.

Employee Worker Shortage Report: A Civil Service Recruitment and Retention Crisis. www.astdn.org/downloadablefiles/ASTHOworkershortage.pdf A report by the Council of State Governments (CSG) and the Association of Health and Territorial Officials (AHTO) outlining the workforce challenges that public health agencies have in facing future threats.

Omar Ha-Redeye

PART 3

Planning

Chapter 7	Project Planning: Projects and Protocols	123
Chapter 8	Project Planning Using the PRECEDE–PROCEED Model	134
Chapter 9	Planning Human Resources	159
Chapter 10	Planning for Policy Advocacy for Health Promotion	173

Project Planning: Projects and Protocols

Robert MacLennan

Objectives

After reading this chapter, readers will be able to:

- Understand a methodology for students to plan a health promotion investigation
- Write a project protocol and manual for its implementation.

Key terms

goals (or aims) of a program
objectives of a project
plan of action
project manual
project protocol

Introduction

This chapter is an introduction to the conduct of collaborative research projects in human populations. Health promotion programs may consist of many projects, each of which has its protocol and specific objectives. After principles have been described they are illustrated here by projects that could be done by members of a class during an academic year. The principles described apply also to projects carried out by individuals, although health promotion projects usually involve a team with collaborative functions.

Setting program goals and project objectives

Program goals

Goals (or aims) of a program: the broad, long-term, quantifiable outcomes of a program of which a planned project is a part.

Projects are planned in the context of the overall program goals, alternatively termed aims. Goals are the broad, long-term, quantifiable outcomes of a program of which a planned project is a part. The goals are usually defined by an organisation such as a health department (local, state, or national) or other organisation, such as smoking reduction programs of the Heart Foundation or Cancer Society. Programs normally consist of a series of related projects. The overall goals of a program may have been determined by an agency or employer and cannot be changed. But there still may be scope for selection of part of the overall goals that can be addressed in a focused project. Such selection may result, for example, from historical review of a program, from review of the health literature, or from discussion with colleagues.

Project objectives

Objectives of a project: specific, usually short-term, outcomes.

The objectives of a project are usually defined in terms of specific, short-term outcomes. The objectives specify the population (community) in which the project is to be implemented, and the scope and extent of the observations and/or interventions. The community is a major stakeholder in programs and projects, and must be consulted in planning and implementation, with provision for communication and interaction. The statement of objectives consists of a concisely worded paragraph. The plan for the project that is expressed in the project protocol and manual is logically derived from the statement of specific objectives. The objectives influence the choice of population, project design, data variables, and so on. The formulation of objectives is potentially the most creative and possibly the most difficult part of the project. Great care and thought are needed to express the objectives precisely.

Prerequisites for developing projects

Identifying a problem

The purpose of many investigations in health is the collection of information that will provide a basis for action, or for assessment of the results of interventions. Before planning can start, a problem must be identified. Data from the needs assessment can be used for identifying the problem (see Chapter 3). It has been said that 'if necessity is the mother of invention, the awareness of problems is the mother of research' (Geitgey & Metz, 1969). The formulation of the research problem involves a clear, brief statement of the problem, with concepts defined where necessary. If the problem cannot be stated briefly and in clear, simple language, there is likely to be more than one project embedded in the statement.

Feasibility

There may be many important questions that could be answered by an investigation in some circumstances, but which may not be feasible in the given situation. For example, records may not have the information needed (or no records may be kept), the health system may not be suitably structured, the population may not have the relevant variation such as in immunisation rates, antenatal care, in infant feeding practices, in extended midwifery services, and in hair colour (for study of the risks of skin cancer and melanoma associated with red hair). Other aspects of feasibility are having a team with the knowledge and skills to work on a particular project. For a project to be feasible, it may be necessary to train staff or recruit people from elsewhere.

Significance of the problem

Health data can be used to support the significance of a problem. For example, data on the incidence of skin cancer in Australia indicate its importance as the most common cancer, with high total health care cost. It is believed that appropriate health promotion through reduction of intense sun exposure, together with early detection and treatment, will reduce incidence and increase quality of life. Through absence of data, pain relief and palliative care of patients has only recently been recognised as an important problem. There is little relief of severe pain in the majority of the world's populations, even among relatively affluent populations. For example, Centeno and colleagues (2000) report from Spain that 'Of the patients who die from cancer each year in our country, 21.2% receive palliative care during

Robert MacLennan

the final weeks of life'. Recognition by cancer societies and health departments of the problem of pain relief for many cancer patients is relatively recent in Australia. At least solving the problem, or answering a question, must be considered to be worthwhile by the investigator or by funding sources. General recognition that there is a problem is a major factor.

Is the problem soluble?

It should also be shown at this stage that the problem is potentially soluble. As Nobel Laureate Sir Peter Medawar (1967) has said: 'If politics is the art of the possible, then science is above all the art of the soluble. Scientific investigation is an immensely practical affair.' Some problems may be potentially soluble, but not in a particular region or country. Some questions cannot be answered at all by science, such as whether there is human existence in some form after death. But the effect of prayer on recovery from an illness could be investigated.

Induction or intuition?

Background information is a prelude to formulating a hypothesis. More than induction based on such information is necessary. Health promotion theories or models are reviewed and selected in order to provide a framework for the project (see also Chapter 2). Intuition may also be needed. In other words, hypothesis formulation is often a creative process stimulated because something unusual has been observed, something which does not accord with previous experience or expectations.

A hypothesis is a postulate about what may be found in a research project. In science, it must be able to be falsified or rejected. If shown to be false, the hypothesis may be completely rejected or, more commonly, modified. People are usually reluctant to completely abandon their hypotheses, and try to retain them after falsification. An example is a hypothesised relationship between dietary fat and colon cancer.

Note that good practice is fostered by health workers being observant and devoted to quality practice. Questions will arise that need investigation in order to improve practice. Improvement of preventive practice is the important potential outcome. Rarely, observations will be made which lead to significant advances in the understanding of disease and its prevention, and often these are chance observations. For example, Fleming was doing routine microbiology when he made the observations that led to the discovery of penicillin. *Helicobacter pylori*, bacteria that cause peptic ulcer and gastric cancer, were discovered because an alert resident in pathology in Perth kept gastric biopsies over a weekend, longer than routine, before examining them by microscopy (Marshall & Warren, 1984).

Project design

Broadly, projects may be qualitative or quantitative. Chapter 3 describes both types of research methods. Many programs include projects of both types. Many health promotion projects have qualitative designs with interaction between the investigator and a small sample of members of the community. Such projects are frequently followed by related quantitative projects.

The preparatory work for a qualitative study is similar to that for a quantitative study. You must identify the problem you wish to study, and generate questions concerning the problem. Finally, you will choose a project with data collection, processing, and analysis. Even the format for the final write-up should be considered in the early stages of the project (Bailey, 1997).

Often, the only data collection 'instruments' used during qualitative research are the investigators themselves, who collect data via observation, interviewing, and tape recording in the field. Qualitative data analysis is the process of systematically organising the field notes, interview transcripts, and other accumulated materials until you understand them in a way that addresses the research questions and you can present that understanding to others (Bailey, 1997; Liamputtong & Ezzy, 2005).

For an example of a qualitative project, an ethnographic project could describe the culture of a hospital, an aged-care facility, or beliefs about health and illness held by the target population. Unbiased observation is difficult. If the observers are members of the group being studied, they may miss important insights because they are common and part of the routine. If the observers are from outside the group being studied, they are less likely to overlook everyday behaviour, but may miss the less common because they do not understand and hence fail to observe subtle indicators. Qualitative research is of great importance in obtaining new insights into the functioning of health systems, but requires great skill and experience (Liamputtong & Ezzy, 2005). It may be difficult to avoid biased data collection (examples of bias are reported to be found in Margaret Mead's field work: the anthropologist was unaware of being misled by young women in Samoa who invented stories about their precocious and promiscuous sexual behaviour in response to questions from the anthropologist (Freeman, 1983)).

Quantitative designs are used in epidemiological studies, for example to assess prevalence of risk factors or health conditions. Such studies may be repeated over time in different samples of the population to assess changes, possibly following a health promotion intervention. More complex are follow-up (or cohort) studies where the same individuals are followed over time (Bonita et al., 2006).

The project protocol

Project protocol: the rationale of the project, specific objectives, the procedures that it will follow, ethics review application, plans for data analysis, and plans for reporting.

Plan of action: the proposed chronology of the various stages of a project. It may be a part of the project manual.

Health promotion research, whether qualitative or quantitative, requires the systematic collection of information. This needs to be documented in advance in a written protocol. To do this involves many steps. A protocol is a document summarising how a research study is to be conducted in practice, including the rationale, objectives, methodology, a plan for analysing the results, and a budget. The protocol logically flows from the statement of objectives. The study design and methods should be stated, including the population, how subjects are to be selected and recruited, the data to be collected and by whom, and a broad chronology of the project. Methods of data processing and analysis must be outlined, together with plans for reporting the results. It will contain a budget, a time line, and a plan of action for the project. An application for ethical approval must also be submitted and approved before funding is granted. The protocol is different from the project manual (below), which has more practical details and assists in management and quality control of the project. Protocols have much in common with grant applications and submissions for ethics approval.

Development of the protocol in itself may involve substantial effort, often iterative. The latter implies that in developing a protocol it is often necessary to go back to the beginning several times and change some aspects as a result of changes to the later stages, or to accommodate the results of pre-tests or full-scale pilot studies. Such modifications may involve refining the question, the purpose of the study, and the hypothesis. The input of colleagues is invaluable, especially in formulating a clear and concise statement of objectives.

The project manual

Project manual: document with all the detail needed for planning the project, and for the collection and analysis of data. It includes correspondence and decisions (such as changes to procedures) made throughout the project and forms a permanent record of its implementation.

Once funding has been obtained for a project, the next phase is detailed planning and the preparation of a written project manual. Having received a grant, investigators are impatient to begin implementation and data collection. An approximation is that they should divide the time for a project into thirds—a third for the protocol and project manual, including development and testing of data collection instruments with instructions for their use, a third for project implementation and data collection, and a third for analysis and reporting.

Manuals of procedures are commonly found in industry, the military, and in franchises. In the franchise business model, now common, they are essential for training, maintaining quality control, and monitoring performance by the franchisees, many of whom may have had little experience in the particular type of business. Project manuals are especially needed in health research in populations, even for apparently simple projects. They are of great value for programs that may continue over months or years. Without such documentation, investigators may have forgotten details when projects are analysed, especially where they are responsible for several concurrent projects. Collaborative projects have an even greater need for project manuals, especially where they are done in several centres or where there are several team members involved in data collection.

The lack of a project manual in single-centre projects may cause problems in analysis of long-term projects, where undocumented modifications may have been made in aspects of data collection for various reasons, including changes in personnel. Unless such changes are documented in a manual, analysis may be impeded, especially some years later when further analyses of the data may be attempted.

The project manual includes a summary of the project proposal, pro-forma letters to be sent, forms and schedules with detailed instructions for their use, and instructions for coding and data entry. Examples from such a manual are included in Appendix 2.

Forms are designed to help organise a project and to monitor its progress. They may be numbered from 1. Examples of forms are information about the project sent to government departments, health practitioners, consent to approach subjects, lists of subjects approached, informed consent forms that explain the aims and objectives of a project and seek informed consent, lists of subjects who have consented and from whom data have been collected and on what date, date of data processing (checking, coding, data entry), and planned follow-up (if any).

Schedules are used to record data. Examples are questionnaires, whether self-administered or by interview, and records of data extracted from records or from instruments etc. They may be numbered alphabetically from A. Each form and schedule must have a title, and record the date when created or modified.

Each form and schedule must have *instructions* for its use, including how it is to be used, definitions of each item therein, and, if changes are made to the definition of items, relevant details including dates.

The addition of new items must be fully documented. Projects in human populations are often complex, of long duration, and involve many staff who may change during the course of a project.

Data collection schedules must be pre-tested before use. This should be done on a sample of subjects similar to, but not the same as, those later selected. The project manual will include the results of the pre-tests, and preferably also of a pilot ptudy, which is a full-scale rehearsal of data collection conducted in a sample from the target population. The manual will have flow diagrams with a chronology of whom to contact and when.

The manual will also describe procedures for drawing the sample of people to be recruited. Possibilities are a completely random sample using a complete listing

Robert MacLennan

of the population as a sampling frame, a cluster sample with randomly selected people forming the nucleus of a cluster, or a proportional sample. Expert advice is recommended.

Staff training is an important issue often neglected. All staff must be made aware of the purpose of the project, the meaning of variables, and the importance of asking questions as instructed in the manual. Provision should also be made in the schedules for open-ended questions, which may reveal unforeseen data. The manual also deals with the processing of data—checking, coding, data entry, and analysis.

Quality control and monitoring

Monitoring of data from different interviewers may reveal systematic differences caused by an interviewer not following instructions. Fabrication of data by interviewers or data collectors does occur, and can be monitored by asking a sample of subjects simple questions such as 'Were there any aspects of the interview upon which they would like to comment?' A project requires a plan of monitoring (part of the plan of action) to assess compliance with the plan (objective measures), by the community with the intervention (qualitative measures), independent interval analysis to detect unfavourable outcomes (quantitative), adherence to budget (quantitative), and to schedule of data processing and analysis. Other contingencies requiring remedy may involve relationships of personnel with each other or with community members.

Check list prior to implementation and collection of data

1. Have you considered theories or models to be applied in your project? Have you stated the objectives of your project precisely?
2. Have you listed all the variables you wish to measure, including those needed to evaluate the outcome? Will your instruments (such as questionnaire schedule) collect the required data with the details necessary for analysis?
3. What are the logistical considerations for efficient data collection? Have items of questionable importance or those that are unnecessarily redundant been eliminated? Hill (1962) states that a long and rambling set of questions is to invite disaster. He quotes a proposed questionnaire on the causes of prematurity that 'ran to a trifle of 180 questions, which covered a catholic range. For instance, it seemed that the author was confident that some person or persons could accurately inform her for each of the woman's previous confinements of the time interval between the birth of the child and the placenta; the incidence of congenital malformations in her blood relations; whether she wore high- or low-heeled shoes; how often she took a hot bath; the state of health of the father

at the time of conception; and the frequency of sexual intercourse which was engagingly included under the sub-heading *social amenities*.' He suggests that 'of every twenty-one questions, the investigators should ask themselves twenty and the subjects one'. Questions for themselves would include 'Is it necessary? What do I hope to learn from it? Will the respondents understand what I mean?'

4 Have you pre-tested the research instruments? Can you evaluate their validity and precision?
5 How will data be collected, for example by direct (face-to-face) interview, or part by mail, telephone, or other means?
6 Who will be responsible for collecting the data and maintaining quality control? Who will have responsibility for the daily supervisory staff?
7 How will you cope with non-response (unavailable and refusals) and response error?
8 Does the data collection instrument lend itself to pre-coding?
9 Have you established that you and your team have (or will have) the appropriate skills and expertise to complete the project satisfactorily?

CASE STUDY

Fast foods, exercise and body weight in primary school children in Brisbane

Background

The prevalence of overweight and obesity in children has increased in Australia. This may lead to increased chronic diseases such as heart disease and diabetes later in life. Although descriptive, this project will provide a baseline for a subsequent intervention program whose goal would be to reduce the prevalence of overweight and obesity in school children. This project will be undertaken by a group of twenty health promotion students over an academic year.

Objectives of the baseline prevalence project

The objectives are to assess the frequency and type of intake of fast foods and the level of physical activity in primary school children in Brisbane, and their relation to body mass index by gender and age.

Comment

Although apparently simple, these objectives may not be specific enough, and, depending on how data are to be collected, they may need to be limited

Robert MacLennan

by age and type of school (public or private school). 'Fast foods' will need to be defined (with advice from a dietician), as will the type and frequency of physical activity (with advice from a human movement expert). Data on food and exercise could be collected in classrooms with self-administered questionnaires completed by pupils under the guidance of a team member (implying that only children who are literate would participate). Body weight in kilograms (with normal school clothing) and height (in metres) without shoes are to be measured to calculate the body mass index (weight divided by height squared).

The project would require the following (see also Appendix 2):

- authorisation to approach schools by the Queensland Department of Education or relevant non-government denominational authority
- agreement by school teachers to obtain written authorisation from a parent or guardian for a child to participate (through letters taken home and returned by each child)
- consent by the children and guardians, and
- approval by the researcher's institutional ethics committee.

The project would have to be limited to a sample of schools and classes, and this requires a sampling frame and a method of selection. Measurement of height and weight would not require physical examination, so direct physical contact does not occur. A decision would be needed at the outset whether the baseline project would be part of a follow-up study of individual children or would be followed by cross-sectional prevalence surveys in the future. The above considerations would need to be elaborated in a written project proposal and in a project protocol and manual.

The team may consist of five to eight students. All members should be involved in writing the project protocol and the project manual. If needed, this should describe what additional knowledge and skills are required to implement the project successfully. Students could use the examples in Appendix 2 to assist in planning their project.

Conclusion

Health research in populations, including health promotion projects, has increasingly become a collaborative, often multidisciplinary, enterprise requiring large budgets. Applications for funds are competitive and must be in writing. Other than auditing that the funds are broadly used as applied for, little attention is paid by the funding agency and the investigators to the details of implementation once funding has been given. This chapter has offered advice on more efficient planning and quality control of the implementation phase of projects in human populations.

CRITICAL THINKING EXERCISES

Write statements of specific objectives for the following projects.

1. You are leading a project to prevent falls among elderly people. There are five key project members. You need to plan how you can work as a team with the others. How are you going to decide who is doing what? Think through the process and work with the team members. The final outcome of your working with the team is that the objectives for the project are written. Write these objectives.

2. Skin sores are believed to increase the risk of rheumatic fever and glomerular nephritis in Aboriginal children. Write a statement of objectives to investigate the prevalence and bacteriology of skin sores in an Aboriginal community.

FURTHER READING

Abramson, J.H. (1974) *Survey Methods in Community Medicine*. Churchill Livingstone: Edinburgh.

Miller, D.C. (1983) *Handbook of Research Design and Social Measurement*, 4th edn. Longman: New York.

WEBPAGE RESOURCE

The National Office for Summative Assessment: http://www.nosa.org.uk/information/audit/npms/trainers.htm. This website describes the training of general practitioners in the United Kingdom.

Robert MacLennan

8

Project Planning Using the PRECEDE–PROCEED Model

Peter Howat, Graham Brown, Sharyn Burns & Alexandra McManus

Objectives

After reading this chapter, readers will be able to:

- Discuss how planning models can be used to develop health promotion programs
- Describe the steps involved in program planning using the PRECEDE–PROCEED model
- Apply the planning process to a health promotion program to develop a program goal and objectives ready for the selection of appropriate strategies.

Key terms

enabling (facilitating) factors
predisposing (motivating) factors
protective factors
reinforcing (maintaining or rewarding) factors
risk factors

Introduction

As discussed in previous chapters, effective planning is critical to the success of any health promotion program. Program planning can be enhanced by following a systematic process. Before deciding what you will actually do in your program, it is often helpful to carry out a needs assessment (see Chapter 3), to determine the focus of your program. Once the focus of the program has been determined and the target group described in detail, the program goal (based on the health issue) and the objectives (based on the risk and protective factors) can be developed. Strategies to achieve your goal and objectives can then be devised. A clear and well articulated plan ensures that collaborators and stakeholders have a consistent understanding of the program expectations and approaches, thus supporting an ongoing and effective partnership.

Protective factors: those factors that produce resilience to, or reduce the probability of the development of, a disorder, disease or specific cause of death.

This chapter explains the process of program planning up to the setting of goals and objectives using the PRECEDE–PROCEED model. This is one of the most influential models of health promotion planning, with more than 900 published applications describing its use. It provides a useful format for the systematic assessment of priority health issues and identification of factors that should be the focuses of health promotion interventions.

The intent of the model is consistent with the following definition of health promotion (see also Chapter 1):

> Health promotion can be regarded as a combination of *educational, organisational, economic* and *political* actions designed with genuine consumer participation, to enable individuals, groups and whole communities to increase control over, and to improve their health through *knowledge, attitudinal, behavioural, social* and *environmental* changes. (Howat et al., 2003: 83).

The PRECEDE–PROCEED model

PRECEDE is an acronym describing the planning and developmental phases of the model:

- *Predisposing, Reinforcing* and *Enabling Constructs* in *Ecological Diagnosis* and *Evaluation*. These phases refer to the 'diagnosis' (Green & Kreuter, 2005: G-6).

PROCEED is an acronym describing implementation of strategies and evaluation:

- *Policy, Regulatory* and *Organisational Constructs* in *Education* and *Environmental Development*. These phases expand on the implementation aspects and include evaluation steps (Green & Kreuter, 2005: G-6).

Peter Howat, Graham Brown, Sharyn Burns & Alexandra McManus

The PRECEDE–PROCEED model can be summarised by five planning and five evaluation questions, as detailed in Table 8.1.

TABLE 8.1 Research questions related to the PRECEDE–PROCEED model.

Phase	Planning questions	
1. Social assessment	How serious is the health problem?	Health Issue and risk/protective factors to set goals and objectives
2. Epidemiological, behavioural and environmental assessment	Which health-related behavioural and environmental factors are involved?	
3. Educational and ecological assessment	What are the determinants of those behavioural or environmental factors?	
4. Administrative and policy assessment and intervention alignment	Which combination of health promotion interventions might change these determinants and behavioural or environmental factors? How can those interventions be implemented?	Selection and development of strategies
	Evaluation questions	
5. Implementation	6. Has the implementation been carried out as intended?	Tracking program progress and implementation
6. Process evaluation	7. Have the interventions been executed as planned?	
7. Impact evaluation	8. Have the determinants of behaviour changed? 9. Has the behaviour changed?	Short-term impact
8. Outcome evaluation	10. Has the problem lessened?	Long-term outcome

Source: Green & Kreuter (2005)

A desirable feature of the PRECEDE–PROCEED model is that it encourages the planner to conduct comprehensive and effective preliminary work before setting clear goals and objectives. The identification of these goals and objectives, in turn, informs the systematic development of intervention strategies and appropriate evaluation measures.

Figure 8.1 illustrates the phases of the PRECEDE–PROCEED model and how they link to the research questions associated with the model.

PRECEDE–PROCEED model — FIGURE 8.1

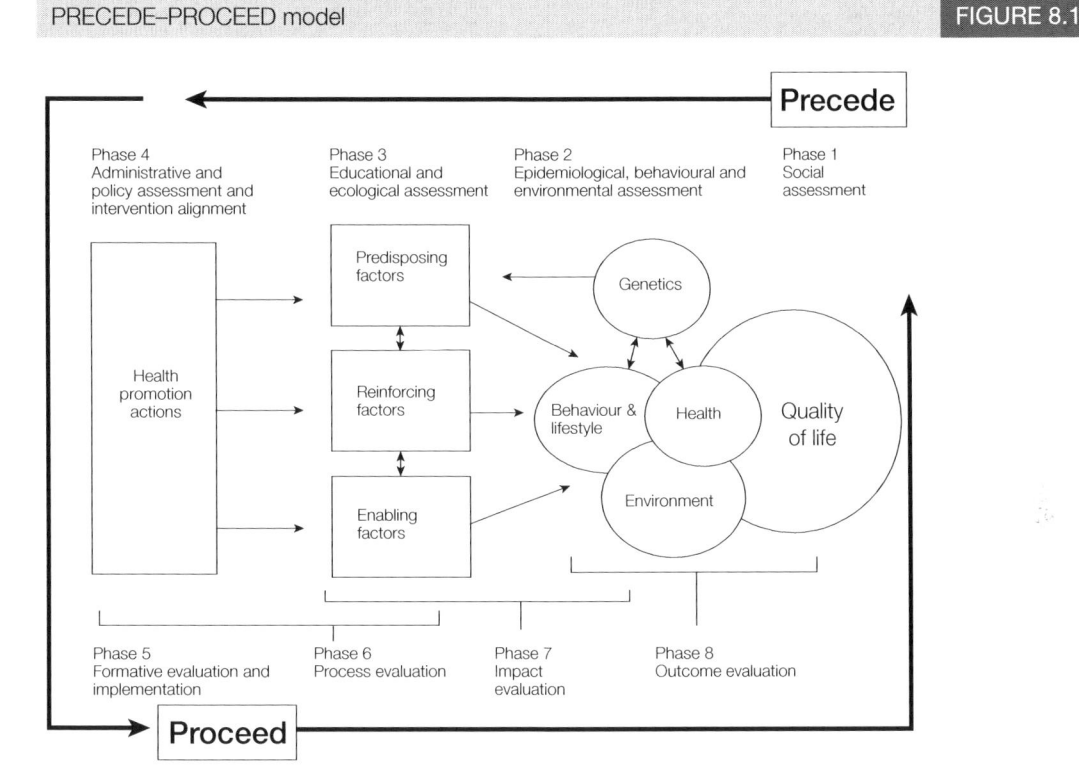

Source: Green & Kreuter (2005)

This chapter provides a brief discussion of the phases of the PRECEDE–PROCEED model and how they can be used as a guide for program planning.

Program planning and the PRECEDE–PROCEED model

The basic premise of the PRECEDE–PROCEED model emphasises that:

> the determinants of health must be diagnosed *before* the intervention is designed; if they are not, the intervention will be based on guesswork and will run a greater risk of being misdirected and ineffective (Green & Kreuter, 1999: 37).

The determinants of health that Green and Kreuter refer to are the forces that predispose, enable, and reinforce life styles, or shape environmental conditions of living in ways that affect the health status of people. These predisposing, enabling, and reinforcing factors are discussed in more detail in later section (see Phase 3, below).

Peter Howat, Graham Brown, Sharyn Burns & Alexandra McManus

To help illustrate the phases of the PRECEDE–PROCEED model, examples from Case Study 1, the Child Pedestrian Injury Prevention Project (CPIPP) will be referred to throughout this chapter. In addition, to illustrate different types of health promotion programs, other examples, including local, state, and national projects, will also be given.

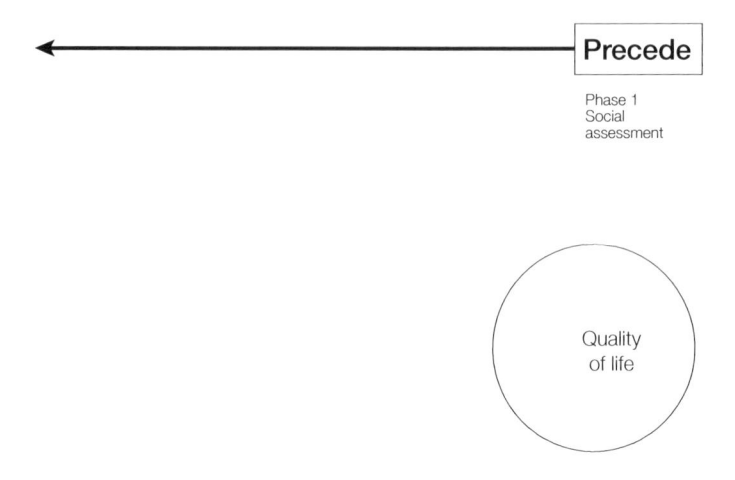

FIGURE 8.2 Phase 1 of PRECEDE: social assessment and situational analysis

Precede

Phase 1
Social assessment

Quality of life

Source: Green & Kreuter (2005)

Phase 1 (see Figure 8.2) identifies quality of life indicators and consists of three main steps:

➤ self-study by the community of its problems, needs, aspirations, and resources, and barriers to dealing with the problems (for example, employment opportunities, violence)
➤ documentation of the presumed causes of the problems, needs or determinants of the problems, and
➤ selection of the priorities from the list of problems or needs, based on their perceived importance and presumed changeability, and on formulation of quantified goals and objectives (Green & Kreuter, 2005).

This phase involves a range of information-gathering processes within a community. It is also an ideal time to establish new partnerships or build upon existing ones.

It should be noted that many localised health promotion programs may be implemented based on the identification of regional or national health problems. Therefore, this phase may have already been completed. For example, in Australia, the National Alcohol Strategy was implemented at a local level without individual communities needing to conduct their own social assessment, as this was conducted nationally as part of the development of the national approach. Although this national social assessment provided significant direction, direct participation in the local strategy selection and implementation was also deemed important to ensure strategies were appropriate to specific local needs (Department of Health & Ageing, 2001).

The Child Pedestrian Injury Prevention Program (CPIPP) in Western Australia is an example of a health promotion program that developed from community-identified needs (Case Study 1). Like many other local programs in Australia, CPIPP evolved from a need identified from state Health Department data that showed child pedestrian injury was a priority health problem. This was reinforced by the state's Education Department, which had identified concerns among the school community about the safety of children in the road environment.

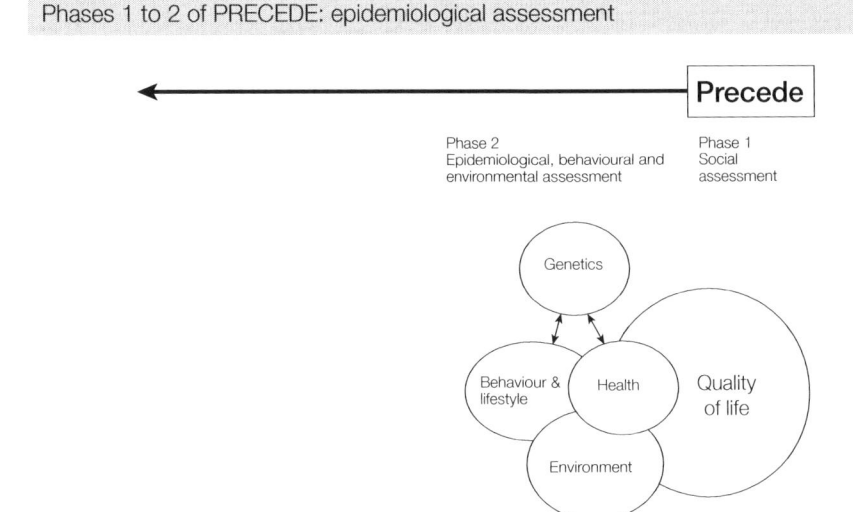

FIGURE 8.3 Phases 1 to 2 of PRECEDE: epidemiological assessment

Source: Green & Kreuter (2005)

Phase 2 (see Figure 8.3) consists of two steps. Step one reviews the significance of health problems through the use of epidemiological data. Step two involves the identification of etiological factors or determinants of health in the genetics, behavioural patterns, and the environment of the population that are linked to the priority problems that were identified in Step One of the epidemiological assessment and in the social assessment phase (Green & Kreuter, 2005).

Epidemiological assessment

Health priorities can be determined through establishing the relative *importance* and *changeability* of various problems, and setting program priorities. Indicators of health problems may include mortality, morbidity, and disability. Other indicators may be used to help assess the prevalence, incidence, and distribution of the health problem or issues (Green & Kreuter, 2005).

The type of information gathered in this phase of planning, combined with the assessment conducted during Phase 1, enables the health promotion practitioner to identify more accurately the principal health issues relating to the community or target group. It is necessary to prioritise these key health issues in order to move towards specifying a program goal.

For example, when this phase was conducted as part of the CPIPP, the incidence of pedestrian mortality and morbidity among children, especially those aged 5 to 9 years in Western Australia, provided justification for funding and enabled the most appropriate target group to be identified (see Case Study 1).

Relevance to planning health promotion programs

The assessment of epidemiological data is a critical step in the planning process, as it is this process which leads to the specific description of the program's *goal*. However, the reality of much of our health promotion practice is that often this phase has already been completed as a part of a commitment to a regional, state, or national strategy. For example, in Australia and many other developed countries, priority health issues may already be set at a national, agency, or organisational level, or through the development of state or national strategies such as the Mental Health Strategy, Obesity Strategy, or Drug and Alcohol Strategy. We may find that the program we are developing will contribute to higher-level goals, which have been already identified. Often our role in this situation is to identify specific target groups within a geographic area or community and develop interventions appropriate to their needs.

Identification of etiological factors

As noted previously, this step identifies the etiological factors or determinants of health in the genetics, behavioural patterns, and the environment of the population that are linked to the priority problems identified in the epidemiological assessment and social assessment phase.

These determinants can be separated into *genetic, behavioural,* and *environmental factors* relating to the health problem. 'Behavioural factors' refers to the behaviours of individuals and groups (together with social circumstances or life styles) that either protect them or put them at risk of developing health problems. They also include behaviours or actions of other people that may influence the health status of the target group. These factors can then be *prioritised* in terms of *causal importance*, *prevalence*, and *changeability*. It is more difficult to base a program on behaviours that are resistant to change. The CPIPP identified key behaviours, such as inappropriate road crossing and failing to seek help to cross roads, that put five- to nine-year-old pedestrians at risk of injuries. In addition, the behaviours of parents who did not supervise their child, did not teach appropriate road-crossing skills, and did not model appropriate road-crossing behaviours, were also identified. This information helped establish the need for parents to become part of the secondary target group (see Case Study 1) (Howat et al., 1997).

In addition, *environmental* influences must be assessed using the same approach as used to assess behavioural influences. Environmental factors are those determinants outside the person that can be modified to support behaviour, health, or quality of life. The influence of environmental determinants on health is significant and complex.

To allow more practical and feasible health promotion planning, it is recommended that readers concentrate on those aspects of the environment that are:

➤ more social than physical (for example organisational and economic)
➤ interactive with behaviour in their impact on health, or
➤ able to be changed by social action and health policy (Green & Kreuter, 1999: 142).

Some of the primary determinants within the social environment include the social network (for example social support), culture, and family history. Some examples of physical environmental influences include housing, food supply, water supply, prices of low-fat food, alcohol availability, extent of open spaces including walking/bike paths for exercise, availability of low-fat food from restaurants, road design, sun shades at playgrounds, and workplace smoking regulations. For example, the CPIPP identified traffic volume and speed, road design, and roadside obstacles as environmental risk factors (see Case Study 1).

Risk factors: those characteristics, variables, or hazards that, if present for a given individual, will increase the probability that they will develop a disorder, disease, or specific cause of death.

Genetic factors are a new addition to the PRECEDE–PROCEED model and are likely to emerge as more relevant in future years as knowledge of applied genetics develops (Green & Kreuter, 2005: 14).

Relevance to planning health promotion programs

The identification and assessment of the behavioural and environmental determinants are critical steps in the planning process, as it is this process that leads to the specific description of the program's *objectives*. While most health issues have both behavioural and environmental risk factors, the main risk factors might be either one or the other.

> **FIGURE 8.4** Phases 1 to 3 of PRECEDE: educational and ecological assessment

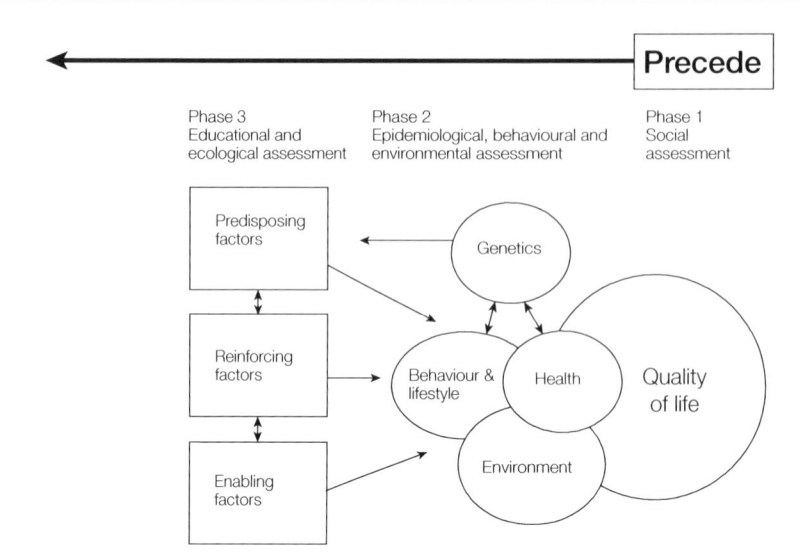

Source: Green & Kreuter (2005)

Enabling (facilitating) factors: factors that facilitate or hinder the desired behavioural or environmental changes, and include availability of and access to health resources and personal health-related skills.

Predisposing (motivating) factors: factors that facilitate or hinder motivation for change and include knowledge, beliefs, values, and attitudes.

Reinforcing (maintaining or rewarding) factors: factors that provide rewards or incentives for the continuation or maintenance of behaviours. Social support and peer influences are examples of reinforcing factors. They also include tangible or imagined rewards.

Types of factors

In the third phase of the model (see Figure 8.4), factors that have the potential to influence the behavioural or environmental determinants (or risks) are grouped according to their type of impact (Green &Kreuter, 2005: 14). The three broad groupings are:

- *predisposing* (*motivating*) factors, such as knowledge, beliefs, values, and attitudes that facilitate or hinder motivation for change
- *enabling* (*facilitating*) factors, such as availability of and access to health resources, and personal health-related skills that facilitate or hinder the desired behavioural or environmental changes, and
- *reinforcing* (*maintaining or rewarding*) factors. These factors provide rewards or incentives for the continuation or maintenance of behaviours. Social support and peer influences from other significant people, such as parents, teachers, and health professionals, are examples of reinforcing factors. They also include tangible or imagined rewards, social benefits, and physical benefits, along with mass media messages.

Tables 8.2 and 8.3 illustrate how these types of factors operate in relation to one health behaviour, smoking.

Factors that may contribute to a person quitting smoking	TABLE 8.2
Predisposing	Knowledge of the harmful effects; beliefs that they could be susceptible to lung cancer
Enabling	Access to Quit programs; legislation that restricts the number of places that smoking is allowed; legislation that influences the cost of cigarettes
Reinforcing	Friends are all non-smokers; smoking is not considered socially acceptable.

Exploring reasons why people continue to smoke	TABLE 8.3
Predisposing	Knowledge of harmful effects but do not consider themselves at risk as they are 'too young'
Enabling	Cigarettes are easy to get; there are plenty of places to smoke
Reinforcing	Friends all smoke; smoking is popular in the community in which they live; parents smoke

These factors are very important when considering behavioural intention. In some cases, a person may intend to adopt a health-enhancing behaviour but may not do so because of the influence of factors such as time, money, equipment, skills, or health service. For example, enabling factors for a family-planning program may include availability of contraception, accessible family-planning services, and the skills to use contraception.

Enabling factors also include *time* to carry out the health-promoting actions. For example, parents are encouraged to take young children to child-health clinics regularly. In many countries, in both the developing and developed world, it is the mother who usually takes on this role. This can be difficult for women who are also responsible for looking after the rest of the family, preparing meals, and working (Hubley, 2004).

These groupings provide us with insight into the educational and ecological approaches likely to be used in a health promotion program to bring about behavioural and environmental change.

Relevance to planning health promotion programs

The identification and assessment of educational and ecological factors is another critical step in the planning process, as it is this process which leads to the specific description of the program's objectives, which in turn inform the selection of interventions, and development of evaluation measures.

CASE STUDY

1. The Child Pedestrian Injury Prevention Program (CPIPP)

This case study, based on Howat et al. (1997), summarises part of the planning undertaken for the CPIPP, a school- and community-based project aimed at reducing the incidence of injury to child pedestrians in the City of Gosnells, Perth, Western Australia.

The CPIPP identified a number of predisposing, enabling, and reinforcing factors, as described below. The identification of these factors facilitated the development of more specific objectives and appropriate interventions. The case study illustrates the planning process based on the PRECEDE–PROCEED model for an injury-prevention program.

Phase 1: Social assessment

Identify the health issue for intervention
Information from the state Health Department, and concerns about traffic safety of children by the state Education Department and parents, identified child pedestrian injury as an important issue.

Phase 2, Step 1: Epidemiological assessment

Identify the target group and program goal
This phase initially involved a review of the Health Department data on injury, which showed that child pedestrian injury rates warranted intervention. Epidemiological details associated with child pedestrian injury in Western Australia were then reviewed, which included the identification of the characteristics of the at-risk groups. In addition, mortality and morbidity data and risk factors identified in an analytic epidemiological study of childhood pedestrian injury were reviewed (Stevenson et al., 1995). This review confirmed that child pedestrian injury was a significant priority problem deserving of intervention, as illustrated by:

- pedestrian mortality as the major injury death for Western Australian children
- Western Australia had a higher rate of such deaths (3.2 per 100,000) than the mean for the country
- child pedestrians hit by vehicles usually sustained serious injuries
- severe head injuries were sustained by 80 per cent of critically injured child pedestrians, and

- five- to nine-year-old child pedestrian injury victims were hospitalised for a mean of thirty days.

Based on this information, the *primary target groups* were identified as five- to nine-year-old children, their parents, and teachers.

The *secondary target groups* were identified as city officials, school administrators, legislators, police, road safety advisory committee members, and drivers.

The *program goal* was to reduce by 10 per cent the incidence of injury to child pedestrians in the City of Gosnells within three years.

Phase 2, Step 2: Behavioural and environmental assessment

Identify risk factors and objectives

Behavioural and environmental determinants (risk factors) of injuries to child pedestrians were identified, and objectives established for each of the main risk factors. The factors were arranged in order of priority based on their relative importance and changeability, according to procedures outlined by Green and Kreuter (1999) and a review of relevant literature and official health statistics, and these priorities were later complemented by baseline data collected as part of the CPIPP

The *behavioural assessment* identified two main risk factors for the *children's* road-related behaviours:

- inappropriate road crossing behaviour, and
- children failing to seek help to cross roads.

Three behavioural risk factors were identified as most relevant to *parental influences* on the road crossing behaviours of their children. These were:

- parents failing to supervise children at road crossings
- parents failing to teach their children appropriate road crossing procedures, and
- parents failing to model appropriate road-crossing behaviours.

Behavioural objectives were formulated for each of these risk factors.

The *environmental assessment* identified the major environmental risk factors for five- to nine-year-old pedestrians as traffic volume and speed, road design, and roadside obstacles. *Environmental objectives* were formulated for each of these risk factors.

Peter Howat, Graham Brown, Sharyn Burns & Alexandra McManus

Phase 3: Educational and ecological assessment

Identify contributing factors and sub-objectives

Factors that contribute to each of the behavioural and environmental risk factors were identified in this step. These contributing factors were then classified into predisposing, enabling, and reinforcing factors. These three groups of factors incorporate both barriers (negative) and facilitators (positive) to action (Green & Kreuter, 1999).

Predisposing factors related directly to child pedestrians included:

- lack of knowledge about safe road-crossing behaviour, and
- a perception of low risk of injury associated with crossing busy roads.

Enabling factors for these children included:

- inability to identify safer road-crossing places
- undeveloped road-crossing skills
- lack of social skills required to ask people to assist them cross roads, and
- insufficient road-safety education in the schools.

Examples of *reinforcing factors* were:

- parents allowing their children to cross roads unaccompanied, and
- parents' perceptions that their children have adequate abilities to cross roads safely, while alone.

Phase 4: Administrative and policy assessment and intervention alignment

Includes identification of suitable interventions

The main intervention developed for CPIPP was school-based, with links to the community via the parents. It also involved a community environmental component via road safety committees established by the participating schools and local community representatives (see Stevenson et al., 1999; Cross et al., 2003).

School strategies included:

- road crossing curriculum for Grades 2, 3, and 4 students
- home education component aimed at parents and
- review of school policies.

> Community strategies included establishing school road safety committees (actions included advocating for improved road environment and traffic management around their schools, and reduction of speed limits to 40 kmh in proximity to schools).
>
> Refer to Appendix 3 for details of objectives and strategies developed for CPIPP.

CRITICAL THINKING EXERCISE 1

This activity gives you the opportunity to apply the first three phases of the PRECEDE–PROCEED model. You may wish to use the table below to guide your work.

1. Identify a *health issue* of interest to you. Your health issue should be significant from a public health perspective.

2. Identify two major risk or protective factors relevant to your health issue.

   Risk factors are those characteristics, variables, or hazards that, if present for a given individual, will increase the probability that they will develop a disorder, disease, or specific cause of death (adapted from Mrazek & Haggerty, 1994; Green & Kreuter, 2005).

   Protective factors are those factors that produce resilience to, or reduce the probability of the development of, a disorder, disease or specific cause of death (adapted from Spence, 1996).

3. Now consider what contributes to each risk and protective factor and identify if this factor is a predisposing, enabling, or reinforcing factor. Try to think of both a behavioural and an environmental risk or protective factor.

Health issue:
Identify behavioural and environmental risk/protective factors and their contributing factors
Risk/protective factor: Contributing factors (predisposing, enabling or reinforcing):

Peter Howat, Graham Brown, Sharyn Burns & Alexandra McManus

> Risk/protective factor:
>
> Contributing factors (predisposing, enabling or reinforcing):

Re-defining the target group

It is useful at this stage of the planning process to review your target group, particularly because of the importance of the relationship between the style of intervention and the target group (both primary and secondary).

The social, epidemiological, behavioural, and educational diagnoses may have indicated a need to change or modify the target group. For instance, it might be appropriate to target a person or organisation with influence over the primary target group (for instance parents, employers, teachers). For example:

➤ a program aiming to improve the nutrition of small children may target parents and caregivers, or

➤ a program that aims to reduce the number of children injured as pedestrians by reducing the speed limits around school may target organisations such as town or city councils and government agencies.

Thus, it is important to consider at this early stage whether there is a need to include a secondary target group in addition to the primary target group. Other reasons to consider modifying the target group at this stage may be because the target group is too large, or perhaps because of limitations on available funding or resources.

For example, in the CPIPP, the primary target group was six- to nine-year-olds; however, the behavioural risk factors showed some parents were not supervising children, were not teaching appropriate road-crossing behaviour, and were failing to model appropriate crossing behaviours. Given the importance of parents' attitudes and beliefs for this age group, it was essential to also target parents as a secondary target group. The CPIPP also included school administrators, legislators, police, road-safety advisory committee members, and drivers, as secondary target groups as they had direct influence on the children, driver behaviours, and environmental and legislative changes, and hence child pedestrian safety.

Prior to finalising the target group(s) and the setting, program planners need to make a number of decisions regarding:

- program focus (that is, what audience should the program be aimed at—individuals, groups, populations or a combination of these?), and
- program setting (that is, would the program be implemented more effectively in a specific setting such as school, worksite, or hospital?).

Determining goals and objectives

Chapter 7 addressed the issue of formulating goals and objectives. In this section, goals and objectives will be described in the context of the health promotion planning process, and will provide clear and logical links with the relevant phases of the PRECEDE–PROCEED model.

Setting goals and setting objectives are essential steps in the planning process. Until they are stated clearly, it is not possible to plan appropriate strategies or evaluation methods. The program goal describes what the program aims to achieve, while the objectives describe the changes you want your program to bring about in your target group (and/or in the relevant environment).

Setting goals

The information gathered from a needs assessment (the social and epidemiological assessment; phases 1 and 2 of the PRECEDE–PROCEED model) will provide sufficient detail to enable clarification of the priority health issue or problem. It is at this stage that a program *goal* can be formulated (that is, what do you ultimately want to achieve by running the program?). The goal needs to describe a change in your target group, related clearly to the priority health issue. What you state as your goal relates directly to what you measure in the evaluation (for example, did the program, in the longer term, achieve its goal?).

If your program is very small, with limited resources, and of a short duration, the goal might relate to a change in the short term. For example, your program may be one of many programs contributing to a broad agency or even state goal, or it may be that your program is only of twelve months' duration, but the outcomes will not be known for four or five years or longer. In these circumstances, it may only be feasible for your program to measure the impact (behavioural or environmental change) of the program, not the long-term outcome (change in the health status). In the latter case, the long-term program goal may be outside the parameters of your program; it will, however, still show the intent of your program to *contribute* to an improvement in the health issue (such as a reduction in mortality, morbidity, or disability). It is essential in these situations that the theoretical or medical link between achieving your objectives (the change in behaviour or environmental risk factors) and the intended goal is clearly articulated and supported by evidence.

Some examples of program goal statements include:

- to reduce the proportion of overweight children aged 14 to 15 years in community X from 20 per cent to 15 per cent within two years
- to reduce by 10 per cent the proportion of Indigenous people injured in car rollovers while travelling in open load spaces in the Midwest area within two years, and
- to reduce by 10 per cent firearm injuries among 18- to 35-year-old males in North Region within 12 months.

Setting objectives

Objectives describe the changes you would like your program to bring about in the target group. They are the immediate steps that must be accomplished if the goal is to be reached. Objectives correspond to the determinants or risk (or protective) factors, and are measured by impact evaluation. You may wish to refer back to phases 2 and 3 of the PRECEDE–PROCEED model to revise the process of identifying risk factors, and categorising these into behavioural and environmental factors where appropriate. Your objectives are devised directly from the identified risk factors; thus your program may or may not have both *behavioural* and *environmental* objectives. It is important to make sure that your objectives are measurable and reflect realistic levels of change.

Examples include:

- to increase by 10 per cent the proportion of children aged one to five years in community X who report eating a healthy diet by the year Y (behavioural)
- to reduce by 20 per cent, on current levels, the proportion of adults aged 18 years and over from Midwest Aboriginal communities who report that they drive while intoxicated by alcohol, by year X (behavioural)
- to improve roadside lighting in community Y to a specified criterion (for example at least one street light at every 50 metres of road) by the end of the program (environmental), and
- to increase by 20 per cent the proportion of firearms stored securely in locked cabinets in North Region by 2008 (behavioural).

In order to write goals and objectives in measurable terms, it is desirable for the statements to reflect the place, person, time, and amount. This will also facilitate your evaluation plan.

The *place* refers to the geographical location, organisation, or setting in which the program is to take place. The *person* usually refers to the target group. If the change is to be legislative, environmental, or organisational, specify which organisation or which aspect of the environment instead of which person or group of people. Provide details, including the age group, gender, and interest group if relevant.

Time refers to the point by which you expect to see the desired change. This is usually expressed as a period after the beginning of the program (for example, within six months of beginning the program) or a period after the end of the program (for example, within one year after the end of the program, or by the end of the program). It may also be expressed in terms of milestones, for example 'by 2010' (Hawe et al., 1990).

The *amount* is expressed as either:

➤ increasing or decreasing the proportion of people carrying out the behaviour, for example, increasing the number of mothers who breastfeed for at least six months from 50 per cent to 60 per cent, or
➤ increasing or decreasing the average frequency of a behaviour, for example, increase the amount of fruit children eat from one to two pieces per day (Hawe et al., 1990).

An acronym that is useful in ensuring effective and useful objectives is SMART objectives (specific, measurable, achievable, realistic, and time-specific).

To determine the proportion of change you expect from your program, you will need to review the literature to find out what type of changes other programs that have focused on your health issue have been able to achieve. This will provide a guide. However, the proportion of change for your program will depend on the health issue, the current prevalence and behaviours in your community or a similar community, the amenability to change, the number of people involved in your program, and the characteristics of your target group.

An effective pilot program that undertakes strong process evaluation is often used to determine how much change is achievable under certain circumstances, and can often provide data for a reasonable estimate in replicating the program elsewhere. However, this will not be feasible for many small-scale programs you plan.

Case study 2 illustrates how the program and behavioural and environmental objectives have been formulated based on the process recommended by the PRECEDE–PROCEED model. It also shows how more specific objectives (sub-objectives) have been used. These are optional and may be useful for large-scale programs and where there are adequate resources for more detailed planning and interventions.

CASE STUDY

2. The Seniors Pedestrian Injury Prevention Program (SIPP)

The project *goal* is to develop, implement, and evaluate a community-based intervention that will lead to a reduction of pedestrian injuries incurred by seniors in selected communities in Western Australia. This will be achieved by conducting a community education and environmental intervention trial over a three-year period.

Program goal

By the end of the program there will be a 10 per cent reduction in pedestrian injuries among men and women 60 years and older in the intervention communities.

Behavioural objectives

Primary target group

By the end of the program there will be a 15 per cent increase in the proportion of seniors in the intervention communities who report:

- using safe road-crossing procedures
- crossing at safer places (such as at pedestrian signals and traffic lights when appropriate)
- walking and crossing roads during less busy periods
- obtaining assessments for their sensory and motor abilities, and
- reporting pedestrian hazards to their local council.

Sub-objectives

By the end of the program there will be a 15 per cent increase in the proportion of seniors in the intervention communities who:

- can list safer crossing procedures
- believe they are susceptible to pedestrian injuries
- believe that pedestrian injuries can be of high severity
- can demonstrate safer crossing procedures (for example, in relation to traffic lights, roundabouts, busy roads)
- can describe safer places to cross
- can describe how medications may affect their road-crossing ability

- can describe physical and sensory limitations of seniors that affect road-crossing safety, and
- can describe how decreased judgment of traffic speed and distance increases road-crossing risks.

Environmental objectives

By the end of the program there will be, in the intervention communities:

- a 10 per cent reduction in hazards relating to safe road crossing, and
- a 10 per cent increase in environmental changes that facilitate pedestrian safety.

Note that environmental objectives will depend on the cooperation of city councils in the intervention communities and Main Roads WA.

Strategies

Community-based seminars:

- Safe road crossing seminars held in seniors' centres (seniors in the program invited to attend)
- mailed materials
- specially produced safe road crossing booklet (sent to seniors in the program), and
- specially produced safe road crossing DVD (Iredell et al., 2004).

CRITICAL THINKING EXERCISE 2

Reflect on the PRECEDE part of the PRECEDE–PROCEED model and complete the parts of the table that are relevant to your proposed program. Refer back to what you did in Critical thinking exercise 1. You do *not* need to complete boxes that are not relevant. Note that you can adapt the table to suit your health issue. For example, you may have only one behavioural objective but may have both environmental and behavioural objectives, or you may have one objective that relates to more than one contributing factor. You may now want to change some of the things you wrote in Criticical thinking exercise 1. This is all part of the planning process!

Peter Howat, Graham Brown, Sharyn Burns & Alexandra McManus

Statement on severity/type of health issue:	Goal:
Identify behavioural and environmental risk/protective factors, contributing factors and their corresponding objectives	
Risk/protective factor: Contributing factor (predisposing, enabling or reinforcing):	Objectives (and if appropriate relevant sub-objectives):
Risk/protective factor: Contributing factor (predisposing, enabling or reinforcing):	Objectives (and if appropriate relevant sub-objectives):

Intervention alignment and administrative and policy assessment

Intervention alignment and administrative and policy assessment is phase 4 in the model (see Figure 8.5), and follows the selection of priorities, targets, and objectives. The previous phases of the PRECEDE–PROCEED model have enabled you to identify factors that need to be modified or changed in your target group and the environment in your proposed program (for example, in CPIPP, road-crossing behaviours of six- to nine- year-old children, and traffic speed and volumes around schools).

In this phase of the model, selection of your intervention strategies occurs. (Refer Chapters 11 to 13 in Part 4 for details relevant to implementation of strategies.)

Some of the key administrative and policy factors that need to be addressed during phase 4 include an assessment of available resources (time, personnel, and money), and an assessment of the organisational barriers and facilitators that can affect program implementation as well as the policies that may need to be developed or modified in order to support the program. It is important to address these factors prior to finalising program strategies to ensure that the strategies selected are appropriate and feasible in relation to available resources. Once these

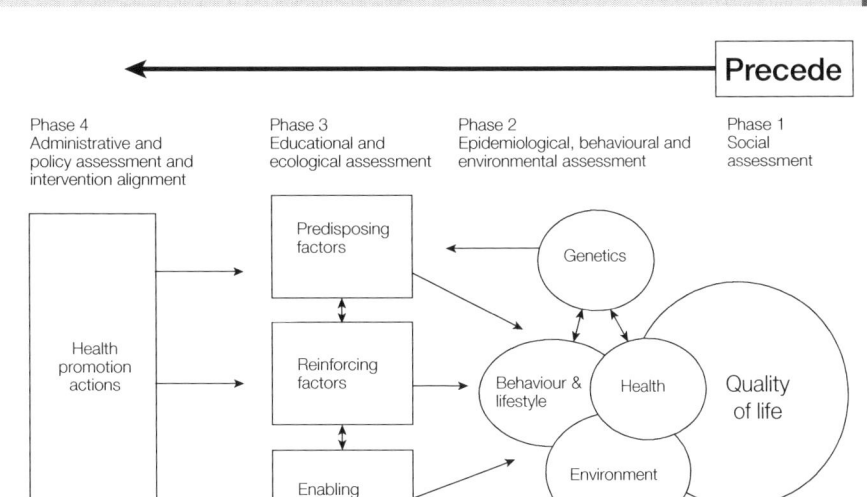

FIGURE 8.5 Phases 1 to 4 of PRECEDE: intervention alignment, administrative and policy assessment

Source: Green & Kreuter (2005)

factors have been addressed, the final components can be added. These include formalising the plan with a timetable, assignment of resources and responsibilities, and a budget (see also Chapter 7).

The specific *settings* in which the health program's strategies and activities will occur also need to be identified during this phase. The setting (community, schools, clinics, worksites) will determine the actual methods and materials to be used in the intervention. Once this level of planning is complete, the program is ready to PROCEED to the implementation phase (see Part 4) and evaluation phase (see Part 5).

The process of selecting strategies is critical, and requires a comprehensive and multi-faceted approach.

Settings may be:

1. physically bound spacetimes in which people come together to perform specific tasks (usually related to goals other than health), for example, church groups, sport groups, and so on, or
2. places of sustained interaction with pre-existing structures, policies, characteristics, institutional values, and both formal and social sanctions on behaviour, for example, schools, workplaces, hospitals (Poland et al., 2000).

Traditionally, settings have been considered to be face-to-face settings, with the key settings including the workplace, schools, universities, neighbourhoods or communities, and primary health care centres and hospitals (Naidoo & Wills, 2000; Poland et al., 2000; Baum, 2008). In today's society, however, it is important to consider also the implications of virtual settings, for example, the internet (Liamputtong, 2006). In addition, less traditional settings such as nightclubs, pubs, and street corners are also important to consider (Poland et al., 2000).

Implementation

Implementation is referred to as the act of converting program objectives into actions (Green & Kreuter, 2005). In finalising any implementation plan, it is important to consider some of the possible obstacles or barriers that may hinder progress of the program. For example, staff commitment and attitude, community circumstances, and quality assurance, training, and supervision can significantly influence program implementation. Green and Kreuter (2005) have identified an additional five core components for more effective program implementation:

- a well thought-out plan
- adequate budget
- solid organisational and policy support
- constructive training and supervision of staff, and
- careful monitoring in the process evaluation stage.

Prior to implementation, the planner should have made a decision as to whether the program is a pilot project, a phase-in, or a fully implemented program (O'Connor-Fleming & Parker, 2001: 92). It is also important at this stage to complete a final strategy check to ensure that there is an appropriate combination of intervention strategies. The specific type of program setting will have a strong influence on the final strategy mix. It is, therefore, important for the planner to be familiar with the various settings in which health programs are commonly implemented (refer to Part 4, Chapters 11 to 13 for details relevant to implementation).

Conclusion

In this chapter, we have discussed a summary of planning procedures for health promotion programs based on the PRECEDE–PROCEED model. We have also provided a step-by-step framework that can be used as a systematic guide to effective planning for community health and population-based health programs.

This is just one of the many 'models' of planning that are available. We strongly recommend that you use a model that is appropriate for the health issue and the setting or community in which you are working.

Acknowledgments

We acknowledge the thousands of students who have studied health promotion planning in a Curtin University degree or continuing education course. Their interaction and feedback has been valuable in influencing the way we teach and the way we present our educational materials, including this chapter. We thank our colleagues who have also contributed to the material presented in this chapter, including Jenny Collins, Donna Cross, John Fisher (deceased), Greg Hamilton, Steve Jones, Tony Lower, Bruce Maycock, Julie Rose, and Lorraine Telfer. Special thanks to Professor Lawrence Green and Professor Marshall Kreuter, for sharing their great scholarship with us during their visits to Perth and during our sojourns in the USA and Canada.

CRITICAL THINKING EXERCISE 3

While we have not discussed strategy selection in any detail, you may find it useful to add some strategies to the table. Refer to other chapters for more details about strategy selection.

Rationale/needs assessment	Program goal and objectives	
Statement on severity/type of health issue:	Goal:	
Identify behavioural and environmental risk/protective factors, contributing factors and their corresponding measurable objectives		**Strategies to achieve the objectives**
Risk/protective factor: Contributing factor (predisposing, enabling or reinforcing):	Objectives (and if appropriate relevant sub-objectives)	

Peter Howat, Graham Brown, Sharyn Burns & Alexandra McManus

Risk/protective factor:	Objectives (and if appropriate relevant sub-objectives)	
Contributing factor (predisposing, enabling or reinforcing):		

FURTHER READING

Gielen, A.C., & McDonald, E.M. (2002) Using the PRECEDE/PROCEED Planning Model to Apply Health Behavior Theories. In: K. Glanz, B.K. Rimer, & F.M. Lewis (eds), *Health Behavior and Health Education: Theory, Research and Practice*, 3rd edn, 409–36. Jossey-Bass: San Francisco.

Gielen, A., & Sleet, D. (2003) Application of Behavior-Change Theories and Methods to Injury Prevention. *Epidemiologic Reviews*, 25: 65–76.

Green, L.W., & Kreuter, M.W. (2005) *Health Program Planning: An Educational and Ecological Approach*, 4th edn. McGraw-Hill: New York.

WEBPAGE RESOURCES

Homepage of Professor Lawrence Green: www.lgreen.net. This website is the homepage for Professor Lawrence Green, the principal author of the PRECEDE–PROCEED model. It will give you links to case studies, and references about the model.

Planning Human Resources

9

Lee Stewart, Rusieli Taukei & Kim Usher

Objectives

After reading this chapter, readers will be able to:

- Discuss the rationale for ensuring local leadership capacity in planning human resources
- Describe the advantages of ensuring local champions are key members of the human resource team
- Identify the necessary components of an active partnership
- Identify at least four factors that maximise the sustainability of a health project
- Apply the key elements of human resource planning to a health-related project.

Key terms

active partnership
human resources
mentoring
stakeholders
sustainability

Introduction: Leadership

The focus of this chapter is to help readers appreciate the crucial role that people play in the success of a project. Many readers who are students are obviously involved in their undergraduate studies at present, but many registered nurses choose to work in developed or developing countries coordinating or being involved in worthwhile project activities. We will direct this chapter to readers as if they are considering pursuing such an option.

During the planning stage of a public health project, human resources are carefully identified, selected, and invited to take part in the project. The best possible people will facilitate the achievement of the project's goal and objectives. Dwyer and others (2004) suggest that a health practitioner must make a plan, and be flexible enough to recognise that plans change. Planning for human resources means that sensible questions have to be asked at the outset of a project. Some of these questions include:

- What is the project aiming to achieve—what is the major goal?
- What sort of technical skills are needed for this project—what sort of knowledge is needed about the actual project?
- What sort of complementary skills and knowledge (cultural sensitivity, local knowledge, negotiation skills, and facilitation skills) are needed for this project?
- Do local people have these skills and knowledge?
- Are potential local project team members known and respected by the community? Do they have credibility?
- What sort of skills and knowledge will have to be 'brought in' to undertake this project and achieve its aims?

Human resources: the people who are required in order to plan for, undertake, and evaluate the project.

Sustainability: the continuation of activities related to the project after the project team has officially concluded its input.

There is an absolute requirement for good leadership to facilitate the asking and answering of these sorts of questions in the planning phase of a project. It has been claimed that 'the most significant contribution leaders make is … to the long term development of people and institutions so they can adapt, change, prosper and grow' (Kouzes & Posner, 2002: xxviii). Leaders can be either formal or informal. In a hospital or community health service there will be a formal nursing leader. Importantly, others will also take on leadership activities informally because of their interest or capability in a particular area. Hence, good leadership in planning human resources is about choosing the appropriate people for a project and developing them so they can achieve project goals. In addition, it is about ensuring that, once the project is complete, those people have the knowledge, skills, and motivation to continue with the work required to ensure sustainability.

As Dr Lee Jong-wook (2006: 11), the late Director General of the World Health Organization, pointed out, leaders ensure that three priorities form the basis for any health care imperative: 'acting now, anticipating the future, and acquiring critical competencies'.

Our project was about planning for and implementing a clinical governance framework for the Fiji Ministry of Health. Clinical governance is 'a system through which … organizations are accountable for continuously improving the quality of their services and safeguarding high standards of care by creating an environment in which excellence in clinical care will flourish' (Scally & Donaldson, 1998: 2). The necessity exists in clinical governance for human resource management practices that not only motivate people and develop their confidence, but also provide them with the necessary technical skills so that they are competent in their work (Vanu Som, 2007). Further, a key component of successful clinical governance is effective clinical leadership (Degeling et al., 2004) and a key component of successful planning for human resources is effective project leadership. We have recognised the importance of leadership education for nurses in Fiji, given the clinical governance agenda and other health reform activities in the region. We have been involved in further developing the nurse leaders of Fiji (Stewart et al., 2006b) so they can continue to guide health reform at all levels within the Fiji Ministry of Health. Additionally, the International Council of Nurses (ICN) developed the Leadership for Change (LCF) program to prepare nurses to provide leadership during the health reform programs that were being instituted in many developing countries (McMurray, 2007). This brings us to the need for local leaders.

Stakeholders: those groups and organisations having an interest or stake in a program.

Local champions, key stakeholders

With any project, there will be key stakeholders. These are individual people, groups of people, and/or organisations that will be affected by or who will influence the success or otherwise of the project. Mistakes that sometimes occur are about not taking time in the planning stages to recognise these people and include them as members of the 'human resource team'. They will not necessarily be formal team members, but if individuals, organisations, or community groups have a stake in what is happening with the project, if it is going to affect their lives in some way, then they must be included in the plan. Obviously, not every consumer of health care is going to be on the project team, but consumer representation is vital so that local knowledge comes not only from local health professionals, but also from the general community. Readers need to be aware that 'good public-health practice encourages people and communities to take part in decisions about their own health' (Macfarlane et al., 2000: 841). This means inclusion in any project that is going to affect the structure and organisation of health services, as well as actual health care practices. Appointing a local champion in the planning stages means there will be somebody on the project team with local knowledge at the outset of the project. A local champion can range widely depending on the project and its setting. In a traditional community, a local champion may be an elder, a teacher, or a nurse. Countries differ, and communities within countries can differ also. Taking account of the social, political, cultural, and religious conditions, beliefs and practices within the country or community where the project occurs is a precondition of ethical and, indeed, successful project outcomes. One may read about a country or talk to people about a country, but, in our experience, the nuances of life that make up the lifeworld of that country cannot be captured in books or from general conversation. At issue here is the cultural safety of the community who are going to be affected by the project work. Cultural safety can be described as:

> a manner, which affirms, respects and fosters the cultural expression of the recipient. This usually requires nurses to have undertaken a process of reflection on their own cultural identity and to have learned to practice in a way, which affirms the culture of clients and nurses. Unsafe cultural practice is any action, which demeans, diminishes or disempowers the cultural identity and well being of an individual.
>
> New Zealand Nurses Organisation, 1995: no page number

A local person who is known by the community, and, just as importantly, respected by the community, will be able to assist the project team to avoid 'cultural harm' and achieve success with a project or task that involves working with Indigenous communities. Sometimes a problem occurs where a local project officer is not appointed early enough in the process, with consequent unnecessary delays in implementing some of the key elements of the project. As McMurray (2007) points out, one of the keys to a socially just environment is to minimise power differences between professionals and consumers. The early appointment of a local project officer serves this end. It is crucial to learn from the possible mistake of not appointing locals early enough, and to take account of the fact that 'workforce solutions require stakeholders to be engaged in both problem diagnosis and problem solving' (Lee, 2006: 8). A local champion is the key stakeholder in this sort of situation, and should be on board during planning. He or she will assist the project team to navigate the local situation, and to employ the best local people for the human resource team. Local champions are in fact local *leaders*, because leadership is what they provide. An external person may be *managing* a project, and may have leadership responsibilities, but the goal of ensuring sustainability will not come from the person who is an external consultant and is often only in a region or a country for a relatively short period of time. This brings attention to the vital issue of working together in genuine partnership in the planning stages of a project.

Partnership, collaboration, and sponsors

The declaration of Alma-Alta includes the notion that public health:

> requires and promotes maximum community and individual self-reliance and participation in the planning, organization, operation and control of Primary Health Care, making fullest use of local, national and other available resources, and to this end develops through appropriate education the ability of communities to participate (cited in Talbot & Verrinder, 2005: 246).

Major concepts from Alma-Alta that will need to guide the role of the project team in the field are about equity, community self-reliance, and cooperation between countries. In planning for human resources, particular challenges are around establishing a balance between local personnel and foreign personnel. Project teams will often need people from other regions or countries who have the technical expertise required for the project and which might not yet be locally available. The sort of partnership necessary here is termed an 'active partnership' (McIntosh & McCormack, 2001). As opposed to a 'passive partnership', where the technical expert may give advice but not listen to or take account of local knowledge, an active partnership means that all project team members share their knowledge and skills so that the *team* benefits from such collaboration. The issue of 'partnership' is vital here. Unfortunately, the world has a history of colonisation, where countries like Fiji have had 'Western' culture imposed upon them over decades (Murray & Storey, 2003). There remains a danger that international consultants will go to work in developing countries and will (often inadvertently) attempt to impose their own values and practices on local people (Stewart, 2006). Similar problems occur in Australia, where, for example, external project consultants work with Indigenous communities and fail to empower community members through not engaging in equitable collaboration. Partners listen to and hear each other; they share equal power about decision-making; they do not give in to temptations to force their views on others at the expense of collaborative, creative problem-solving. One example of such a project occurred in relation to introducing clinical governance

Active partnership: partners having an equal role in decision-making.

Lee Stewart, Rusieli Taukei & Kim Usher

in the Fiji Islands, and the primary partnership involved a small team of people with particular roles around clinical governance, and comprised both locals (called *kai viti* in Fiji) and foreigners (known as *kai valagi*). A key aspect of the success with this project involved having *a kai valagi* technical expert who lived in Fiji, and worked in partnership with the local project officer over several years. This may not always be possible, but this continuing relationship is to be encouraged (as opposed to occasional visits by a technical expert) as very desirable in terms of human resource planning. Having a *kai valagi* consultant visit at intervals to not only provide support and advice, but also to evaluate project outcomes, was another aspect of human resource management that proved invaluable.

In addition, in any project in either a developed or developing country, the role of a powerful *local* sponsor is paramount. Project teams are not going to progress well unless they have the backing of someone who supports what they are doing. This person also needs the power to influence others, including local government agencies, to enable teams to do their work. The local sponsor can ensure the project team receives necessary resources. More importantly, they can facilitate the team's ability to network with all of those people who could either enable or stop a project, often depending upon the project team's communication with them. At issue here, in terms of establishing the project, is that 'there is commitment to the proposed action from the leaders in the group you are working with, so that the program is seen as legitimate' (O'Connor-Fleming & Parker, 2001: 83). The perceived legitimacy or otherwise of the project can be the difference between success and failure. Planning human resources to include someone in a formal leadership position as project sponsor is a key imperative to project success. This person has the role of 'sponsoring' the project team's efforts. Obviously, clearly identifying various roles and responsibilities for the different people on the team is yet another critical element of project planning.

Roles and responsibilities

The people who do the work in any project need a clear idea of what it is they are supposed to be doing. Where 'blurring' of roles exists, this must be clearly identified, so that certain elements of the project do not get 'missed' because somebody thought it was somebody else's job! Developing clear role descriptions with performance indicators attached to the various aspects of each role allows each individual to determine both theirs and other people's responsibilities concerning the project. Developing role descriptions should be undertaken, where possible, as a team, to enhance the possibility of collaboratively arriving at a situation where the most appropriate person does the job that best suits their interest as well as knowledge. Motivation is enhanced if people can spend at least some of their time (or most of it, if possible) doing the things that most interest them, and where they are most skilled.

Training

Education and training for the people involved in a project commences before the project does. It involves a number of stages which can be summarised as:

- Identify technical knowledge and skills, and complementary knowledge, skills, and attitudes (for example, negotiation skills or teamwork, local culture and conditions) required for the project
- Undertake a needs assessment with personnel who will be involved in the project to assess their current levels of required knowledge, skills, and attitudes
- Identify learning gaps among the different personnel
- Develop or purchase required education and training materials to meet learning gaps
- Implement education and training
- Evaluate new knowledge and skills levels following education and training
- Implement remedial education and training as necessary.

Undertaking needs assessment with communities has been referred to as problematic, because it can highlight deficits that might be present rather than determining both strengths and gaps (Talbot & Verrinder, 2005). Therefore, training-needs assessments should be inclusive of both learning gaps *and* the knowledge and strengths that various personnel will bring with them to the project team. In this way, existing knowledge can be shared among the team in the spirit of active partnership. Also of critical importance here are the attitudes of various personnel towards the project, and towards working together to achieve project outcomes. While education and training concerning technical aspects of the project and communication are important, values-clarification about issues of racism or lack of cultural sensitivity are also vital. Arrogant people who arrive in an Indigenous community in Australia, or in a developing country such as Fiji, and who lack sensitivity towards local conditions, values, and beliefs, can ruin a project. The best solution here would be to remove them from the project, but if this is impossible, there may be the necessity to include aspects of cultural education in the education and training programs.

Initial education and training is, however, only the beginning. Project work in health care rarely proceeds exactly as it commenced, or indeed as planned. Needs change, conditions change, and the necessity for further education or training tends to occur throughout the life of the project. The skilled project facilitator knows this, and incorporates elements of *performance review* into various stages of the project, so that continuing requirements for learning can be discussed and implemented. As we are reminded: 'Lifelong learning should be inculcated in the workplace. This may include short-term training, encouraging staff to innovate, and fostering teamwork' (Lee, 2006: 10). Hence, all of these elements of education and training then become part of a continuing learning process within the team throughout the life of the project. Some team members will certainly be able to assist others, through either supervision, collegiality, or mentoring of less experienced team members.

Mentoring and supervising

Mentoring: taking an interest in, coaching, and supporting another person in their career.

Mentoring is very similar to long-term coaching that occurs in a planned way (Smeltzer, 2006) throughout the life of the project and beyond. Mentors tend to value the use of education to assist their protégé to achieve the same knowledge and skills that they themselves have. A good definition of mentoring is that of a partnership between two or more people, where one assists the others in terms of career development (Postlen-Slattery & Foley, 2006). The idea of mentoring rather than 'supervising' is probably preferable in these particular projects.

Mentoring involves 'time out' for both mentor and protégé to discuss what worked well, what did not work, and what needs to be changed. For our project, the local project officer provided mentorship in terms of acting as a 'cultural broker' for those people involved in the project who were not from Fiji. Cultural brokers assist others to act in ways that 'minimize behaviours that might be misunderstood or might offend' (Stewart et al., 2006b: 50) local personnel. On the other hand, the consultant mentored the local project officer by sharing specific knowledge about the technical aspects of clinical governance. Because this was an active partnership, the goal was that everyone on the team had access to the same literature about clinical governance. In this way, the whole team could discuss and debate project goals and processes as partners. Providing extensive literature about the technical aspects of the project was vital, as the aim is for the local project officer to have the same information as the external consultant. As such, the risk of dependency on 'external' knowledge is significantly reduced, and the local community becomes increasingly empowered.

Our experience included the local project officer having a period of time experiencing a different environment where a similar project was underway. She had the opportunity to visit a hospital in Australia where the elements of clinical governance, such as risk management and customer focus, had been in place formally over an extended period of time. The external consultant had also worked with the host hospital, providing literature about clinical governance and assisting with policy decisions (Stewart et al., 2006a) to support best patient outcomes. This exposure was invaluable, because it also enabled the project officer to learn from a range of different people rather than having more limited contact with only one or two people with technical knowledge. One example that illustrates this learning well concerns a hospital's goals to reduce the number of adverse events for patients, specifically hospital-acquired or nosocomial infections. A program of education, monitoring, and evaluation of appropriate handwashing by health professionals serves to reduce this risk for patients. The local project officer's experience in terms of the Infection Control Unit's activities in the Australian hospital had direct parallels with quality improvement projects in Fiji. Thus, local project officers can experience an increased sense of confidence and empowerment concerning health care practices in their own communities. We would recommend that mentoring be both a supportive and educative process, and that all personnel engaged in the project have an opportunity for this to occur. Good mentoring is one of the keys to a project's goals being sustained over time.

Sustainability

McMurray (2007: 23) describes sustainability in community health as 'a type of health–illness carrying capacity—that is, all the health resources it needs and capacity to respond to all the illness it produces'. This lofty goal should be considered in terms of human resource planning. Sustainability in terms of planning for human resources is about having the right people still there when the project ends. What this means is that there is a long-term commitment by those who fund a project, such as international aid agencies or government bodies, to continue to support workers for the length of time required for the project to meet its initial goals. Then, depending on the nature of the work, there needs to be continued support for personnel to continue to undertake the activities necessary to sustain what was achieved, or to improve it. As already discussed, sustainability also means that local people have acquired, and are provided with the capacity to continue to acquire, the knowledge and skills necessary to do their work.

The challenges we encountered with the project were those that face many health workers. There had been a history of advisers coming to Fiji, sharing their expertise, and then leaving the country. Importantly, sustainability means

Lee Stewart, Rusieli Taukei & Kim Usher

everyone involved in the project being there for the 'long haul' in an appropriate way. Having interested and knowledgeable local people who have 'ownership' of a project is the key to sustainability from a human-resource perspective. The local project officer in our situation took an increasing leadership role as she gained in confidence and knowledge about what was required for the complexities of good clinical governance. Again, the reader should be reminded of the notion of an active partnership, where local people are mentored until they know as much or more than the mentor at the conclusion of their mentor relationship. This is a crucial issue, because a major challenge for the novice worker in this area is to commence a project with very good intentions but to continue to provide effective leadership themselves throughout the project instead of acting in partnership with the rest of the team. This is such a temptation because people will admire project teams and often give them very positive feedback, and it is so easy to get 'caught up' in such compliments at the expense of eventual project success. Real success is concerned with empowerment of local people and the long-term sustainability of project outcomes. This is a similar concept to that of the difference between teacher-focused education and student-focused education. Teacher-focused education occurs where an educator is an expert and 'performs' to the admiration of students—the educator feels very valued but the students might learn little. Alternatively, educators who are student-focused have student learning as their main goal. Of course, they still have expertise in their area, but all of their activities with students are about the students rather than themselves. If readers do choose to pursue a nursing career where project work such as has been described is part of a career path, it is vital to pay careful attention to the importance of sustainability. The key role for the project team is to build capacity in the area where they are involved. Building capacity means people can do things for themselves; project teams are usually short-term facilitators for that capacity building. Not building capacity might mean that 'holistic, community based health programmes are generally undermined by narrowly selective interventions and ... the sustainability of people-owned initiatives can be put in jeopardy' (Macfarlane et al., 2000: 843). The goal for any project is that stakeholders, the people who really own the activities, have the resources for sustained continuation of the work.

Examples and case studies

We have thus far made reference to some of our experiences with the Clinical Governance Project in Fiji. To address this more comprehensively, we now present a summary of the various processes and outcomes that occurred between 2004 and

2007 in Fiji. Although the described project occurred in Fiji, there are immediate parallels for human resource planning in Australian communities, be they metropolitan or rural and remote communities. In addition, we have provided an example of how these principles have also been applied in a different way in an Australian hospital.

1. Introducing clinical governance in Fiji

The Director of Nursing/Director of Health System Standards and her colleagues in Fiji had several years' experience with working to create a culture of continuous quality improvement throughout the Fiji Ministry of Health.

They employed various external consultants to provide workshops to staff about quality improvement programs.

The consultants came to Fiji, conducted workshops which staff were enthusiastic about, and then went home to their own countries.

We became involved then, and the following processes happened:

- The first workshop about clinical governance occurred with the Executive of the Head Office of the Fiji Ministry of Health.
- A workshop occurred with various stakeholders (doctors, nurses, and administrative and housekeeping staff) from different hospitals and health centres throughout the Fiji Islands. At this workshop, each of the three Divisions that comprise Fiji Health decided together on a particular quality improvement project they wished to engage with during the ensuing twelve months.
- The Fiji Ministry of Health appointed a National Risk Management Adviser at the Head Office in Suva. The Adviser is an Australian with technical expertise in risk management, who would live and work in Fiji for the next several years.
- An Australian academic was appointed as clinical governance consultant to the Fiji Ministry of Health.
- Further clinical governance workshops were held with staff throughout Fiji.
- A local (Indigenous Fijian) project officer was appointed as clinical governance coordinator for a twelve-month period.
- Pamphlets and information booklets for all staff were developed by Health System Standards (the department in which the National Risk

Lee Stewart, Rusieli Taukei & Kim Usher

Management Advisor, Clinical Governance Coordinator and Consultant worked), and distributed throughout Fiji.
- Risk-management officers were appointed in each major hospital.
- Customer-service officers were appointed in each major hospital.
- Patient-satisfaction surveys were conducted, collated, and responded to.
- Risk-management education was developed and delivered to staff, and the reporting of critical incidents in hospitals increased. Root Cause Analysis of adverse events (Vincent, 2001) began in the hospitals.
- Consumer groups were included in planning for health care policy and practice.
- A 'Year of Patient Safety' was declared, with various projects developed within hospitals and community health services to increase consumer involvement and enhance patient safety.

The Project continues…

2. Development of human resources in rural Australia

Between 2002 and 2003, a health promotion program was funded by the Australian Federal Government to reduce the impact of chronic diseases among population in four Queensland rural communities (Jirojwong & Savage, 2003). The members of the Advisory Committee of this program comprised representatives of different community groups. During an initial stage of the community-needs assessment, it was found that the members of the Advisory Committee needed knowledge about the management process of an organisation and its governance. It was agreed that a formal workshop could be useful for the conduct of the program. However, the participants of this workshop would include other key community leaders, as it could provide long-term benefits to the communities. These key community leaders would also be important influential human resources of the program. Through out the two-year period of the project, the workshop participants described the benefits of the workshop to the governance of the project and other organisations within the communities (Jirojwong & Savage, 2003).

Conclusion

Effective human resource planning is crucial to the success of any project. Successful human-resource planning begins with asking key questions at the outset, including questions about the project's major goal(s), required technical and complementary knowledge, skills and attitudes, availability of local skills and knowledge, credibility of local members of the team, and the possible necessity for importing technical skills and knowledge. A project's success depends upon good leadership, particularly local leaders, and the involvement of local champions and key stakeholders. Active partnership and real collaboration are requirements of all team members. The necessity for a powerful local sponsor will facilitate successful project outcomes. Roles and responsibilities must be clearly stated, and are best decided upon by the team themselves. Knowledge about not only technical requirements but also optimum communication skills should be assessed, and education and training provided throughout the project. Mentoring of team members is vital, and increases the possibility of sustainability of the project aims through building capacity for local people. Sustainability is the major aim of any health care project and is clearly linked with the empowerment of local stakeholders.

CRITICAL THINKING EXERCISES

Using each of the elements in this chapter—leadership, local champions/stakeholders, partnership/collaboration and sponsors, roles and responsibilities, training, mentoring and supervising, and sustainability:

1. Choose a human resource team to respond to a problem you are having as a group of students (for example students arriving late to lectures, lecturer delays in returning marked assignments).

2. Pick out your least favourite television program and identify who should be on a team to improve the program.

3. Identify a health problem in a local community and design the best human-resource team that should be involved in improving the health problem.

4. Choose an unsatisfactory health policy in the state where you are a student. Discuss the policy as a group and plan the finest team of people to rewrite the policy.

Lee Stewart, Rusieli Taukei & Kim Usher

FURTHER READING

Best, R.G., Hysong, S.J., Pugh, J.A., Ghosh, S., & Moore, F.I. (2006) Task Overlap among Primary Care Team Members: An Opportunity for System Redesign? *Journal of Healthcare Management,* 51(5): 259–307.

Haroon Akram-Lodhi, A. (ed.) (2000) *Confronting Fiji Futures*. Asia Pacific Press: Canberra.

Nankervis, A., Compton, R., & Baird, M. (2005) *Human Resource Management*. Nelson: Melbourne.

Nayacakalou, R.R. (1975) *Leadership in Fiji*. Oxford University Press: Melbourne.

Rodriguez, H., & Aguirre, B.E. (2006) Hurricane Katrina and the Healthcare Infrastructure: A Focus on Disaster Preparedness, Response and Resiliency. *Frontiers of Health Services Management*, 23(1): 13–24.

Zairi, M. (1998) Building Human Resource Capability in Health Care: A Global Analysis of Best Practice—Part III. *Health Manpower Management,* 24(5): 166–9.

WEBPAGE RESOURCES

Fiji Ministry of Health: www.fiji.gov.fj/publish/m_health.shtml. This website provides a comprehensive outline of the Ministry's health priority goals. It provides students with an excellent context for the major case study.

World Health Organization: www.who.int/. This website is the gateway to World Health Organization (WHO) activities globally. Students are able to use the search function to access information about WHO projects worldwide, including in Fiji.

AusAID: www.ausaid.gov.au. This website provides information about the Australian Government's overseas aid program AusAID. Students who may be considering a career in this area can explore the numerous opportunities and programs funded by this body.

10

Planning for Policy Advocacy for Health Promotion

Vivian Lin & Prue Bagley

Objectives

After reading this chapter, readers will be able to:

➤ Understand advocacy as a strategy for affecting policy change
➤ Identify the critical steps in planning advocacy for policy change.

Key terms

advocacy
policy

Introduction

The Ottawa Charter (WHO, 1986) proposes that implementing a healthy public policy is one of the essential actions needed to promote the health of the population. The need for policy action is often identified during the problem-analysis phase that is the first step in planning a health promotion project. This is because policy action is often needed to address the social, economic, and environmental determinants of health. However, incorporating policy action into a project plan is not easy. Public policy decisions are usually made at the population or societal level, while health promotion projects are implemented at the level of local community or health service. Advocacy for healthy public policy is, thus, one of the core activities in a health promotion project.

In this chapter, planning for advocacy will be discussed with reference to advocacy for policy change. Advocacy is one of the principal means by which environmental change is achieved. Advocacy for policy change, however, is not simply a matter of stating what should be changed. Decision-makers are confronted daily with many competing interest groups who all want to have something changed, and they often have to trade one issue off against another. The role of the health promotion practitioner in advocacy is to mobilise interested parties and build partnerships, to get messages through to decision-makers at all levels about the need to take action, to articulate what actions are possible, and what benefits can be gained from acting.

This chapter will begin by discussing the concepts of policy, advocacy, and policy advocacy. It will then introduce the main principles for advocacy. Steps in planning for advocacy will be outlined, along with the most commonly used tools. The chapter concludes with discussion about critical success factors for an advocacy campaign.

> **Advocacy**: an action directed at changing the policies, positions, or programs of government or any other institution.
>
> **Policy**: a program of action adopted by government, or the set of principles on which it is based.

Key concepts

In order to advocate for policy change, it is important to understand what policy is. Policies come in many forms, and can be represented by a government document that states action intent, a piece of legislation, budget allocations, or promises made by ministers. It is essentially a program of action adopted by government, or the set of principles on which they are based.

Policy development, according to Colebatch (1998: 89–90), will always involve:

1 *authority*—there will be an identifiable person (such as a minister) or group (including cabinet) who will make the decision, which will occur through specific procedures, and be supported by officials
2 *expertise*—decision-makers will seek advice from a range of people (such as academics, business and community groups, lobbyists, consultants), and
3 *order*—policy development will entail a process of creating shared understanding leading to a new order that may entail altered practices.

Advocacy is an action directed at changing the policies, positions, or programs of government or any other institution. This action is usually undertaken on behalf of community interests, and it attempts to bring to the attention of decision-makers important community concerns with a view towards making positive change. In health promotion, advocacy is usually designed to create conditions for living and working that support healthier life styles. Advocacy may take many forms—be it demonstrations, letter-writing campaigns, petitions, editorial comment in the mass media, or lobbying in the corridors of power. It is a process of winning the support of key constituents and decision-makers. It also involves enabling people to participate in the decision-making processes that affect their lives.

There are two commonly contrasted approaches to advocacy. One approach sees advocacy as top-down prescription for environmental and policy change. The other approach sees advocacy as empowerment at the community level (Kar, 2000). They are interrelated insofar as top-down prescriptive change seldom happens without grass-roots demands, and community empowerment may be a prerequisite for communities to mobilise in their own interest. Thus, these approaches are both concerned with addressing power imbalance.

Basis for health advocacy

Being armed with the facts is an important starting point for successful advocacy, so it is the first step of planning policy in health promotion. Basic information would include the evidence base that is already useful for program planning purposes, such as:

- human costs—morbidity and mortality
- economic cost—health care, lost productivity
- distribution—whether the problem impacts on some groups more than others, and
- current programs and policies—what exist and whether they are inadequate.

Vivian Lin & Prue Bagley

Advocacy involves securing political action for health gain. So, the starting point for gathering knowledge is not only having a good understanding of the problem, but also the appropriate policy responses. Hence, as Heyman (2000) suggests, advocates for health should particularly understand three critical points:

- how the problem or issue is experienced by different groups of people and in different places (what is the average impact and who is affected), including both common and uncommon experiences
- the extent to which social and economic forces impact on the problem, and
- the appropriate policy solutions that are effective, given diverse social and economic conditions.

In undertaking policy planning, health promotion advocates should be very familiar with available information about the specific issue they want to focus on. They also need to be aware of how different local circumstances might contribute to how problems are experienced. In particular, they should be aware of the attitudes and practices of people towards the health condition and/or the risk behaviour. While access to information is vital, local information may be difficult to obtain, usually because the information is not gathered. If this is the case, then working to improve information systems or improve access to information may be a preliminary or concurrent function for advocates. Using information from relevant communities, states, or countries may also be considered. It is important to keep in mind that it is not always sufficient to understand the problem solely from an international or national perspective—advocates must also understand how people think about the problem in their own locality and the local context. Testimonials and human-interest stories can also be used to supplement statistical data, and have the advantage of making the situation more meaningful to non-professional groups and audiences.

Principles for policy advocacy for health

Policy advocacy for health is not a one-off event. It requires sustained action with multiple players. Advocacy needs to be well planned. Previous advocacy efforts provide well-worn tracks, and it is important to take the lessons from earlier endeavours. The most important questions to consider before starting planning for policy advocacy are:

- Can a 'win–win' outcome be engineered?
- Who do the decision-makers answer to, and how can these people be influenced?

- What are the strengths and weaknesses of an advocate's, or their team's, position compared with the position of their opposition?

The answers to these questions will help determine the strategies and tactics to be adopted. For all types of advocacy efforts, it is also important to keep the following principles in mind:

- Be focused and relevant.
  - Be clear about what is being advocated for.
  - Establish common themes and messages.
  - Do not stray from the message.
  - Make it local and keep it relevant.
- Work in partnership.
  - Target individuals and organisations that can get the message across.
  - Use other people's forums to advocate for the desired policy change.
  - Recruit corporate allies.
  - Develop media contacts (including those outside medicine and health).
- Be credible and appealing.
  - Know the facts and the numbers.
  - Research the issue and document the findings.
  - Find 'attractive' spokespeople.
  - Use icons who have credibility.
  - Use interesting stories.
- Be tactical.
  - Start by assuming the best of others (but know people's interests and arguments).
  - Do not take no for an answer.
  - Be passionate and persistent.
  - Set realistic goals.
  - Plan for small wins.
  - Take the high ground.
  - Be opportunistic and creative.
  - Employ multiple strategies.
  - Be willing to compromise.

(adapted from Cowal, 2000; and WHO, 1999)

Defining the desired policy objectives

Often, many different policy changes would be desirable, but it may not be realistic to try to change the world in one go. This means that it is important to focus on key aspects of policy that, if changed, will make a difference to the issue. This could be budget allocation for a new program, or amendments to existing legislation. It could be a ministerial statement in support of a certain position, or a group of policy announcements that go across several portfolios.

Approaching a policy-maker with a lengthy wish list is unlikely to be effective. Having a careful and realistic sequencing of policies to be targeted for change is usually more effective.

Where should the policy advocacy effort go?

Decision-making results from a complex process and reflects the interplay between many forces. Advocacy needs to be directed at both policy makers and those who influence policy, depending on where the advocate sits within the system. Successful campaigns recognise the interplay between forces, as illustrated in Figure 10.1. The

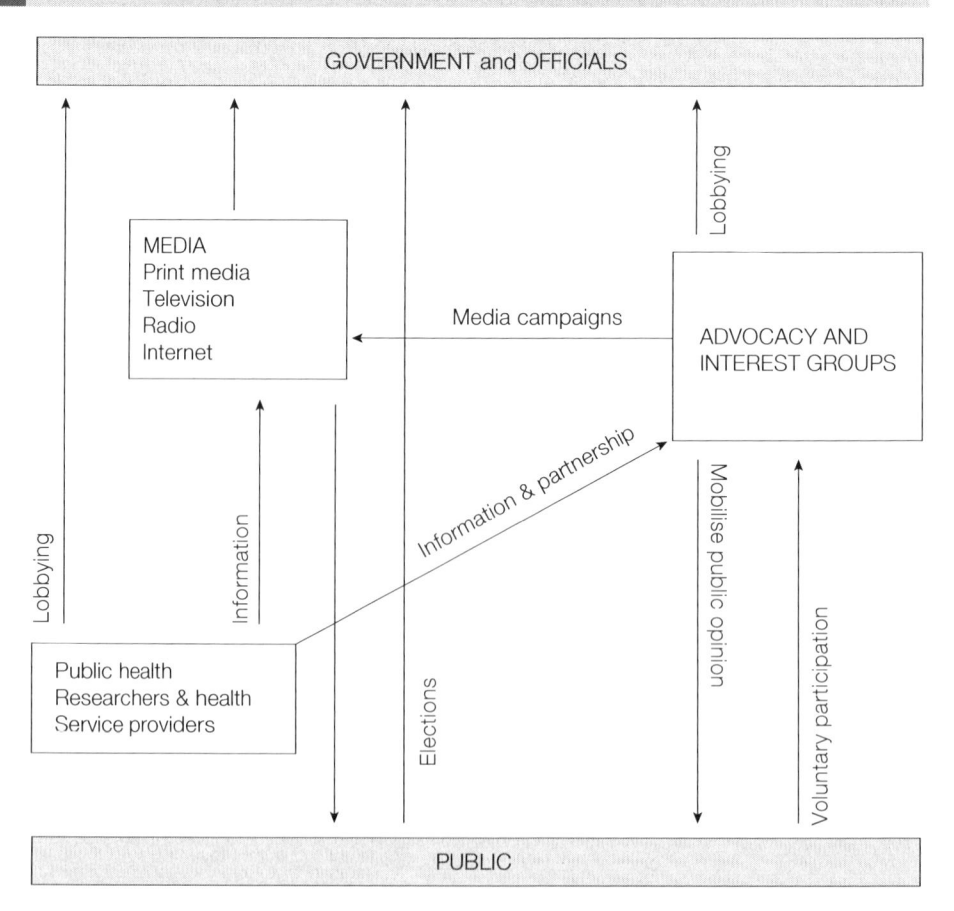

FIGURE 10.1 Factors affecting advocacy

Adapted from Heyman (2000: 376)

exact nature of the relationship between these forces differs from place to place, and from government to government. In some, policy makers may be influenced by direct lobbying from interest groups, or by alliances between interest groups and those working within government. In other places, they may be less amenable to the will of the people.

Planning advocacy

How to get started

Advocacy depends on presenting compelling arguments that convey a sense of urgency for action. It requires presenting decision-makers with proposed actions that are irresistible. Advocacy efforts need planning. The key steps include:

1. Researching the problem.
2. Defining the policy outcomes desired.
3. Knowing the target audience.
4. Deciding on the advocacy approach.
5. Deciding on key messages and key audiences.
6. Making contacts and assessing the climate for change.
7. Building constituency and building alliances.

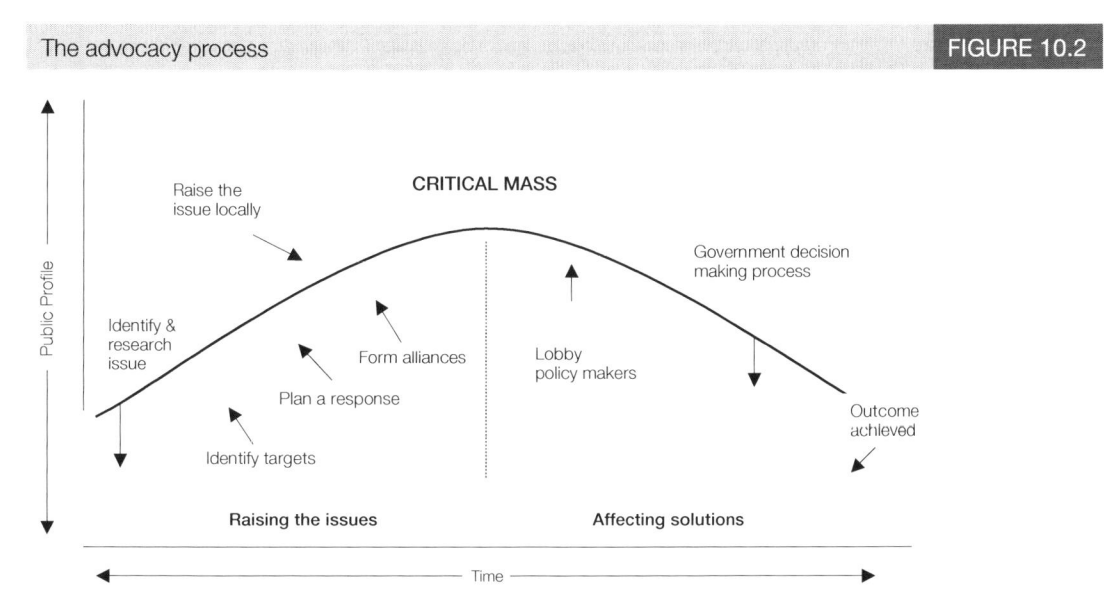

FIGURE 10.2 The advocacy process

Source: Australian Institute of Health and Welfare (2006: 143)

Vivian Lin & Prue Bagley

Advocacy campaigns will vary greatly from issue to issue, and from place to place. However, most campaigns will follow a similar trajectory, as seen in Figure 10.2—although the action at each stage will vary.

Making contacts and assessing climate for change

Timing and targeting are critical features of advocacy efforts, so doing a stakeholder analysis is crucial for choosing subsequent strategies and tactics. The first step in deciding who, how, and when to target is to research the issue. Some of the things should be considered include:

- Who are the people or groups sympathetic to the issue?
- Who are hostile?
- Who are the other players involved?
- What issues are about to become topical?
- When will these issues become topical? and
- Who are likely to be influential?

As part of this process, advocates will often undertake the following tasks:

- make a list of key people—this may include elected representatives, advisers, government officials, political party policy committee members, key professional organisations and leaders, key industry organisations and leaders, health reporters and political journalists
- talk to the people identified and make a table of their position, their interests, and their priorities
- sort the people identified into groups (for example 'friends', 'possible to win over', and 'hostile' camps).

It is also important to make a calendar of when critical events are occurring and an approximate timetable for decision-making. The budget cycle and budget announcements must also be considered. Other aspects, including sitting dates for parliament and election dates, are noted. The advocate needs to be aware of competing policy priorities and their timing.

Mapping out the policy landscape by the information from various activities will help decide whether the issue is ready to be addressed, how much effort needs to be spent on constituency development, who needs to be spoken with, and when to strike. An analysis of the stakeholders should result in adoption of strategies for mobilising their support or in managing their opposition. A stakeholder management strategy might resemble Table 10.1.

TABLE 10.1 A stakeholder management strategy

	Supporters	Opposition
Very important people	Mobilise their interest and enthusiasm; keep them informed and involved	Develop strategies to manage or reduce their antagonism
Less important people	Keep them on side and ensure they remain supportive	Monitor their position to contain opposition

TABLE 10.2 Examples of key stakeholders to consider for common health promotion action areas

Action area	Key stakeholders	
Tobacco	Ministers responsible for communications/media, industry, and trade Medical associations Tobacco farmers Tobacco wholesalers and retailers	Minister esponsible for health and education Treasury
Nutrition	Ministers responsible for agriculture and industry The food industry (including manufacturers, wholesalers, retailers, transport) Bodies representing primary producers Bodies representing consumers	
Physical activity	Minister responsible for sport and recreation Local government officials responsible for recreation, parks, and planning Urban planners Education sector Sports teams and clubs	
Mental health promotion	Groups representing those with mental health problems Social welfare groups Education sector Human rights groups	

Vivian Lin & Prue Bagley

Targeting and framing the messages

In targeting messages for key audiences—that is, the points that should be communicated in each message that is developed—there are two key points to bear in mind. The first is that the human and economic costs of the health issue are enormous. The second is that the problem is manageable.

In selecting advocacy messages, it is important to focus on simple messages that can be repeated. Criteria for selecting messages can be aligned with key health indicators and key policy proposals. Some of the criteria may be that:

- the general public, opinion leaders, and the health and medical communities can easily interpret and understand the message
- they reflect topics that affect the people's health in important ways
- they address problems that can be changed and will have a substantial impact on the health of the population, and
- they can be used in directing public policies and programs (Institute of Medicine, 1999).

It is crucial to focus on communicating in the simplest way possible about the nature of the problem, the desired action, and the potential benefits.

Choosing the advocacy approach and the tools

There are many approaches to advocacy, including public campaigns, private lobbying, meetings, petitions, letter-writing, and media events. The choice of approach depends on the findings from the research undertaken on the issue and on the stakeholders. Consider the following:

- Is it best to work from within (by getting policy papers approved or by lunching with the power brokers)?

or

- Would it be more productive to work from the outside (by creating public outrage or by having media and community events)?

and

- What is the best mixture of internal and external campaigning?

Most advocacy campaigns will require multiple approaches, and the selection of approaches depends, in part, on the targets, the allies, and the spokespeople. The maturity of the issue will help shape the approach. Often, when an issue is new, the primary goal is to raise public awareness. This requires 'making noise' in the public arena. With a mature issue, the goal may be policy change. This may require lengthy negotiations—achieved within the corridors of power. The most common approaches adopted are government relations, media advocacy, and coalition building. Useful tools for these activities are discussed in the next section.

Advocacy toolkit

Lobbying and government relations

Effective government relations require an understanding of how government works and what drives government decision-making. This means, first, understanding the legislative processes and structures of government administration. Effective advocates will research the governmental system and be aware of how the processes work and where the points and people of influence are. In all systems, however, governments like to have good news and to take credit for positive outcomes. Effective government relations will ultimately allow governments to feel successful.

Law-making and budgetary processes are two key political activities in which advocates should take an active interest. The mechanics of each process may vary depending on the government structures of particular jurisdictions, and so it is important to understand how the system operates. The way the 'system' operates can often be complex, and may not always work through formal channels. For example, some politicians may regard the opinions of friends and relatives highly when making policy decisions, so that if advocates are able to influence those friends and relatives, the issue may be more likely to enter the political agenda. In multicultural and multi-faith societies, politicians may bond on the basis of common places of origin or ethnic group or belief systems. In decentralised systems, local and regional interests may have greater responsibility for decision-making, and advocacy efforts will need to be directed more broadly.

Not all policy comes into effect through the law-making process, but it is the ultimate expression of a government's intent. The following table outlines the different stages of the legislative process in Australian jurisdictions. This model points to where an advocate could have the opportunity to exert influence including:

➤ contributing to relevant commissions and parliamentary committees, when they are the source of new legislation
➤ making comments on discussion papers released by the government, to support appropriate legislation, recommend modifications or challenge inappropriate proposals, and
➤ lobbying backbenchers to request changes to the proposal at the party approval stage.

Vivian Lin & Prue Bagley

TABLE 10.3 Legislative process

How laws are made in a Westminster system	
Legislation is proposed	Legislation may come from different sources, including ministers, their staff, backbenchers, from recommendations of commissions, and from parliamentary committees
The proposal is refined	Government agencies and ministers will be involved Public input may be sought through the release of Discussion Papers
It goes to Cabinet	Usually Cabinet approval is needed for the proposal to proceed
Party approval is sought	This is a good point of influence for advocates because backbenchers (who support the health issue) can request changes to the proposal
The bill is introduced	The bill is read a first, a second, and a third time During the second reading the bill may be debated in detail and amendments are presented and voted on
Royal approval is given	The Governor General (on the Queen's behalf) gives royal approval to the bill—it is now an Act of Parliament

Source: Public Interest Advocacy Centre, 1996

Being involved in the budgetary process is another key activity for advocates seeking policy and program solutions to their issues. While the process may vary between states, there are two areas to investigate:

1. What is the timing of the process (that is, when is the most effective time to feed ideas into the process)?
2. What are the costs and pay-offs for the proposed solution by the advocate; that is, in what economic terms can the proposed solution be sold?

The following points should be kept in mind:

- Typically, proposals are developed six to nine months before the budget. Advocacy in this early period should target ministers and departmental officials.
- Three to six months before the budget, the proposals are with senior members of government (Cabinet or a Cabinet sub-committee). They will be considering the possible trade-offs between different sectors and within sectors. This is an important consideration in the health sector where funds may be withdrawn from one area to support another.

- Advocacy during this budget period should target Finance and Treasury as well as key members of Cabinet or the Cabinet sub-committee.
- Policy ideas that are not expensive (or that generate revenue) are popular.
- Potential budget savings will have to be determined for policies and programs that are expensive to be considered.
- In budget submissions, it is important to have a convincingly costed proposal.

Lobbying politicians is an important part of advocacy. This involves attracting the support of those with the influence to promote or resolve the issue. When the opportunities for advocacy within the political process have been identified, there are a number of techniques that can be used to develop effective relationships with the key players. Face-to-face meetings are a necessity at some stage, but it requires planning about timing, with whom, what the core message is, and who will attend. The following list outlines some questions to consider in planning a lobbying effort. Another common means of influencing policy makers is through a letter-writing campaign. Again, planning is required about timing, to whom, and what the core message is. Increasingly, the internet can be used creatively to build relationships and gather public support.

- Identify the right target (governments may produce directories to help identify the correct minister or agency to deal with your issue):
  - What level of government (local, state, or federal)?
  - Which government agency or minister?
  - What piece(s) of legislation?
- Ask the politician to:
  - raise your concerns with Cabinet or Caucus, or in policy committees
  - ask questions in parliament
  - provide access to government information that might otherwise be difficult to obtain.
- Target ministers: they usually have more power to influence policy than other politicians.
- Use ministerial staff: staff in the minister's office usually know what she or he thinks about an issue and they may be able to influence how the minister sees the issue.

Media

Social marketing and media advocacy is often used in health promotion for raising awareness and promoting behaviour change. Media advocacy can also be used to shape public discussion in a way that increases support for healthy public policy proposals (Wallack, 1994).

Media advocacy, according to Wallack (1994), has three broad functions, which are:

▶ *Setting the agenda*: getting access to the media and attracting coverage for the issue. Media coverage raises public concern and, in turn, increases political sensitivity to an issue. Issues that fail to attract media attention are unlikely to be advanced.
▶ *Shaping the debate* involves the definitions of the issues being highlighted. How a problem is defined is critical because the cause suggests the solutions. In advocacy for health, shaping the debate may involve broadening the definitions of health issues so that problems (such as smoking and drug taking) are seen as more than individual pathology.
▶ *Advancing the policy*: after attracting attention and defining the problem, the final step is to advance a solution—usually in the form of a particular approach or policy (Wallack, 1994).

Effective media advocacy requires careful planning. When planning for this kind of advocacy, the GOTME (goal, objective, target, message, evaluation) approach, as outlined in Table 10.4, provides a useful set of guidelines.

TABLE 10.4 Media advocacy planning

Goal	Setting specific goals is particularly important when groups are working in coalition with others.
Objective	Objectives support the overall goal established in the first planning step. There are different levels of objectives, including program, policy, and media campaign objectives.
Target	Identify the three target audiences: • those with the power to make the desired change • those who can be mobilised to apply pressure to this group • the general population.
Message	This may be seen in three parts: • statement of concern (what the situation is at present) • value dimension (why that situation should be changed) • policy objective (how that change might be effected).
Evaluation	Assess the value of the effort. Identify any lessons that could be learned for future efforts.

Source: Wallack & Dorfman, 1996

The media—radio, television, newspapers, magazines—can be an important ally for health promotion advocates. This is because these media have the potential to deliver an advocacy message to a large number of people. Sometimes, advocates will use the media with the intention of swaying public opinion around a health issue (such as smoking), intending that this changed public opinion will pressure politicians and organisations to introduce policies that will lead to improved health outcomes. However, advocates should be aware that the media is not merely a passive tool to be used for advocacy. Indeed, media organisations (and the people who work in them) will often have their own agendas and interests, which may directly oppose the goals of health promotion advocates. Even when the media support the health promotion goals, an advocacy message may be changed substantially by the media to suit their own perspectives regarding what is interesting and important. This may occur not because the media deliberately set out to undermine health promotion advocacy, but because the ultimate objectives of health promotion and the media are very different.

Journalists and other people working in the media are often in search of interesting health stories, so advocates can often 'help them out' by providing journalists with updates on recent developments in research, or by drawing their attention to new programs with interesting facts or stories that might provide the basis for a media article.

It is always important to remember that *timeliness* is one of the key characteristics of news media. When a new story or issue hits the headlines, journalists are expected to work very quickly to gather as much information about that issue as they can, and quickly prepare that information for presentation through their media—be it in print, on television, on radio, or via the internet. For this reason, the advocate must be able to provide journalists with information as soon as they need it—and, if possible, *before* they need it—so that the views on a particular health issue will receive free media coverage through news items.

Coalition building

Coalition building with community organisations is important in advocacy for health. Policy makers will respond more readily when there is substantial community support for an issue. Good public health policy can be advanced through such coalitions in two ways. First, community organisations can be encouraged to adopt good practice within their own organisation. For example, local schools and industries can be encouraged to promote nutritious lunches, and local authorities encouraged to increase access to recreational facilities. Second, community organisations can lend support during specific campaigns. Potential groups include churches, schools, social service and consumer organisations,

Vivian Lin & Prue Bagley

professional organisations, and women's, youth, or older people's organisations. Not everybody is a potential ally, however, and it is important to think about who supporters and enemies might be on particular issues.

There are some general principles that may help when the advocate is trying to build alliances with different organisations. The World Health Organization (1999) suggests the following:

- Choose unifying issues.
- Understand and respect institutional self-interest.
- Help organisations to achieve their self-interest.
- Recognise that contributions from member organisations will vary.
- Structure decision-making carefully, based on level of contribution.
- Clarify decision-making procedures.
- Agree to disagree.
- Play to the centre with tactics.
- Achieve significant victories, and
- Distribute credit fairly.

Be warned, however, that making coalitions work takes time and effort. Prior to embarking on extensive efforts to build coalitions, it is important that the right partners have been identified, that there are sufficient interests in common, and that the coalition can work or be made to work on the shared interests or health issue.

Critical factors for success

Achieving sustainable change in the health of the population requires a combination of personal skills, community action, health services, and good policy. Advocacy is a pathway to successful policies and programs. It is a key ingredient for attaining high-level political support and a multisector approach including different levels and sectors of government, the community, families, and workplaces.

The effects of advocacy efforts may not be apparent immediately. Very often during the process of health promotion advocacy, small changes to the 'environment' will be achieved by advocates, but there will be no perceivable effects produced from those changes—the same number of people will smoke, diabetes admissions to hospital will not decrease, and, despite winning over key politicians to participate or act on your health issue, there still be no new legislation passed into law. This can be disheartening to advocates, who may feel as though they are not making progress.

Patience is required in all aspects of health promotion, and particularly in advocacy. Gladwell (2000) suggests that, while the effects of people's efforts are not immediately apparent, change is not gradual. Rather, there comes a point at which people's efforts finally tip the balance, and dramatic change occurs.

Gladwell (2000) describes three special qualities that can affect the point at which sudden change occurs, and an 'epidemic' of a given phenomenon occurs—whether it be a disease, a sudden jump in crime, sales of a popular book, or even a successful health program. These qualities are what Gladwell calls the 'law of the few', the 'stickiness factor', and the 'power of context'.

The 'law of the few' describes the principle whereby the activities of a few people will have a greater effect than the combined efforts of everyone else. These people have a greater effect because they possess characteristics that make them different from everyone else. They may be celebrities or people who have a wide circle of friends. Health promotion advocates are examples of this principle because they champion their cause, make contact with people who can help to influence others, and persist in their efforts until the 'tipping point' (that is, a critical mass of opinion for change) for their issue occurs. They are joined in their efforts by other health professionals, and if they are successful, by people with influence in society, such as politicians or celebrities. Tobacco use and its negative impact on the health of Australians provides an example of an issue's tipping point. The harm caused by tobacco has been recognised by researchers since the 1950s. However, for years after this it attracted very little public interest. Health advocates in Australia mounted a number of campaigns in the 1970s and 1980s. These campaigns raised public awareness to such a level that a tipping point was reached. This allowed a number of policy changes to be made, including the ban on small packs of cigarettes, tax increases, and the replacement of sponsorship (Chapman & Wakefield, 2001).

The 'stickiness factor' refers to the 'agent' of a particular 'epidemic', and, once again, the tipping point is reached when this agent acquires some characteristic that makes it more 'sticky'. Examples are the increasing virulence of an infectious disease or when a particularly memorable slogan is devised for a health campaign. In health promotion, this factor applies to the key ideas and proposals advocates use when trying to champion their cause. If these do not appeal to the people advocates approach, such as the media or policy makers, the tipping point may never be reached. For this reason, it is essential that advocates are able to communicate their ideas effectively, and tailor those ideas and proposals to suit the interests of key people—while taking great care not to compromise the ultimate aim of health promotion.

Finally, the 'power of context' highlights the importance of the environment on the effectiveness of health promotion advocacy. Occasionally, small changes in the environment may be all that is required for the tipping point to be reached. The environment in this sense means the social context in which arguments and strategies for *advocacy* occur, including the cultural context and the considerations that affect decision-makers and decision-making. The timing and the targeting of advocacy efforts also depend on sound analysis of political context. Health promotion advocates should try to tailor strategies and solutions with cultural context and decision-making contexts in mind.

CASE STUDY

The Penrith Food Project

Penrith is a local government area (LGA) in Sydney's west that has a high rate of cardiovascular disease. The availability of, and access to, nutritious food was identified as a significant issue (Hawe & Stickney, 1997). The Penrith Food Project was launched in 1991 with the intent 'to work primarily, by modifying the policies and practices of Council and other organisations, for a better food system in the community' (Penrith Food Project, 1998: 2). The project was jointly funded and overseen by the Penrith LGA and the Area Health Service (of the state Health Department). It involved partners in the community, academic, and business worlds.

The project has three stated goals: to increase and improve the supply of affordable, acceptable, nutritious, and safe food, to increase and improve the demand for, and consumption of, nutritious food, and to create an ongoing local system for improving the health impact of the food supply and monitoring population food habits (Penrith City Council, 2001).

Over time a range of diverse strategies has been employed to improve the access and availability of nutritious food. These have included changes in bus routes, the development of policy guidelines for food access in new housing developments, and Open Farm days to increase awareness about agriculture.

Not all local governments have been as successful as Penrith in instituting policy change. Yeatman (2003) identified barriers/facilitators of policy change, which included the political and organisational environment. She noted that public health professionals can, with the right knowledge and skills, be very influential in the policy process (Yeatman, 2003).

The success of the Penrith Food Project provides a number of lessons:

➤ Epidemiological research indicated that nutrition was a issue affecting the community's health (Cumming et al., cited in Hawe & Stickney, 1997).
➤ Further research identified barriers to people making healthy food choices (Brierley et al., cited in Hawe & Stickney, 1997).

> - Advocates used the evidence to highlight the issue with decision-makers.
> - Advocates used the research to identify points of possible action and to push for policy change.
> - Multiple strategies were employed.
> - The project encouraged the participation of both the general community and the decision-makers.
> - The health sector can not work alone. Success required working effectively with a number of diverse sectors, including agriculture, environmentalists, food industry, politicians, and tourism, and
> - Projects must be sustainable.

Conclusion

Successful advocacy work requires planning—to ensure that all the factors discussed here have been considered. Advocacy work also requires an investment—to develop skills, identify and obtain resources, undertake research, and monitor progress. It requires that people involved in advocacy think seriously about the range of factors and contexts that affect the ways different health issues are regarded in society. It also requires that health promotion advocates be innovative, forthright, and strategic in the way they approach improving the social, cultural, economic, and physical factors that determine health. Finally, health promotion advocates must be aware of what their colleagues are doing towards changing life styles and reorientating health services, so that all efforts can be coordinated and organised effectively. With these things achieved, the health promotion advocate will be prepared to become a true champion of health for the community.

CRITICAL THINKING EXERCISES

1. Identify what policy changes would be needed in your local area to encourage residents to increase their level of incidental physical activity.

2. Using the information supplied in this chapter, develop a policy advocacy plan for improving health care access for refugees and asylum seekers.

Vivian Lin & Prue Bagley

FURTHER READING

Calvert, G., & Smith, R. (2004) A National Framework for Promoting Health and Well-Being in the Early Years. *Health Promotion Journal of Australia*, 15(2): 99–102.

Chapman, S., & Wakefield, M. (2001) Tobacco Control Advocacy in Australia: Reflections on 30 Years of Progress. *Health Education Behaviour*, 28: 274–89.

Ewles, L., & Simnett, I. (2003) *Promoting Health: A Practical Guide*, 5th edn. Baillière Tindall: Edinburgh.

Jones, L., Sidell, M., & Douglas, J. (eds) (2002) *The Challenge of Promoting Health*, 2nd edn. The Open University/Palgrave: Basingstoke.

Lewis, J. (2005) *Health Policy and Politics: Networks, Ideas and Power*. IP Communications: East Hawthorn.

Loue, S., Lloyd, L., & O'Shea, D. (2002) *Community Health Advocacy*. Kluwer Academic/Plenum: New York.

Milio, N. (2005) Ideology, Science, and Public Policy. *Journal of Epidemiology and Community Health*, 59(10): 814–15.

Wallack, L. (2000) The Role of Mass Media in Creating Social Capital: A New Direction for Public Health. In: B. Smedley & L. Syme (eds), *Promoting Health: Intervention Strategies from Social and Behavioral Research*, 337–65. National Academy Press: Washington DC.

World Health Organization (2004) *Advocacy Guide: HIV/AIDS Prevention among Injecting Users*. World Health Organization, UN AIDS: Geneva.

WEBPAGE RESOURCES

'A' Frame for Advocacy—Bloomberg School of Public Health, Johns Hopkins University Baltimore: www.infoforhealth.org/pr/advocacy/index.shtml
Basic information relating to advocacy can be used as a starting point for students who are interested in this field.

California Centre for Public Health Advocacy: www.publichealthadvocacy.org/
It contains research, reports and strategies used by the Centre. Information can be used as a guide for a large project team.

The Policy Project. Networking for Policy Change: An Advocacy Training Manual: www.policyproject.com/pubs/AdvocacyManual.pdf
It is a very good advocacy training manual.

The California Wellness Foundation—The Policy and Public Education Program of the California Youth Violence Prevention Initiative: www.tcwf.org/pub_evaluations/youth_violence_prevention.htm
It is a good example of a project with an advocacy as its major component.

PART 4

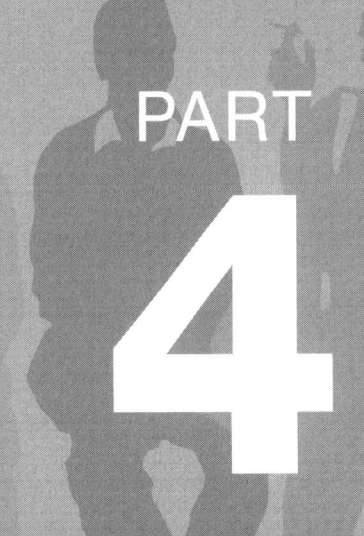

Implementation

Chapter 11	Health Promotion: How to Build Community Capacity	195
Chapter 12	Community Development and Empowerment	215
Chapter 13	Health Promotion and Health Education for a Multicultural Community	232

Health Promotion: How to Build Community Capacity

Glenn Laverack

Objectives

After reading this chapter, readers will be able to:

- Understand the definition of community capacity
- Understand the interpretation of the 'domains' of community capacity
- Describe a tool to build and measure community capacity
- Describe a method to visually represent community capacity.

Key terms

capacity domains
community capacity building
measurement

Introduction

This chapter addresses why some communities have more ability than others—why some communities are more capable at accessing resources, at influencing decision-makers, are better organised and are better at mobilising themselves to address their concerns and needs. The chapter also discusses the key characteristics (or 'domains') of community capacity, and describes a tool that can be used by practitioners to build and measure this concept in health promotion programs.

The definition of community capacity

Community capacity building: increasing the assets and attributes of a community through improvements in skills, knowledge, and competencies.

There is a broad body of literature in regard to the definition of community capacity. For example, Labonte and Laverack (2001a: 114) define capacity building as the 'increase in community groups' abilities to define, assess, analyze and act on health (or any other) concerns of importance to their members'. Community capacity is seen by several authors (Goodman et al., 1998; Bopp et al., 2000) as a process that increases the assets and attributes that a community is able to draw upon. The capacity of a group is also dependent on the resource opportunities or constraints (social, political, and economic) and the conditions in which people live. Community capacity is not, therefore, an inherent property of a particular locality, nor of the individuals or groups within it, but of the interactions between both.

Interest in community capacity building as a strategy for sustainable skills, resources, and commitments in various settings has developed because of the requirement to prolong the gains from health promotion programs (Gibbon et al., 2002). These qualities exist in relation to specific people and groups, specific issues and concerns, and specific activities or programs. For a health promotion organisation or health promoter, the task is not to create a new program called 'capacity-building'. Rather, the task is to examine how its practice can support the development of capacity building (Laverack, 1999). Capacity building becomes the process by which the end result of increasing community control and program sustainability can be achieved through, for example, increasing knowledge and developing skills and competencies.

Capacity domains: areas of influence that enable a community to organise and mobilise itself better towards increasing its assets and attributes.

The 'domains' of community capacity

The process of community capacity is influenced by several characteristics or 'domains' that contribute significantly to its development. In particular, the organisational characteristics that influence community capacity provide a useful means to build and measure this concept (Labonte & Laverack, 2001b). The 'capacity domains' represent those aspects of the process of community capacity that allow individuals and groups to better organise and mobilise themselves towards gaining greater control over their lives. They also provide a link between the interpersonal elements of community capacity, such as individual control and community cohesiveness, and the contextual elements such as the political and economic circumstances (Laverack, 2001). The existence of functional leadership, established community structures, the level of participation and the ability to mobilise resources are indicative of a community with both strong organisational and social abilities. The 'capacity domains' are robust and collectively capture the essential qualities of a capable community. The domains have been cross-checked against the literature to ensure their validity (Laverack, 2001) and have been successfully implemented elsewhere within a program context (Laverack, 1999; Jones & Laverack, 2003).

The 'capacity domains' provide a predetermined focus through nine areas of organisational influence such that a health promotion program:

1. improves stakeholder participation
2. develops local leadership
3. builds organisational structures
4. increases problem-assessment capacities
5. enhances stakeholders' ability to ask 'why?'
6. improves resource mobilisation
7. strengthens links to other organisations and people
8. creates an equitable relationship with outside agents, and
9. increases stakeholder control over program management.

The following is a brief description of each 'capacity domain', including examples that illustrate their relevance to health promotion practice.

Improving stakeholder participation

Community participation occurs when people become actively involved in a broad range of common needs by sharing their ideas and experiences to identify concerns (Rifkin, 1990). Participation is often based on representation, as it is not usually possible for all community members to be involved in this process. Participation describes the involvement of individuals in groups and in 'communities of interest' that share and have the capacity to begin to address their needs. Individuals are able to influence the direction and implementation of a program through their participation, and this can involve the development of their skills and abilities.

Developing local leadership

Participation and leadership are closely connected because, just as leaders require a strong participant base, participation requires the direction and structure of strong leadership (Goodman et al., 1998). Karina Constantino-David (1995), a writer in community development, discusses the experiences of community organising in the Philippines and the success of utilising local leaders or 'organic organisers'. Competent leaders were developed by Civil Society Organisations among poor people, who offered a more insightful understanding of the community problems and culture. However, it was found that a lack of skills training and previous management experience of these people created limitations in their role as leaders. Leadership style and skills can, therefore, influence the way in which groups and communities develop and in turn this can influence capacity building.

Examples of leadership qualities that can be enhanced in a health promotion program include:

➤ an empowerment style of leadership that encourages and supports the ideas and planning efforts of the community, using democratic decision-making processes and the sharing of information
➤ the ability to collect and analyse data, evaluate community initiatives, facilitate the activities undertaken by groups and sommunities, and solve problems
➤ skill in conflict resolution, and
➤ the ability to connect to other leaders and organisations to gain resources and establish partnerships (Kumpfer et al., 1993).

Building organisational structures

Organisational structures in a community include committees, faith groups, social and sports clubs, and women's associations. These are the organisational elements that represent the ways in which people come together in order to address their concerns. They are also the way in which people come together to interact and to connect, for example to organise sporting and cultural events. In a program context, it is also the way in which people come together to identify their problems, to find solutions to their problems, and to plan for action to resolve their problems.

The characteristics of a functional community organisation have been found to include a membership of elected representatives that meet and participate on a regular basis. The members have an agreed membership structure (chairperson, secretary, core members, and so on) that keeps records such as previous meetings and financial accounts. A functional community organisation is also able to identify and resolve conflict quickly, and its members are able to identify the resources available to them (Jones & Laverack, 2003).

Increasing problem-assessment capacities

Problem assessment involves the identification by the community of problems, of solutions to the problems, and of actions to resolve the problems. The success of a health promotion program depends to a great extent on the commitment and involvement of the intended beneficiaries. People are more likely to be committed if they have a sense of ownership in regard to the problems and solutions being addressed by the program. This means that the problems being addressed need to be identified by the community concerned rather than by an outside agent.

Outside agents obviously do often have new and useful information to offer, for example, the latest information on how to prevent disease. The point is that this information should not be imposed over the expressed needs and concerns that reside among community members. The best approach is to use a 'facilitated dialogue' between the community and the outside agents to allow the knowledge and priorities of both to decide an appropriate direction for the program (Laverack, 2004).

Enhancing the ability of the community to ask 'why?'

Generally, small groups focus inwards on the needs of their members, but as they develop into community organisations, they must be able to broaden outwards to the environment that creates those needs in the first place (Goodman et al., 1998). Fundamentally, 'asking why' is a process of discussion, reflection, and collective action that is also called 'critical consciousness'. The key term here is 'critical', in which the community members take a long, hard, and analytical look at their situation. It is also the ability of the community to be able to develop strategies to bring about personal, social, and political change based on an understanding of their own circumstances. This is achieved through group dialogue to share ideas and experiences, and to promote critical thinking by posing problems that allow people to uncover the root causes of inequality and powerlessness. Once they are critically aware, the community can then begin to plan actions to change the circumstances that influence their lives (Freire, 1973).

Improving resource mobilisation

The ability of the community to mobilise resources from within and to negotiate resources from beyond itself is an indication of a high degree of skill and organisation.

Glenn Laverack

Goodman and colleagues (1998) discuss resources in terms of 'traditional capital', such as property and money, and 'social capital', which includes a sense of trust and the ability to cooperate with one another and with other communities. The outside agents may be expected to provide assistance to mobilise resources at the beginning of a program, but control over these must be increasingly carried out by the community, otherwise a paternalistic relationship can occur. Resources that health promoters might expect to mobilise from a community are traditionally based on voluntary labour (participation), materials, local knowledge, and implementation insights, as well as some small financial contribution. That communities possess both traditional and social capital is sometimes ignored by outside agents who believe that they can bring with them the necessary resources for the health promotion program (Goodman et al., 1998).

Strengthening links to other organisations and people

Links with other people and organisations include partnerships, coalitions, and health alliances. These relationships demonstrate the ability to network, collaborate, and cooperate, and to develop relationships that promote a heightened interdependency among its members. They may involve an exchange of services, pursuit of a joint venture based on a shared goal, or an advocacy initiative to change public or private policies.

Partnerships, coalitions, and health alliances have become a popular theme within health promotion and are seen to be a two-way process incorporating both top-down and bottom-up principles of programming. It is implicit that the process is fully participatory and that government organisations do not merely consult or engage with the 'community'. People are involved in the decision-making processes of the program, which also has the aim of being a capacity-building experience (Laverack, 2007b: 66–7).

Creating an equitable relationship with the outside agent

Outside agents such as health promotion practitioners have an important role in linking the community to resources or assisting them to mobilise and organise themselves through building their capacity. This can be especially important at the beginning of a program when the capacity of the community is low. The role of the outside agent is then essentially one of developing the knowledge, skills, and competencies of the community, for example, training in conflict management and specific skill areas such as self-evaluation (Laverack, 2004: 97).

Increasing stakeholder control over program management

At the heart of management is who controls the way in which the program is designed, implemented, managed, and evaluated. Constantino-David (1995) argues that the priorities of outside agents have shifted towards the expectation of better program management, including financial planning systems. As program management becomes more sophisticated, the outside agents are less willing to transfer responsibility and skills to the community, who are perceived as having poor capacity. To build capacity, the community must first have a sense of ownership of the program, which in turn must address their needs and concerns. The role of the outside agent is increasingly to transfer responsibility to the community through a systematic process of capacity building (Laverack, 2007b: 68).

Building and measuring community capacity

In practice, health promotion is implemented as a set of activities within the context of an intervention, a project, or a program. The 'program' is conventionally managed and monitored by, for example, a health promotion practitioner, and commonly includes a period of identification, design, implementation, management, and evaluation. The basic question planners and practitioners need to ask themselves is 'How has the health promotion program helped to increase community capacity in each of the nine "domains"?' A participatory tool (referred to as 'the tool') that uses the nine 'capacity domains' to build community capacity in a program context has been developed and is discussed next (Laverack, 2003).

How is the 'tool' implemented?

Rather than being a substitute for program objectives, community capacity creates a separate set of goals that run parallel to the specific purpose of the health promotion program (Laverack, 2003). The tool is implemented in three phases as a part of the health promotion program: preparation, measurement of each domain, and developing a strategic plan for community capacity.

    Phase 1 involves the use of simple qualitative techniques. Phases 2 and 3 are implemented as a participatory workshop. Figure 11.1 provides an overview of the design of the 'tool' for building and measuring community capacity.

Measurement: the collection and comparison of information.

FIGURE 11.1 The design of the 'tool' to build and measure community capacity

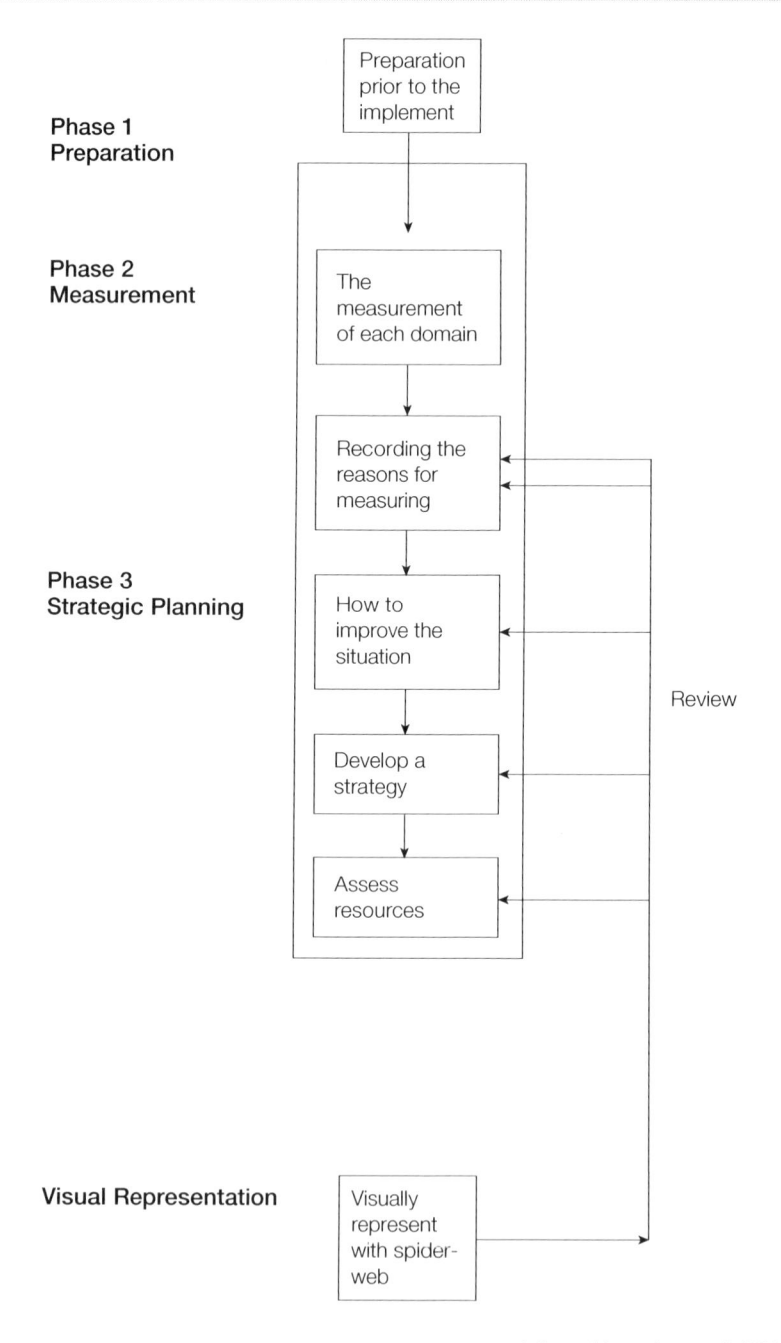

Phase 1 Preparation

- Preparation prior to the implement

Phase 2 Measurement

- The measurement of each domain

Phase 3 Strategic Planning

- Recording the reasons for measuring
- How to improve the situation
- Develop a strategy
- Assess resources

Review

Visual Representation

- Visually represent with spider-web

Adapted from: Laverack (2003: 101)

Phase 1: Preparation

A period of observation and discussion is important to adapt the 'tool' to the social and cultural requirements of the participants in the program. For example, the use of a working definition of community capacity can provide all participants with a more mutual understanding of the program in which they are involved and towards which they are expected to contribute. In Fiji, the use of simple qualitative techniques has been shown to identify the key terms in regard to power and empowerment. Unstructured interviews were used first to identify the headings for power or '*lewa*' and '*kaukauwa*'. Then, through semi-structured interviews, the term '*lewa*' was further identified to refer to chiefly power, the control of the village chief, and the power-over bestowed at work or in the home. The term '*kaukauwa*' is the closest concept in a Fijian context to empowerment. It refers to community strength and unity, which can be developed and assisted by its members and can be used to describe the right a person has to do something (Laverack, 2005: 90).

Phase 2: A measurement of each domain

Using the nine domains (whose meaning can be altered or changed if the context under Phase 1 warrants this action), the participants of the workshop first make a measurement of their community's capacity. To do this, they are provided with five generic statements for each domain, each written on a separate sheet of paper. The five statements represent a description of the various levels of capacity related to that domain (see Laverack, 2005: 99–101). Taking one domain at a time, the participants are asked to select the statement that most closely describes the present situation in their community. The statements are not numbered or marked in any way, and each is read out loud by the participants to encourage group discussion. The descriptions may be amended by the participants, or a new description may be provided to describe the situation for a particular domain. In this way, the participants make their own measurement for each domain by comparing their experiences and opinions.

Recording the reasons for the measurement

It is important that the participants record the reasons why the measurement for the domain has been made. First, it assists other people who make the re-measurement and who need to take the previous record into account. Second, it provides some defensible or empirically observable criteria for the selection. The 'reasons why' include verifiable examples of the actual experiences of the participants taken from their community. This illustrates the reasoning behind the selection of the statement, for example, 'leadership is weak in our community because we have no chief, the last chief having died six months ago'.

Phase 3: Developing a strategic plan for community capacity

The measurement in Phase 2 is in itself insufficient to build capacity, as this information must also be transformed into actions. This is achieved by building community capacity through strategic planning for positive changes in each of the nine 'domains'. The strategic planning for each domain consists of three simple steps: a discussion on how to improve the present situation, the development of a strategy to improve upon the present situation, and the identification of any necessary resources.

A discussion on how to improve the present situation

Following the measurement of each domain, the participants will be asked to decide as a group how this situation can be improved in their community. If more than one statement has been selected, the participants should consider how to improve each situation. The purpose is to identify the broader approaches that will improve the present situation and provide a lead into a more detailed strategy. If the participants decide that the present situation does not require any improvement, no strategy will be developed for that particular domain.

Developing a strategy to improve the present situation

The participants are next asked to consider how, in practice, the measurement can be improved. The participants develop a more detailed strategy based on the broader approaches that have already been identified by:

- identifying specific activities
- sequencing activities into the correct order to make an improvement
- setting a realistic time frame, including any significant benchmarks or targets, and
- assigning individual responsibilities to complete each activity within the program time frame.

Assessing the necessary resources

The participants assess the internal and external resources that are necessary and available to improve the present situation, for example technical assistance, equipment, land, finance, and training. This includes a review of locally available resources and any resources that can be provided by an outside agent.

The visual representation of community capacity

The measurement of community capacity has traditionally used qualitative information to provide 'thick' descriptive accounts, based on the experiences of the 'community', to produce a large quantity of data such as transcribed interviews. This type of data is difficult and time consuming for practitioners to interpret. The visual-isation of such a complex concept, therefore, presents an attractive option to make an analysis of the measurement of community capacity by using the nine domains.

Several authors have used visual representations to compare changes in community capacity. For example, Roughan (1986) developed a wheel configuration and used rating scales to measure three areas—personal growth, material growth, and social growth—for village development in the Solomon Islands. The rating scale had ten points that radiated outwards like the spokes of a wheel for each indicator of the three growth areas. Each scale was plotted according to a measurement by the village members and the points joined together to provide a visual representation of growth and development. However, the approach did not promote strategic planning and used a total of eighteen complex interrelated indicators, such as equity and solidarity, to measure village development. These ethnocentric and complex indicators were difficult to conceptualise by the participants, especially in a cross-cultural context, which introduces some ambiguity into the measurement. Rifkin, Muller and Bichmann (1988) in Nepal, and later Bjaras, Haglund, and Rifkin (1991) in Sweden, were the first commentators on the use of the 'spiderweb' configuration for the visual representation of community participation. Their approach identifies five factors—leadership, needs evaluation, management, organisation, and resource mobilisation—and uses a simple rating scale. However, the approach was not designed by the researchers to be carried out as a self-evaluation by the community or to promote strategic planning. Instead, it was used as a check list by an external agent to measure community participation, a process that does not necessarily promote self-improvement.

These early experiences of evaluation have provided the basis for the subsequent development of a method to represent community capacity visually. As discussed in Phase 2, a set of descriptors are identified for each domain and a rank assigned for each descriptor, from 1 (low) to 5 (high). This qualitative evaluation of each domain then provides a set of rankings that can be quantified and plotted, in this case onto a spiderweb configuration. Different stakeholders in the same program use the interpretation of this visual representation to compare the domains at different times in the life of the program. The spiderweb configuration offers a visual representation that can be understood by all the program stakeholders.

The spiderweb configuration in Figure 11.2 illustrates how this method provides a quick picture of the strengths and weaknesses within a community. The representatives of the Tokbai-Talaa village decided to combine two domains, 'project management' and 'the role of the outside agent', because they saw these two areas as overlapping. This gave a total of eight domains to measure. Community members can then determine more accurately a plan of action, to strengthen the weakest domains over a specific time frame, as detailed in Phase 3 of the tool. The domains are measured again every six months and a strategic plan developed for the weakest domains using the tool. In Figure 11.2, the first and second measurements have been recorded and visually represented on the spider web. In this way, the capacity of the community is gradually built up and the assistance of the outside agency involved is detailed clearly in the strategic plan.

FIGURE 11.2 Measurements for the Tokbai-Talaa village

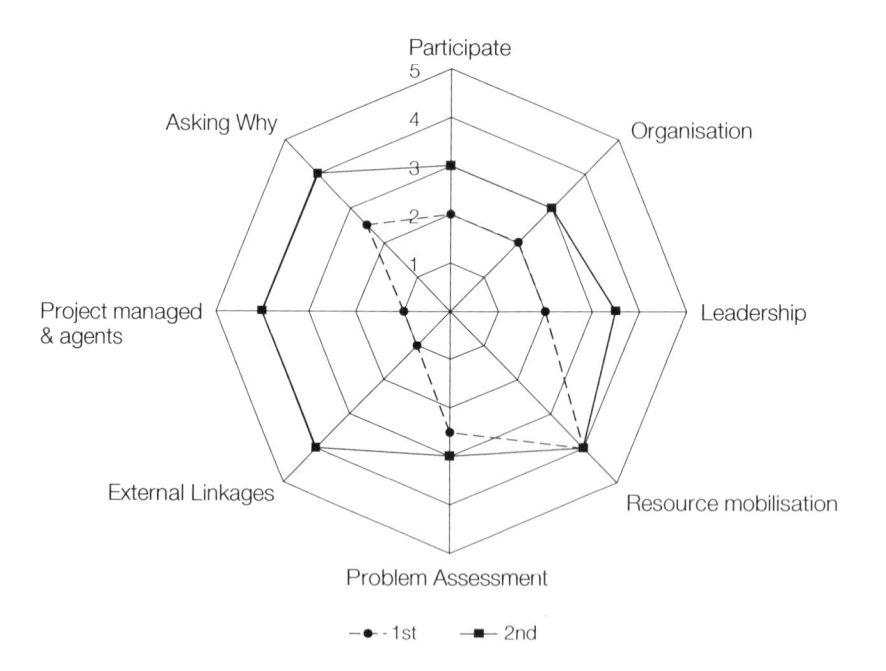

Source: Sustainable Livelihoods for Livestock Producing Communities Project (2004)

1. Building community capacity in Fiji

CASE STUDY

The village of Naivicula is in the Naloto tikina in Fiji, situated on the main island of Viti Levu. A tikina typically represents three or four communities who share the same needs and interests. The spider graph in Figure 11.3 is based on the measurement of community capacity in the village of Naivicula and displays a distribution of high and low ratings for the seven domains, illustrating a range of strengths and weaknesses in capacity in the community (Laverack, 2007a). In this community, an outside agency had not been identified and it was not part of any on-going program. The representatives of the Naivicula community therefore decided to delete the two domains 'program management' and 'the role of the outside agency'. This illustrates the flexibility of the 'tool', which can be adapted to suit the circumstances of the community.

Participation, given a low ranking of 1.0, was identified as being weak because of the failure of local leaders to communicate information to

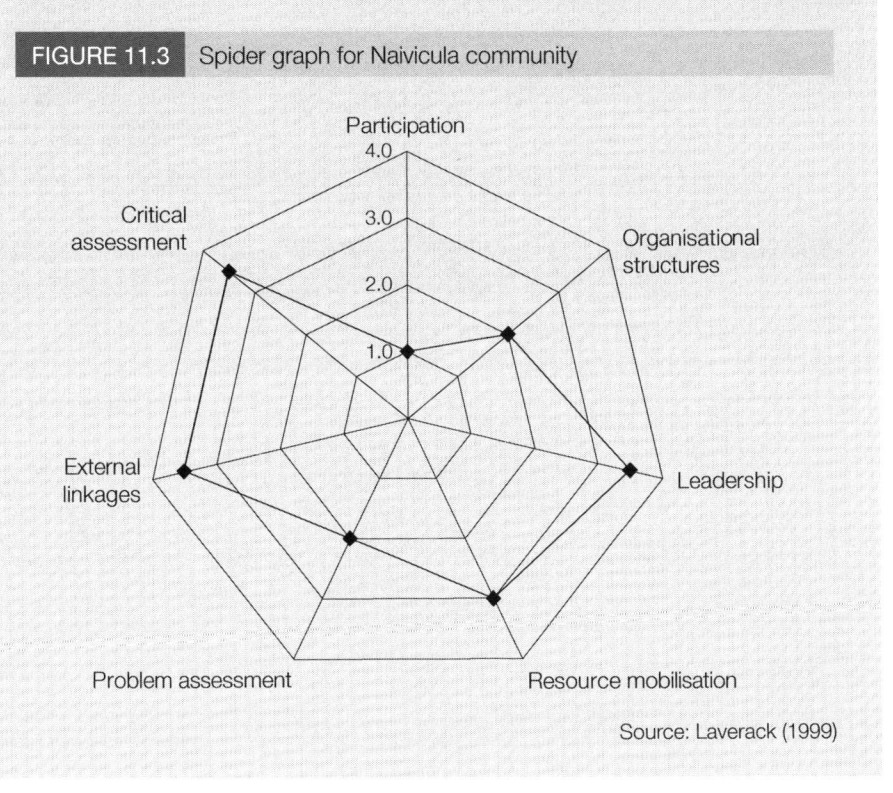

FIGURE 11.3 Spider graph for Naivicula community

Source: Laverack (1999)

Glenn Laverack

other members of the community. Traditional protocol maintains that the approval of the village chief must be sought before holding a community meeting. An individual may be reluctant to defer to the chief or to ask for a particular favour, such as organising a meeting, if he/she lacks respect for the chief or if he/she is not on good terms with the chief at the time. In the community, this situation had led to a reduction in the number of village meetings and in a poor level of participation in decision-making between its members.

Interestingly, the interpretation of the spider web in Figure 11.3 gives 'leadership' a high ranking of 3.5. A Fijian chief is always accorded the outward signs of respect. Even though a person may gain prominence, respect, and authority within the community because of his/her personal qualities or through the acquisition of wealth, he/she would have to defer to the chief on matters of tradition and culture. Local leaders are rarely challenged, and community members can be influenced by traditional views. In these circumstances, it is important that the participants engage in a 'facilitated dialogue' to reach a consensus on the selection of each domain that represents the actual situation in their community.

To build their capacity, the community members decided first to gain the approval of the village chief to meet on a regular basis and on predetermined dates. This overcame the difficulty of having to follow traditional protocol to obtain approval for every meeting while maintaining respect for local customs in their community. Problem assessment was also identified as being weak, with a ranking of 2.0. Following the measurement of community capacity, the Tikina Health Committee requested that a local non-government organisation organise skills training for community leaders in the area of 'problem assessment'. This was supported by the outside agency that was funding the health promotion program. The 'tool' had been used to engage the community members in a process of logical thinking and critical assessment, and had allowed them to identify the areas of influence (the domains) that required strengthening. This helped to improve the efficiency of the delivery of resources to areas that were felt by the community to have the greatest need. In this way, the tool had allowed the community members to take more control of issues that were important to them and was, at the same time, an empowering experience.

2. Building community capacity in a remote Aboriginal community in Northern Australia

Aboriginal people experience a health status well below the Australian average, for example, for indicators of child survival rates, birth weight, and the growth and nutrition of babies. This has been related to their poor psychological health resulting from cultural disintegration, dispossession from their lands, unemployment, and poverty (O'Connor & Parker, 1995).

This case study describes how a remote Aboriginal community decided to build its capacity to improve the health and well-being of its members (Laverack, 2000). To protect the privacy of the members of the community, the names of individuals and the exact location have not been identified. The community is situated in a rural location approximately eight hours' drive east of Darwin in the Northern Territory of Australia. It has an estimated population of 970 residents, predominately Aboriginal. Following a discussion between the community council and the elders and with the support of the Environmental Health Services (the outside agents or 'practitioners'), the community decided to engage in a program to improve housing standards by promoting health and hygiene (Laverack, 2007b: 115–22).

The Ottawa Charter for Health Promotion (WHO, 1986) describes an empowered community as one in which individuals and organisations apply their skills and resources in collective efforts to address health priorities and meet their respective health needs. In practice, this means the community increases control over, and improves, the health of its members through a process of capacity building. This can be best achieved by using a 'domains approach' to strengthen community capacity. What follows is a brief description of how the community decided to build its capacity through each of the nine 'domains'.

Participation

All the representatives from the different clans in the community participated in group discussions during the preparation of the program. Every year, a survey of the state of repair of tenanted houses is carried out in many rural communities in the Northern Territory. The survey provides a crude rating of each house in terms of its 'functionality', and identifies the repairs

Glenn Laverack

and improvements necessary to maintain the housing stock. In some communities, a standardised questionnaire has been used to record the state of repair of each house and the number of occupants. The findings of the survey were shared with the community members, who are encouraged to take an active interest in the program. Regular meetings facilitated by a practitioner, such as an Environmental Health Officer or Aboriginal Health Promotion Officer, are held in the community centre to discuss the program.

Leadership

At the beginning of the program, the leadership is guided by the practitioners, who hold regular consultations with community representatives. The Council of Elders and other local leaders are involved in the planning and administration of the program and receive training and instruction in management skills to build their capacity. The leaders increasingly make decisions concerning the program, with the purpose of devolving responsibility to the community.

Problem assessment

The leaders are encouraged to map and prioritise the immediate 'problems' involved in promoting domestic hygiene. These include a lack of participation, money, and low skill level in managing a program of this size. These issues then become the basis for the planning of strategies for decision-making activities and for the identification of the resources necessary to support these new roles.

Asking why

The participants begin to identify the underlying causes of their powerlessness and poor health through a facilitated process of small group meetings. The practitioner can stimulate the participants' sense of critical awareness by using techniques such as photovoice (Wang et al., 1998; see also Chapter 3). The leaders soon realised that the unsanitary conditions in many households were caused by social and cultural constraints such as the breakdown of authority of the head of the household. The Council of Elders recognised that it was essential to set in place systems for cleaning in each household that depended on the nature of occupancy. To assist, the leaders prepared a schedule of materials required for routine domestic hygiene to help guide each household.

Organisational structures

It is important that an existing organisation has the overall responsibility to implement the program. In this case, it was the Community Management Board. Other organisational groups within the community were also involved in the discussion of key issues; for example, the local store would need to be consulted to ensure that sufficient cleaning materials were available at an affordable price. To enable people to increase control of, and improve health through, the management and supervision of the program, it is necessary to develop an understanding of the key issues.

Resource mobilisation

The community has access to only limited resources, but still has to raise finances to provide cleaning materials, for example, detergents and soap. These can be made available at the local store at subsidised prices, or a special pack of materials can be delivered to each household free of charge. However, the community members are less likely to value materials that have been provided as government 'handouts', and goods that are available in the store at discounted prices are unpopular because people think they are of an inferior quality. The community can start to raise additional internal resources on a small scale through fund raising, and raise external resources through seeking government funding, assisted by the practitioner. The community was able to access funds from the Regional Health Service for the provision of plastic baby baths for families with children less than two years old. Some households had been using the kitchen sink to bathe small children, which had resulted in accidents.

Links to others

The community can use strategies to develop links with other communities and arrange for visits to exchange experiences. The members of the Community Management Board may develop a working agreement with the local store, which is privately owned, to ensure that certain cleaning materials such as soap and detergents will be available at an affordable price.

Glenn Laverack

Outside agents

The practitioners can play an important role in helping the community to raise resources, develop skills and capacities, gain access to policy makers, and support the program through their own 'expert' and legitimate power, for example by raising the concerns of the community with government officials.

Program management

The purpose of program management is to give increasing control to the Community Management Board. This includes management, decision-making, administration, fund raising, and liaison with government officials. The role of the practitioner should diminish to provide assistance and resource support at the request of the Community Management Board. The support of the practitioner is especially important at the beginning of a program when the confidence and skill level of the community members may be low and capacity building has to be developed.

Conclusion

Building and measuring community capacity by using the nine domains in the form of a participatory tool offers a workable approach for health promotion programs. The approach allows communities to scrutinise the achievements that they, in partnership with an outside agency, have identified as being important. It also enables the communities to measure the effectiveness of programs and uses an innovative method of visual representation, the spider web configuration. Being able to demonstrate success in building community capacity and to identify the areas of influence that require strengthening provides a mechanism through which people can develop their knowledge and skills.

The approach to building and measuring community capacity described in this chapter is intended to be an empowering experience for communities. It enables people to participate, to organise themselves better, and to reflect critically on their individual and collective circumstances. More importantly, it enables people to plan strategically for actions to resolve their circumstances, to measure and to represent this process visually as outcomes that are conducive to health promotion programming. It is hoped that this will provide greater clarity to the students of health promotion who are interested in working with individuals, groups, and communities to build their capacity.

CRITICAL THINKING EXERCISES

1 Using each of the nine 'capacity domains', develop a health promotion strategy to address:
   (a) domestic violence
   (b) the empowerment of women living in low income housing.

2 Develop other culturally appropriate methods to represent visually the nine domains in a health promotion context. Refer to readily available computer spreadsheet packages that allow quantitative information to be displayed graphically, usually using the chart wizard option. These are selected from the standard type chart, and then follow the chart wizard steps to set the data range, the chart options, and the chart location.

FURTHER READING

Labonte, R., & Laverack, G. (2001) Capacity Building in Health Promotion, Part 1: For Whom? And for What Purpose? *Critical Public Health*, 11(2): 111–27.

Labonte, R., & Laverack, G (2001) Capacity Building in Health Promotion, Part 2: Whose Use? And with What Measure? *Critical Public Health*, 11(2): 129–38.

Laverack, G. (2006) Improving Health Outcomes through Community Empowerment: A Review of the Literature. *Journal of Health Population and Nutrition*, 24(1): 113–20.

Laverack, G. (2006) Using a 'Domains' Approach to Build Community Empowerment. *Community Development Journal*, 41(1): 4–12.

Laverack, G. (2007) Health Promotion Practice: Building Empowered Communities. McGraw-Hill: London.

WEBPAGE RESOURCES

CommunityBuilders. NSW: www.communitybuilders.nsw.gov.au. This site is an interactive electronic clearing house for everyone involved in community-level social, economic and environmental renewal.

Photovoice: Social Change Through Photography: www.photovoice.com. This website provides details and case studies of 'Photovoice', a participatory

Glenn Laverack

tool designed to bring about social change through photography and social action.

Taking Control In Your Community: www.communitiestakingcontrol.org. This site is about communities in England setting up community initiatives to tackle issues important to local communities.

Family Wellbeing Empowerment program: www.faess.jcu.edu.au/sias/research/empowerment_research_program.html. Reports, publications, and other resources relating to the Family Wellbeing Empowerment Program are available at this site.

Community Development and Empowerment

12

Komla Tsey

Objectives

After reading this chapter, readers will be able to:

- Understand the theory of community development and empowerment as strategies that acknowledge and build on people's existing strengths for working with them towards achieving health and well-being, and appreciate ways in which such understandings can be used to enhance or add value to health promotion projects in a holistic way
- Appreciate how the health development projects provided as case studies to highlight some useful tools for practical empowerment and related community development
- Explain how the attributes of empowerment as an ecological or multidimensional construct provide a useful framework for monitoring and evaluating the interventions' outcomes.

Key terms

Aboriginal Community Controlled Health Service
community development
community engagement
empowerment
power

Introduction

Community development and related concepts, such as community engagement, capacity building, community control, and participation, are all strategies of empowerment (Campbell et al., 2007). These concepts are critical to promoting health and well-being in ways that are relevant, meaningful, and sustainable for the intended beneficiaries.

The terms 'community development' and 'empowerment' have sometimes been used too loosely and by different people to mean different things over the years. A recent review by Campbell and colleagues (2007: 157) found 'a great deal of confusion and contention in the literature about the term "community development" and its constituent concepts of "community", "participation", "involvement", "power", "capacity" and "empowerment". There is also scepticism as to the value and efficacy of community development and empowerment in promoting health. The practitioner needs to address and clarify four important issues prior to using the community development and empowerment:

1. The practitioner must clearly define and explain the main theoretical constructs and approaches being used.
2. The practitioner must describe and explain the ways in which the theoretical concepts and approaches are put into practice.
3. The community development and empowerment initiative must be located in the relevant socio-economic contexts.
4. The criteria by which to monitor and determine the effectiveness of the empowerment outcomes need to be made explicit.

Empowerment and health

A major challenge facing the public health profession in the twenty-first century is how to develop appropriate strategies and interventions to reduce growing health inequalities that reflect the increasingly unequal socio-economic status of populations. Internationally and within Australia, there has been extensive academic and policy interest in social determinants of health. However, there remains a chronic lack of understanding about the causal pathways linking social disadvantage and health, and a serious lack of evidence-based public health interventions that aim to address health inequalities (see Turrell et al., 1999). Evidence from social gradient research indicates a need for micro level studies that explore issues of control of destiny and empowerment (Syme, 1998). A better

---

Community development: a process of organising or supporting community groups in identifying their priority health issues, and planning and acting upon their strategies for social action and change, thereby gaining increased self-reliance and decision-making power.

Community engagement: the ability to establish a meaningful contact, conversation, or discussion with individuals and groups with the aim of maximising their participation and decision-making in issues that are of concern to them.

Empowerment: a process whereby individuals and groups of people become stronger and more confident in controlling or exerting influence over the issues affecting their lives.

understanding of strategies that enhance people's capacity to take greater control over their circumstances is imperative in the context of Indigenous health. As a group, Indigenous Australians experience higher levels of illness and premature death than the rest of the population. They are also more likely to be incarcerated, experience family violence, have lower levels of education and employment, and suffer from excessive use of alcohol and other substances. Recently, community leaders using language that resonates with notions of empowerment and control in the emerging public health literature have called for more innovative and creative research that would assist Indigenous people take greater control and responsibility for their situation (Pearson, 2000).

Empowerment is central to the Ottawa Charter for Health Promotion and subsequent WHO health promotion strategies. As a theoretical construct, empowerment involves both processes and outcomes that generate change at multiple levels—individual, organisational, and community—strengthening the capacity for collective action to influence social situations positively (Wallerstein, 1992; Rissel, 1994). Although there has been clear global acceptance of these concepts as core principles of health improvement, the translation of this rhetoric into action has remained less clear. Empowerment involves the ability of people to assert and claim their legitimate rights in any given situation, and their capacity to accept and willingly discharge responsibilities towards themselves, others, and society. It entails a special responsibility on behalf of the wider society to consciously work towards creating social environments and relationships that bring the best out of people.

In 2006, twenty years after the declaration of the Ottawa Charter for Health Promotion, the World Health Organization Health Evidence Network published a review of the evidence for the effectiveness of empowerment in improving health (Wallerstein, 2006). The review showed that interventions increasing empowerment were effective in improving health; patient and family empowerment strategies increased patients' abilities to manage their disease, adopt healthier behaviours, and use health services more effectively, as well as increasing care-giver skills and efficacy. The most effective empowerment strategies were those that built on and reinforced authentic participation, ensuring autonomy in decision-making, sense of community, and local bonding, and psychological empowerment of the community members themselves. They recommended that health promotion should address effective empowerment strategies. Government investment in multiple-method research was recommended, and evaluation by collecting evidence systematically on the impact of such empowerment strategies over time (Wallerstein, 2006).

The report also identified pathways through which empowerment is generated at psychological, organisational, and community levels, and links the effect of these

Komla Tsey

Power: the ability to affect change rather than the power to exploit or dominate others.

outcomes to improvements in health. The report concludes that there is evidence that initiatives based on empowerment as a multilevel construct can reduce health disparities, but that successful approaches cannot simply be replicated across populations. It highlights the need for development and evaluation of strategies relevant to the lived experience of populations experiencing social exclusion (Wallerstein, 2006). Thus, the operationalisation of the process of empowerment with marginalised populations and demonstration of its potential in reducing health inequalities remain a major challenge (Laverack & Wallerstein, 2001).

Fundamental to any initiative that aims to enhance empowerment and control is that it is relevant to the needs of its participants, that it starts where people are 'at', and that it engages different people who have differing life experiences and opportunities and who may be at different levels of motivation and ability. Wayne McCashen (1998) has developed a framework that views empowerment/disempowerment in terms of a continuum (Table 12.1).

TABLE 12.1 Spectrum of empowerment

	Disempowered ⟵⟶			Empowered
Present experience	Diminished ability Diminished motivation	Ability Insufficient motivation	Unrecognised ability Sufficient motivation	Recognised ability High motivation
Tasks	Deep listening Validation Provide resources Small steps	Deep listening Validation Rewrite the dominant story Add resources Build a picture of the future Start with small steps	Elicit and build on strengths Work with/enable Strengthen the main story	Facilitate/enable Ensure resources Re-affirm the main story

Source: McCashen (1998).

This framework provides some ideas in regard to the different actions required for working with people at different stages of empowerment. While those at the more empowered end of the spectrum need to be 'enabled' or given opportunities, people at the disempowered end may well first require support to start to build a sense of hope. Differentiation needs to be made between 'power over', whereby individuals, groups, or institutions assume the right to make decisions for others, and 'power with', which involves a commitment to self-determination or capacity of people to determine their own affairs (Ife, 2002).

Where to start: Balancing principles and approaches with narrative

Community development and empowerment strategies, including community engagement, capacity development, and participatory action research, have one thing in common. That is a 'strengths-based approach' for working with people to bring about their own change (McCashen, 1998). This approach takes the philosophical position that, in order to bring about meaningful personal and social change, the oppressed must be heard and the world seen through their eyes; they need access to the necessary physical resources, the opportunity to be the subjects of their own transformation, and the knowledge and skills to participate effectively (Wallerstein, 1992; Campfens, 1997). Community engagement involves strategies that assist communities to understand and use their strengths as the basis for change. It also forms the critical initial steps towards effective community development and empowerment. A number of strategies exist that health workers can use to engage and work with people within the strengths-based approach. These strategies include focusing on people's strengths, knowledge, and resilience, rather than on problems or deficits; an understanding that change is always possible no matter how desperate the situation might look at first, creating vision and hope for the future; and celebrating small steps towards change and using these small steps to build the belief and confidence that change is possible no matter how difficult a situation first appears (McCashen, 1998).

Community development and empowerment are not something that one person, health professional or expert can do to, or give to, another person or group of people, in a neat and uncontested linear fashion. The interventions are multi-layered and constantly changing as the social environment changes. Community development and empowerment are complex and messy interactive processes of reflective learning-by-doing. They are part science and part art. It is part science because there are established principles and approaches, such as starting from where people are at, locating and working through community opinion leaders, and the need for facilitators to be enablers rather than doers (Campfens, 1997; McCashen, 1998). It is part art because community development and empowerment work are not only context specific. However, the social environment changes constantly and requires well-developed abilities of self-examination and expertise to make routine adjustments to practice in response to the changing environment. Narrative and sharing stories are essential to the process of community development. When people feel safe and confident to share stories and experiences with each other, they often develop greater understanding, respect, and empathy among themselves. This enhances social cohesion and stability.

Community development in Indigenous Australian communities

In Indigenous Australian communities, as in many developing countries, the concept of primary health care was developed in response to the failures of traditional curative medical care to address the health needs of the populations effectively. In Australia, Indigenous community-controlled health organisations are a means for people to take control of and responsibility for their own health and well-being. They also mean a broader conception and understanding of health that includes not just clinical care and health education, but also the enhancement of social and economic opportunities for people in the form of education, training, employment, and, above all, pride in cultural identity (Boffa et al., 1994).

It is in this context that Indigenous Australians have built one of the world's most astounding and sustained community development movements, the Aboriginal Community Controlled Health Services (ACCHS) (Scrimgeour, 1997; see details on the National Aboriginal Community Controlled Health Organisation (NACCHO) website, 200: 1). Local Indigenous community control is essential to Indigenous holistic health, and allows communities to determine their own affairs, protocols, and procedures. As of January 2008, there are approximately 130 ACCHS, representing the single most significant employment sector for Aboriginal people. About 70 per cent of the ACCHS workforce is made up of Indigenous people. The ACCHS approach has as its philosophy self-determination and empowerment, which are critical foundations for promoting health and well-being.

Within this context, as a practitioner I develop analysis and understanding of the contemporary Indigenous situation and what this might mean for community development initiatives that are likely to make a difference. I spend a substantial amount of time observing, talking to people, reading, reflecting, and writing. I also explore differences and similarities between colonial experiences in Australia and Ghana (my birth country) and how these may have affected life chances and opportunities differently for the Aboriginal populations (Short & Tsey, 1992; Tsey, 1994a, 1994b, 1994c, 1994d). An example of differences is the settler colonisation in Australia and the crown colony in colonial Ghana. In Australia, the metropolitan power used the land as a place to settle and make a home and reduced the original populations to a minority in their own country. In Ghana, the main aim of the

Aboriginal Community Controlled Health Service: a primary health care service that is initiated and operated by the local Aboriginal community to deliver holistic, comprehensive, and culturally appropriate health care to the community (National Aboriginal Community Controlled Health Organisation, 2006).

British was to set up systems of administrative controls through systems of indirect rule based on the traditional chieftaincy in order to extract natural resources, sell industrial goods, and convert people to Christianity (Short & Tsey, 1992).

The settler colonisation in Australia and recent government policies also severely undermined Indigenous forms of work without replacing them with dependence on wage labour, as is the norm in a market economy. Welfare payment keeps people alive and prevents them from begging, but does little to improve health (Tsey, 1994b: 1). I call for urgent attention to formal education, including basic literacy and numeracy, as a central part of any initiative aimed at improving life chances for Indigenous Australians (Tsey, 1996, 1997). The critical role of education is to build Indigenous capability to function in an increasingly complex and multilayered society. There are limited meaningful opportunities and incentives for Indigenous Australians to participate fully in national socio-economic activities.

At the core of the issue is what Noel Pearson has described as a serious breakdown in Aboriginal social norms and values regarding responsibility, reciprocity, and ideas about what is good and what is wrong (Pearson, 2000; Pearson, 2001; see also Anderson, 2003; Behrendt, 2003; Couzos & Murray, 2003). There is no doubt that colonial dispossession and its resultant social, cultural, economic, and political dislocations clearly continue to affect the health and well-being of Indigenous Australians (Anderson, 2003; Behrendt, 2003). However, as Pearson (2000, 2001) argues, these factors alone cannot fully explain the extent of the social problems currently facing Indigenous Australians. According to Pearson, the availability of welfare payments means they become the main source of sustenance for some Indigenous communities and families. The availability of money through welfare payments, unlimited amounts of negative leisure time due to underemployment, an unregulated supply of alcohol, and a generally permissive alcohol and drug culture in mainstream Australian society, have all combined in varying degrees to create an 'alcohol epidemic' in many Indigenous communities (Pearson, 2001). A combination of complex historical and recent social policies may have created the initial alcohol problem. However, the scale of the problem is beyond the colonisation and related social problems (Pearson, 2001; Anderson, 2003; Behrendt, 2003)). Efforts to improve Indigenous social conditions, therefore, need to tackle issues of alcohol and welfare dependency at multiple levels, including policy reforms that provide appropriate incentives for people to engage in meaningful work and other healthy lifestyle changes. Central to this process is the need to rebuild Indigenous social norms and value systems in ways that allow people to resume greater control and responsibility for their lives (Cape York Institute, 2007). The Family Wellbeing (FWB) empowerment program, described in the following case study, is one approach that helps rebuild Indigenous social norms and values.

Komla Tsey

CASE STUDY

The Family Wellbeing (FWB) empowerment program

In 1993, the Family Wellbeing (FWB) Program was developed in South Australia by a group of 'stolen generation' Indigenous Australians through the Aboriginal Education Development Branch (AEDB) of the Department of Education, Training and Employment. 'Stolen generation' refers to the thousands of Indigenous Australians who were forcibly removed by the state from their families as children and raised in government institutions and foster homes, for the most part between 1910 and 1970. In a national survey released in 2004, four out of ten people aged 15 years or over reported that they or one of their relatives had been removed from their natural family (Whiteside et al., 2006).

As with many of the generations stolen throughout history, members of Australia's stolen generation and their descendants have suffered emotional pain and the destructive behaviours (for example, alcohol and drug misuse, sexual abuse, family violence) so frequently associated with the experience of forced separation from family and culture. Survivors of this experience are playing important leadership roles in Indigenous self-determination, driving developments such as community-controlled organisations for health services, housing cooperatives, legal services, and land and community councils. Despite this focus on what can be viewed as structural empowerment, these community leaders were also aware of the need for personal life-skill development at an individual level, to address appropriately not only the pain and hurt of the past, but also the day-to-day challenges of being a systematically dispossessed and marginalised population within a highly affluent society. As one architect of FWB explained, 'the question we were asking ourselves is: "How did we survive?" If we can understand how we survived then we can help others' (Tsey & Every, 2000). They intended FWB to help people become personally empowered and therefore more able to engage meaningfully with the structural empowerment that both community-controlled organisations and mainstream opportunities provide.

The aim of FWB is empowerment and transformation. It is based on the principles of psychosynthesis and grounded in Indigenous experiences of family survival (Tsey & Every, 2000). Psychosynthesis is a process of personal growth that involves harmonising the physical, emotional, mental, and spiritual aspects of life through learning a range of practical techniques.

Life experiences of FWB facilitators and participants are the main learning resources of the program. The program has developed into a structured but highly flexible 120-hour psychosocial group-learning process. It is structured into four stages, each stage taking 40 hours to complete.

The FWB approach aims to create a healthy social environment for individuals and groups to maximise their life chances. Clearly defined sets of rules, values, and norms that guide day-to-day human behaviour as to what is acceptable and what is not are developed. This requires the existence of appropriate sanctions and incentives that the majority of the people are committed to uphold. The FWB program starts by teaching participants how to develop their own group agreements that create environments in which they feel safe, supported, and motivated to learn. Within these supportive learning environments, the participants are taught to become more aware of their inner human qualities, such as self-awareness, acceptance, empathy, perseverance, and creativity (see the list in Table 12.2, Critical thinking exercise 2 below). The participants then learn to take steps as individuals and communities, irrespective of socio-economic circumstances, to cultivate and use these qualities consciously in their daily lives in order to bring about change for themselves and for their wider community. The safe and supportive learning environment also provides an opportunity for people to reflect on and share stories about important questions for life: Where am I going with my life? Who is benefiting and who is losing out? What can I do to change the situation and what are consequences? (Flyvbjerg, 2001)

Bruner (1990) highlights the role of narrative in social cohesion and stability. One of the most powerful forms of social stability is the human tendency to share stories of human diversity and to make their interpretations congruent with different moral commitments and institutional obligations. Breakdown in culture is connected with limited narrative resources and a total loss of stories. The 'worst scenario' story seems to dominate daily life and the variation no longer is possible (Bruner, 1990).

Since 2000, I have worked as part of a team to adapt this innovative values-based program as a practical tool to empower Aboriginal individuals and communities in improving their health and well-being. The research has demonstrated benefits for program participants and their communities. The FWB program has been implemented in South Australia, Western Australia, Central Australia, and North Queensland. The initial research

Komla Tsey

in Central Australia showed that the participants increased personal empowerment. They described an enhanced self-worth, resilience, belief in their capacity to improve their social environment, and ability to reflect on root causes of problems, find solutions, and address immediate family difficulties (Tsey & Every, 2000). The ripple effect is increased community harmony and capacity to address community structural issues. The participants are active in addressing other issues, including poor school attendance rates, family violence, alcohol and drug misuse, and Indigenous workforce development. There is a sense of urgency expressed across all project sites that the skills learnt are vitally needed not only in Indigenous communities but also across mainstream Australia (see Tsey et al., 2003; Whiteside et al., 2006).

Since 2005, the FWB program has also linked with a range of health and education interventions. Listed below are selected areas in which significant progress has been made. The flexibility of the FWB empowerment intervention enables its use across a broad range of settings and groups. These include:

- promoting better outcomes for mental health consumers
- enhancing the success of alcohol rehabilitation, and
- enhancing parenting skills and approaches.

Personal strength and capability emerge as common elements of social and emotional well-being that must be promoted effectively. The findings also confirm that the process of empowerment is lengthy, taking years to achieve change beyond the individual level. They highlight the process of initial engagement and personal transformation that enhances individual social and emotional well-being. They also provide a critical foundation for broader community and structural change (Tsey et al., 2005a, 2005b).

Monitoring and evaluating empowerment

Community development requires planned action to change or improve human relationships and conditions. Working with people to bring about change is one of the most challenging undertakings because of the complex nature of human beings and their social relationships (see Flyvbjerg, 2001). Theoretical models and frameworks are tools that can help the practitioner simplify and make sense of the complex social realities. Working to change or improve people's social realities is also value laden. An explicit framework allows the practitioner to be more accountable to the communities with whom he or she works, while taking into account of the practitioner's own value systems and political positions. The theoretical models and frameworks should evolve and change as knowledge accumulates based on day-to-day micro-practice. The three domains of empowerment (psychosocial, group, and structural) and their relevant attributes used in this chapter combine Nina Wallerstein's multi-level or ecological approach with findings and observations from my own community development and empowerment research in Indigenous Australia (Wallerstein, 1992; Tsey & Every, 2000; Tsey et al., 2003; 2005a; 2005b; 2006).

Personal or psychological domain of empowerment

Personal empowerment is essentially how individuals feel about themselves and what they are able to do with their lives. It includes:

- the ability to understand and manage constructively emotions such as anger, fear, guilt, and sadness
- the capacity to make a living through meaningful work and other socio-cultural activities of value to their community
- levels of self-esteem
- the extent to which they feel confident and motivated to deal with day-to-day challenges and stresses of life without being overwhelmed by them.

Attributes of the personal domain of empowerment include:

- hope
- goal setting
- communication skills
- empathy
- perseverance
- a level of participation in meaningful work and other valued socio-cultural activities
- the ability to analyse and make sense of the root causes of problems
- the belief that the social environment can change.

Stories that people tell about themselves and their situation that are often full of positive problem-solving attitudes and beliefs about life. The more disempowered may tell stories of negativity or chronically feeling stuck and not being able to see beyond immediate problems.

Komla Tsey

As empowerment increases, we see individuals drawing more and more on internalised personal empowerment attributes to deal better and better with life.

Group or organisational domain of empowerment

Group or organisational empowerment is about groups of people with common interests and aspirations. It means:

➤ working together to overcome differences
➤ developing greater understanding, mutual respect, and solidarity with each other
➤ sharing experiences and committing themselves to working together towards achieving common goals.

The attributes of the group or organisational domain of empowerment are:

➤ being willing to uphold relevant social norms and standards that the community or society value. Such norms might include fairness, respect, human dignity, and other rights and responsibilities associated with being part of the group
➤ ability of people to stand up and say 'no' to behaviours and attributes that violate cherished norms and values, such as abuse and violence, corruption and nepotism, racism and discrimination.

Community or structural domain of empowerment

Community or structural empowerment is about the social structures, laws, and cultural norms within which individuals and groups try to achieve their life aspirations. Structural empowerment is the extent to which the social structures and institutions that shape our lives nurture and provide opportunities for people to realise their human potential. Some social environments can wittingly or unwittingly be oppressive and debilitating for particular sections of society, while favouring and nurturing others.

The attributes of the community or structural domain of empowerment are:

➤ public policies that promote equitable access to education, economic, health, political, and other socio-cultural incentives and opportunities for people, irrespective of race, gender, class, or geographical location
➤ traditional customs, rituals, and belief systems that enhance rather than undermine human dignity and respect
➤ appropriate functioning of the necessary law and order systems that makes individuals, groups, and communities of people feel safe to go about their day-to day business

▶ healthier working and living environments leading to objective improvements in physical, emotional, mental, and spiritual health and well-being.

This and other frameworks can be used to monitor and evaluate community development projects. The practitioner can also use them as an engagement tool to start conversation about where a community might be along the spectrum of empowerment. Canvassing the community's views and attitudes regarding the various empowerment domains and attributes helps participants to reflect more on their own values and norms and how that might affect the effectiveness of projects (see, for example, Tsey et al., 2002).

Semi-structured questions can act as prompts to start conversation. Some of these questions are: How relevant is this framework to your situation? What changes may be required for the framework to suit your needs? The information gathered at this formative stage can serve as baseline data. Given the holistic and interconnected nature of the framework, it helps the community to ask what else needs to be happening in order to maximise the effectiveness of a particular community development initiative. Simple qualitative measurement scales can be constructed to assist the participants to monitor and assess their own progress against the relevant domains and attributes over time (Tsey et al., 2004a; 2004b). Depending on the availability of resources, it is possible to adapt standardised instruments to measure the relevant domains and attributes. It can be concluded that the plan of monitoring and evaluation needs to be carefully thought through due to the complexity of the empowerment concept, the three levels at which it operates, and the many pathways and experiences of empowerment in people's lives.

Conclusion

The WHO Health Evidence Report on the effectiveness of empowerment to improve health (Wallerstein, 2006) found that participatory empowerment interventions with socially excluded populations have produced empowerment across psychological, organisational, and community levels. The interventions lead to improved health outcomes and quality of life. However, the report recognised that effective empowerment strategies could not be standardised. There is a need for the development and evaluation of programs that are locally relevant and address broader social and economic inequalities. The point is to be explicit about the criteria that have been used and the basis of those criteria.

Strengths-based approaches work from a philosophical position that has the participants as the centre of the project (Wallerstein, 1992; Campfens, 1997). A number of powerful strategies can be used by the practitioner. These strategies

Komla Tsey

include using people's strengths, knowledge, and resilience, rather than on problems or deficits (McCashen, 2005). Community empowerment and change are as much about processes as they are about outcomes. The latter can take years and even be inter-generational, depending on the nature of the issues being addressed. Facilitators, therefore, need to develop appropriate skills and tools to sustain the process.

As an ecological construct, empowerment involves a synergy, or interactive changes, at all three discrete but related levels. Consequently, multilevel community and other development initiatives are often required to maximise empowerment interventions through models that incorporate a range of programs and services, rather than an intervention model built around a single program. These may require collaborative partnerships with those working in other contexts, networking, lobbying, activism, and advocacy. Empowerment, according to this model, is not one-way or linear. It can start from, or be fostered at, any of the three levels or domains. It provides both a holistic way of thinking about an appropriate mix of interventions to promote health and reduce inequalities, and a comprehensive framework for evaluating empowerment interventions.

Acknowledgments

The following people and organisations are warmly acknowledged for their contribution and support: the Aboriginal Education and Development Branch; Tangentyere Council; Apunipima Cape York Health Council; Gurriny Yealumackah Health Service; Janya McCalman, Mary Whiteside, Radhika Santhanam, Melissa Haswell, Yvonne Cadet-James, Andrew Wilson, Suzzane Gibson, and Annie Preston-Thomas.

CRITICAL THINKING EXERCISES

1. Read through the following table from the FWB program (Table 12.2), which outlines four broad areas of basic human needs. If you disagree with this broad description of human needs, make changes to the table so that you feel comfortable with it. Now, reflect on your own life in relation to each of the main domains of human needs. Cast your mind back to when you were a child, and an adolescent to the present. Were there any particular times in your life when you felt that some aspect of your basic human needs had not been adequately met? If so, how did that make you feel at the time? What about the present?

Do you feel that all of your basic human needs are being met in a balanced fashion? What are some of the barriers preventing you from being able to meet your needs? Is there anything you can do about them?

TABLE 12.2 Areas of basic human needs

Type of need	Relevant attributes
Physical	Food, water, shelter, sleep, clothing, cleanliness, physical safety, touch, and sexual expression
Emotional	To be loved for who we are; accepted, valued, respected, and recognised; to be deeply understood, treated with tenderness and gentleness, nurtured, cherished, and given attention; to have self-esteem, approval, appropriate touching and nurturing, and confidence and self-worth; to express anger, sadness, and fear freely; to be supported, to give from the heart, and take without guilt; to love others and build trusting relationships; and to love and accept ourselves just as we are.
Mental	To speak freely, think for oneself, question information, show curiosity about the world, and be free to ask about any subject; to have choices, to agree or disagree without restriction; to have one's opinion valued; to continue learning throughout life; to be allowed to make mistakes; to be able to be silent and to change one's mind about an issue or decision.
Spiritual	To be deeply connected with one's inner self; to be deeply connected with others; to be deeply connected with something greater than ourselves, whatever we perceive that to be—depending on the individual, this 'connection' may or may not have a religious association; to express that connection in whatever way is right for us; to have meaning and purpose in our lives, and to value our true self and trust our intuition; to be able to express the higher qualities of our nature, to discover one's life purpose and ask 'Why am I here and what is my life's purpose?'; to be able to grow, change, and fully express who we truly are; to have in our lives beauty, harmony, balance, order, truth, creativity, justice, unconditional love, joy, freedom, and peace.

Source: Tsey (2000).

2   Take a minute or two and think about one person in your family who inspires you. You can define family in any way that suits your circumstances. The person you select may be living or dead. Make a list of some of the things that inspire you about this person. Now, think of another person, outside of your family.

Komla Tsey

This person maybe a friend, somebody you met professionally, somebody you haven't met at all. The person may be from your own country or from another country, and may be living or dead. Again make a list of the things that inspire you about this person. Now, take a step back and look closely at yourself and think about some of the things that inspire you about yourself. Make a list of them. Collate the lists you have made. Is there anything striking about the list? Now, compare your list with the FWB inner qualities below (Table 12.3). In what ways can these qualities help a community of people in their efforts to plan and implement community-improvement initiatives? Which of these qualities do you need to develop further in order to be more successful in your role as community development facilitator?

TABLE 12.3 Some inner qualities

Love	Gratitude	Wisdom	Simplicity
Joy	Openness	Kindness	Cheerfulness
Loyalty	Will	Strength	Peace
Courage	Creativity	Understanding	Calm
Silence	Enthusiasm	Willingness	Determination
Gentleness	Trust	Faith	Spontaneity
Curiosity	Fun	Awareness	Light-heartedness

Source: Apunipima Cape York Health Council (2006)

3 Take a moment to reflect on the following questions. What are our beliefs and attitudes about men, about women, about gay people, about black people, about white people, about alcohol and drug use, about children, about old people, about people unemployed and dependent on state welfare payments, about domestic violence and abuse? Where do these beliefs and attitudes come from? Where as society are we going with current policies and programs designed to address these issues? What is working and what is not working? Which people are benefiting and which people are at the receiving end? By what mechanisms of power is this happening? Is this helping us as society or is this hindering us? What role can you play as a community development facilitator to bring about change for the communities with whom you work? What will the effects of the change be?

FURTHER READING

Labonte, R. (1994) Health Promotion and Empowerment: Reflections on Professional Practice. *Health Education Quarterly,* 21(2): 253–68.

Laverack, G. (2006) Improving Health Outcomes through Community Empowerment: A Review of the Literature. *Journal of Health Promotion and Nutrition*, 24(1): 113–20.

James, P. (1996) The Transformative Power of Storytelling among Peers: An Exploration from Action Research. *Education Action Research*, 4: 197–221.

WEBPAGE RESOURCES

Rural Community Empowerment Program: www.ezec.gov. This webpage describes activities and accomplishments of participating rural communities, and offers access to resources that may be helpful to all rural communities that seek to enhance the quality of their futures.

World Bank: www.worldbank.org. This site is serves as a resource for those interested in the practical and conceptual dimensions of empowerment. On this site, you will find information on the definition of empowerment and on different ways to approach empowerment in practice. You can also access information about the current work of the Empowerment Team.

Taking Control In Your Community: www.communitiestakingcontrol.org. This site is about communities in England setting up community initiatives to tackle issues important to local communities.

National Aboriginal Community Controlled Health Organisation: www.naccho.org.au. This website describes the purpose and programs of the National Aboriginal Community Controlled Health Organisation, a peak organisation for Australia's 130 community-controlled health organisations.

Komla Tsey

13 Health Promotion and Health Education for a Multicultural Community

Myna Hua & Chris Rissel

Objectives

After reading this chapter, readers will be able to:

- Describe the key principles of cross-cultural communication and health education, namely cultural awareness, equity, and access
- Describe community organisations or government services to assist in engaging and communicating with people from culturally and linguistically diverse (CALD) backgrounds
- Identify and describe major areas of planning and implementation of cross-cultural health promotion programs
- Understand research and evaluation issues in developing and implementing a health promotion evaluation plan for programs targeting CALD communities.

Key terms

acculturation
attitudes
cross-cultural
value

Chapter 13 Health Promotion and Health Education for a Multicultural Community

Introduction

In this chapter, three topics are addressed:

➤ principles of cross-cultural communication and health education in a multicultural community
➤ planning and implementing a cross-cultural population-based health promotion program
➤ issues arising from evaluating cross-cultural health promotion programs.

Each of these three topics will include examples or case studies of cross-cultural communication, health education, and health promotion. We will discuss services available and effective tools to facilitate cross-cultural education in primary health care and hospital settings, such as health care interpreter services and a range of functions within migrant health services as well as community organisations. We will highlight national and state policy and guidelines and evidence-based practices in delivering cross-cultural communication, health education, and health promotion to the multicultural community in Australia, such as policies of administering funding for multicultural health promotion programs that ensure the multicultural community has access to mainstream health information. Equity is the underlining principle of cross-cultural access to quality health care. This principle supports equal access to health care for those whose first language may be a barrier to getting medical help or advice.

In this chapter, we also describe the steps in planning, implementing, and evaluating health promotion programs for a multicultural community. Examples from the areas of tobacco control and injury prevention will be used to demonstrate issues related to designing population-based health promotion projects targeting a multicultural community. Research and evaluation issues that arise when working with specific migrant communities will be discussed, such as sampling, designing, and translating questionnaires, bilingual data collection, and understanding the significance of traditional values.

Cross-cultural: pertaining to or involving different cultures or comparison between them.

Value: a conception of the desirable, which may be explicit or implicit, distinctive of an individual or characteristic of a group, that influences the selection from viable modes, means, and ends of action.

The migration context

For a little more than two hundred years, Australia has accepted immigrants and refugees from various parts of the world through skills migration schemes and humanitarian programs. The peak intakes of immigrants and refugees have been linked with wars, such as the Second World War, the Vietnam War, and internal conflicts in Eastern Europe, the Middle East, and African countries, as well as labour

Myna Hua & Chris Rissel

shortages after the Second World War. Understanding the context of migration is a step towards greater compassion, respect for our multicultural population, and awareness of cultural differences.

New South Wales is the state where most of the immigrants settled. Consequently, 18 per cent of the population speaks a language other than English at home. The three most common languages spoken at home, after English, are Chinese (3.2 per cent), Arabic (including Lebanese) (2.3 per cent) and Italian (1.5 per cent). Eleven per cent of the population who speaks another language other than English at home either do not speak English well or do not speak English at all (ABS, 2001). This large percentage of potential clients who would have trouble accessing adequate health care advice should concern professional health care providers.

Both Commonwealth and state governments acknowledge the need for ensuring effective cross-cultural communication and appropriate services for populations from diverse cultural and language backgrounds. To demonstrate government commitment to providing services for clients from culturally and linguistically diverse (CALD) backgrounds, the Commonwealth government developed the Charter of Public Service in Culturally Diverse Society (DIMA, 1998) and the New South Wales government introduced legislation (*Community Relations Commission and Principles of Multiculturalism Act 2000*) along these same lines.

In the context of settlement planning, the principles of 'access, equity, communication, responsiveness, effectiveness, efficiency and accountability' were endorsed by all three levels of government (national, state, and local) in 1998 (DIMA, 1998). They are also used in areas concerning the planning, delivery, evaluation, and reporting of government services in a culturally diverse society.

Definition of cross-cultural communication

Cross-cultural communication is also commonly known as intercultural communication. According to Defleur and colleagues (1992: 378), cross-cultural communication is the 'process of transmitting and interpreting messages between culturally distinct people, in which communicators may encode, perceive and interpret aspects of reality using conventions of meaning unique to the particular group'. In a health service-related context, cross-cultural communication refers to communicating effectively with culturally and linguistically diverse clients in order to achieve accessibility and appropriate program or service delivery. It involves recognising and respecting cultural beliefs, and recognising possible barriers to effective communication that may arise. As highlighted by Pauwels (1995: 3), 'culture can have a substantial influence on people's beliefs and ideas about what constitutes illness, what causes illness and what are appropriate treatments and cures for particular conditions'.

Effective cross-cultural communication requires awareness of 'cultural forces'. As described by Huff and Kline (1999), cultural forces are powerful determinants of health-related behaviours in any group or sub-group. Being aware of personal cultural influences may at times be as important as understanding a client's cultural influences. Openness and respect are crucial for working with CALD populations, as it allows consideration of various possibilities and avenues when developing an appropriate program to meet specific needs. In order to assist readers in this process, several key services can be invaluable resources in helping to understand better a specific community you wish to work with.

Services available in helping health professionals to communicate with people from CALD backgrounds

As a professional health worker, it is important to keep abreast of those services that could assist readers to carry out their duties in the best possible manner. An awareness of services that can facilitate better communication benefits both parties and, importantly, achieves better outcomes in terms of health and mutual satisfaction. The information below serves as an introductory guide.

Government services

Most government services use an interpreting and translating service or employ bilingual staff as part of their overall communication strategies. Type of service and delivery methods may differ, as most are state based, especially in designated language-specific positions or services. These differences are primarily influenced by state government service structures, funding formulas, and population distribution.

The national translating and interpreting service (TIS) was one of the first services developed by the Commonwealth government. It provides qualified interpreters over the phone to assist people who experience language barriers, especially for newly arrived migrants and refugees and those who seek help to overcome language difficulties. TIS (13 1450) is one of the services provided by the Department of Immigration and Citizenship (www.immi.gov.au/tis). It is a fee-based 24-hour phone service to service providers, and covers over 70 languages. TIS also provides a translation service. Over time, state government services have also developed a face-to-face interpreter service. One of the largest state-based interpreter services is the New South Wales Health Care Interpreter Service. They are primarily located in major state hospitals and currently operate in all states except the Northern Territory. The service provides on-site interpreting for medical-related issues. Some state Health Care Interpreter Services provide after-hours service and a limited translation service.

In addition to an interpreting and translating service, most government services employ bilingual or bi-cultural staff as part of their overall communication strategies. In the health sector, bilingual and bi-cultural health workers for larger communities (for example, Chinese, Vietnamese, Arabic, Greek) are appointed to increase their community's access to mainstream health services and therefore achieve better health care outcomes. These include mental health counsellors, migrant health workers, bilingual community educators, multicultural health promotion officers, and obstetric liaison officers. These workers have multiple roles, not solely providing a cultural perspective on health issues. They also provide valuable support to patients in accessing mainstream health services, particularly in reducing stress and facilitating understanding between patients and service providers. Primarily, multicultural health workers aid in understanding cultural values and issues that may affect treatment or the development of programs targeting a particular community. They also conduct health-education talks to groups, and plan, implement, and evaluate multicultural health promotion programs. All these positions, outlined above, are usually under the responsibility of migrant health services located at the level of area health services.

In New South Wales, there are also state services to address particular health issues. The New South Wales Multicultural Health HIV/AIDS and Hepatitis C service (www.multiculturalhivhepc.net.au) and Transcultural Mental Health service (www.dhi.gov.au/tmhc/services/clinical/aboutus.htm) provide support to their clients and families to deal with these specific health conditions. Developing educational and promotional resources and forming support groups are some of their responsibilities.

The New SouthWales Multicultural Health Communication Service is another state service where over 450 on-line multilingual health resources, guidelines, protocols, and policies related to communicating with CALD backgrounds can be accessed (www.mhcs.health.nsw.gov.au). They also conduct research, design health communication campaigns, provide advice to NSW Health, and handle enquiries about all aspects of multicultural communication.

Community-based services

In New South Wales, there are many language-specific community organisations. These community organisations can be the first point of contact for health professionals to learn about cultural practices, reasons leading to migration, language spoken, and social or health issues, as well as possible referral points for your clients. These services are particularly useful for an emerging community or newly arrived refugees.

The more established community organisations, such as Italian, Greek, Vietnamese, Chinese and Arabic, generally also offer services other than those dealing with settlement. They also provide social activities, English classes, aged-care services, counselling, and child-care services. In smaller or emerging communities such as the African or Hmong communities, their organisations may not offer the full range of services found in the more established communities. These organisations might be the only way that health professionals can learn about these communities, as most of the bilingual health professionals are primarily from the larger community groups. Another useful community organisation for helping migrants or refugees to settle in Australia is the Migrant Resource Centre. In New South Wales and Victoria, they are located by geographic area (here are some of their web addresses: www.nhf.org.au (Prahan, Victoria), www.fmrc.net (Fairfield, New South Wales), www.mrcne.org.au (various locations, Victoria), www.mdsi.org.au (Macarthur, New South Wales), www.sermrc.org.au (Dandenong, Victoria).

Engaging with people from CALD backgrounds

In moving from a general understanding of CALD populations and services available to talking to particular clients or patients from CALD backgrounds in direct patient care, or when conducting patient education and health promotion programs, the following points are important to consider.

Familiarity with the culture and conducting culturally inclusive health assessment

During any clinical assessment, it may be useful to include assessment of a client's cultural background. The Centre for Culture Ethnicity and Health in Melbourne, Victoria has developed a useful tool, How to conduct culturally inclusive health assessment (www.ceh.org.au/resources/resbyceh.html). The tool helps to identify things health professionals should find out about their clients, such as country of origin, cultural background (including ethnicity and religion), preferred spoken languages, English proficiency, and preferences for interpreter, literacy in English and in their own language, education, and employment, journey (migration experience, time spent migrating), family and social support in Australia, degree of acculturation or integration, responsibility for decision-making about care, and customs and practices (religious practices, dietary practices, health beliefs and practices).

For example, although Vietnamese is the official language for Vietnam, Chinese dialects are widely used by first-generation Vietnamese Chinese. By identifying a patient's preferred language accurately rather than purely going on the country of origin, this first piece of information can then be followed up by engaging an interpreting service to assist in conducting a thorough culturally appropriate assessment.

Demonstrating willingness and openness

Effective cross-cultural communication relies on willingness and openness on the part of the health professionals to engage truly with their clients. Misconceptions, stereotyping, and simplistic views of multicultural groups limit the effectiveness of health-intervention strategies. An active and inquisitive health professional may break down barriers and create a positive environment for bringing about change.

Developing awareness of and sensitivity to cultural diversity

It is important to note that the mainstream view of a health intervention may differ from culture to culture in complex ways, and this requires the health professional to be flexible in approaching clients from CALD backgrounds. For example, it is common in some cultures to give a full perspective on an illness in terms of its history and the background of symptoms. A feeling of trust is important, and gentle, focused questions by a health professional are recommended to maintain the connection between the health professional and the client. An impatient approach may yield only limited information and may become self-defeating in the long term.

Enhancing skills through cross-cultural competency training

Undertaking professional training and spending time in preparation for an important meeting is invaluable for developing an understanding of the interplay between cultural practice and health issues. Cross-cultural competency requires on-going training and practice through the course of a health professional's working life. The two primary training courses to undertake are *cross-cultural competency* training and *working with an interpreter*. This training is generally available in hospitals, or self-learning materials can be downloaded from the list of websites provided at the end of the chapter.

Planning and implementing a cross-cultural population-based health promotion program

As a health professional, readers may want to advance their skills to promote good health on a population-based level rather than an individual basis. The above guide is a foundation for dealing with a client from a CALD background on an individual basis, but the principles also apply to planning a population-based program.

The majority of health promotion programs targeting minority populations are community-based, and engage members of the community and community organisations through various stages of the project.

Planning and implementing a cross-cultural population-based health promotion program is generally more challenging and resource intensive than working with the English-speaking population. It requires attention to how established the community you are working with is, as this may raise problems in implementing project strategies when there is little infrastructure to support a project. Additionally, community readiness, cultural beliefs and practices, and available communication media are to be considered. Addressing the following issues is essential in setting up a successful program.

Theories, principles, models, and frameworks related to health promotion

It is essential to be familiar with theories, principles, and frameworks of health promotion. Chapter 2 outlines a few theories that are frequently used in health promotion projects. Many books focus on health promotion theories and frameworks. One of these is the book entitled *Theory in a Nutshell: A Practical Guide to Health Promotion Theories* (Nutbeam & Harris, 2004), which can be a good starting point. Theories, principles, models, and frameworks related to health promotion should guide your thinking when planning an effective program, particularly in terms of the most appropriate interventions and evaluation. For example, the transtheoretical 'stage of change' model is widely used in tobacco control projects to assess smokers' readiness to quit. How ready a smoker is to quit will inform the development of appropriate strategies for intervention.

Myna Hua & Chris Rissel

Obtaining relevant data to assist you in defining a health issue

Both Commonwealth and state governments conduct regular demographic and health surveys. The Australian Bureau of Statistics collects basic demographic data in the census every five years. The NSW Health survey has data on health behaviours—smoking, physical activity, nutrition, self-rating state of health, and socio-economic status—and most states have similar data collections. When you use these data for planning your program, you need to be aware of its limitations arising from small sample sizes for particular population groups. However, data for the major CALD backgrounds are collapsed over a period of at least three years and provide some trend data for specific health issues. For example, NSW Health has released its collapsed data on the three major CALD populations (Chinese, Vietnamese, and Arabic). This type of data is extremely useful for writing grant applications.

Literature searches and needs assessments to plan for health promotion interventions

As part of program planning, it is important to search the published literature for evidence of what works or does not with the targeted health issue and population of interest. Most of the published journals are now on line. The outcomes of literature research provide a guide to developing project intervention strategies and evaluation methodology.

In addition to literature searches, it is essential to conduct a needs assessment of some kind. It might be a small-scale survey, focus group, in-depth interviews, or consultation with community leaders (see Chapter 3). This information-gathering can be useful in ascertaining the target population's cultural beliefs, knowledge, practices, barriers, concerns, and communication channels. Methods mentioned above are even more relevant to minority populations, particularly emerging communities where there is no available data from the main data sources.

The concept of acculturation

Acculturation: a process through which migrants and their children acquire the values, behavioural norms, and attitudes of the host society.

The length of time a migrant has lived in Australia may or may not indicate how well he or she has integrated into mainstream society. Acculturation refers to the process through which migrants and their children acquire the values, behavioural norms, and attitudes of the host society (Cortes et al., 1994). Changes can occur in both the host society and the migrant population as a result of migration, and is an on-going process. Understanding the general level of acculturation of a community will help the health promotion planning process to target messages and programs better to match the values and norms of that community.

A standardised acculturation scale has been developed for use in migrant health research in Australia (Rissel, 1997). It has 8 Likert scale items assessing the domains of use of language and adherence to traditions. This scale has identified relationships between low levels of acculturation and poor mental health in the Iranian community (Khavarpour & Rissel, 1997), low levels of acculturation and risky sexual health behaviours in Vietnamese men (O'Connor et al., 2007), and increasing levels of tobacco, alcohol, and marijuana use with increasing levels of acculturation among Arabic- and Vietnamese-speaking high school students (Rissel et al., 2000a, 2000b).

Attitudes: feelings of respect or familiarity, affection or hostility, rights or obligations, by which people feel bound and which will manifest themselves in certain patterns of behaviour.

Formative investigation to inform project design

Formative investigation is driven by the target group of a program (Grbich, 2004), which will help in the design of programs targeting migrants. Qualitative data can provide a richer range of information than quantitative data, and can be especially useful for exploring community beliefs, knowledge, and practices at the early stages of your planning. For example, an environmental tobacco smoke (ETS) project was funded by the NSW ETS and Children Taskforce to extend messages discouraging environmental tobacco smoke in cars and homes to the Arabic-speaking community in the Sydney metropolitan region. During a series of focus groups conducted to explore the understanding of environmental tobacco smoke among Arabic speakers, it was identified that the term 'passive smoking' needed to be explained to most of the group participants. Although participants demonstrated some understandings of the negative health impact of passive smoking on children, this understanding was often not very advanced. There was also a strong misconception about smoke only being harmful if it was visible, and that environmental tobacco smoke was less harmful if children looked healthy. Smoking parents also exhibited a sense of denial of wrong-doing as well as feeling guilty at the same time. Mothers from the focus groups were concerned more about being a good role model than the physical harms of smoking (Jochelson et al., 2003).

Cultural practices, such as allowing guests to smoke indoors to avoid offending guests, and offering cigarettes to visitors, have been identified as the most important barrier in implementing smoke-free homes in the Arabic-speaking community (Jochelson et al., 2003). These qualitative research findings influenced the project team to focus on environmental tobacco smoke among the Arabic-speaking community in the context of Arabic hospitality rather than extending the mainstream campaign 'Smoke-free Zone, Car and Home'.

Myna Hua & Chris Rissel

Forming a project team

As part of project planning, it is important to explore and develop networks with multicultural health or community workers from the target population. Their involvement in the project from the beginning will assist in assessing the needs of the community, and facilitate the development of culturally and linguistically appropriate intervention strategies and gaining community support. Their early involvement in project planning will save time and money, and is particularly important when working with smaller migrant communities, where infrastructure such as language-specific media (newspapers, radio, interpreter or translation services) are not available.

Tips for developing promotional resources

When developing any promotional resources—poster, pamphlet, radio script, or educational DVD—use information gained from formative data collection to develop the concept of the promotional materials. Depending on funding capacity, a social marketing company can be appointed to develop the promotion materials from the concept stage through to the finished product. Testing relevance (imagery and concept), comprehension, and appeal of materials through market testing are strongly recommended; options include running focus groups or circulating materials to community workers or multicultural health workers for feedback.

When using translated materials, a Level III National Accreditation Authority for Translators & Interpreters (NAATI) accredited translator is needed to maintain the standards required by health services. Some language-specific radio stations can develop and produce radio promotions for a reasonable cost. In some communities, a language is spoken in a number of countries. For example, Chinese is spoken by Asians living in China, Hong Kong, Vietnam, Taiwan, Malaysia, and Singapore, as well as by Chinese Australians. Arabic is spoken by people from many Middle-Eastern countries. As a result, there are variations in these languages. These variations need to be discussed and addressed with the translator and multicultural health workers to ensure accuracy and appropriateness with your target groups.

Some multicultural health promotion programs are starting to develop project promotional materials directly in the target language rather than first developing them in English and then translating them into the target language. This direct approach is to be commended, as it brings the culturally and linguistically important elements of an issue closer to the target population. However, this approach requires program developers to possess content knowledge and skills in developing promotional materials, as well as cultural and linguistic fluency.

Disseminating messages and promotional materials

The most effective and economical ways to disseminate multicultural messages are through language-specific radio stations or programs. SBS is a national multicultural radio station. Some language groups, especially the more established communities, have 24-hour radio stations. Other communication media are newspapers, magazines, and cable television. The cost is usually lower than for mainstream media. Community organisations, local libraries, ethnic language schools, bilingual general practice, local pharmacies, religious organisations, and multicultural festivals are also good locations to disseminate promotional resources. Some community organisations are also happy to upload the promotional messages to their service websites.

Cultural relevance in planning and conducting an evaluation

Evaluation strategies and methods need to be included as part of project planning (see also Chapters 14 and 15). Project team members should discuss the objectives, strategies, and desired outcomes of the project so that appropriate evaluation methods can be discussed and agreed upon. Evaluation methods used to measure outcomes of mainstream health promotion programs are generally applicable to multicultural populations.

In planning the evaluation, we suggest several issues that readers should focus on the following areas.

Cultural relevance of indicators

The indicators used to measure an outcome need to be understood by your target groups. For example, when a NSW Health survey tested their translated questions with their target audiences, the indicator of measuring consumption of vegetables ('cup of vegetables') was not understood by some targeted migrant groups, especially in South-East Asian communities. In this case, the term was adapted to 'rice bowl of vegetables'.

Literacy level

In some migrant communities, especially the older groups, written literacy, even in their own language, may be low. It is important to ascertain the level of literacy in the community when a formative investigation is conducted, and decide whether oral or written surveys are more suitable for measuring the program outcomes.

Myna Hua & Chris Rissel

Translation of questionnaires

To translate survey tools, it is essential to have a Level III NAATI qualified translator. It is essential to circulate the translated questionnaire to community workers for feedback or pilot-test the questionnaire to ensure the accuracy of the translation. A more formal way of checking the accuracy of the translated materials is to organise face-to-face back-translation with the original translator, yourself, and another independent translator. This method is used by NSW Health to ensure the quality of their surveys but it is very resource intensive.

Sampling

If a telephone survey is the chosen methodology, one of the tested methods is to develop a list of traditional surnames of the project target population. This technique has been used successfully in other studies of culturally and linguistically diverse communities, including the Vietnamese, Arabic, and Chinese communities (Rissel et al., 2000a, 2000b).

Bilingual data collection

Bilingual data collection can be conducted by a pool of trained bilingual interviewers, such as those surveys conducted by NSW Health on an annual basis. If you do not have expertise in this field, research companies that usually have a pool of trained bilingual interviewers should be explored. A tendering process is required to obtain the most qualified company to conduct the survey.

Budgetary planning

Large-scale cross-cultural health promotion programs are more costly than mainstream programs because of the added expenses involved in resource development and evaluation. Therefore, it is important to budget for these costs. Some small-scale initiatives may be managed with the assistance of multicultural workers.

CASE STUDY

1. 'First Aid for Scalds' campaign
Reaching Sydney's Chinese, Vietnamese, and Arabic-speaking communities

Scalds are a common type of burn injury in children under five. Prevention of scalds involves two strategies: addressing risk behaviours (such as hot water burns) and application of immediate and correct first-aid treatment for the burn (such as running cold water over a burn for up to half an hour). Results from focus groups with three large communities (Chinese, Vietnamese, and Arabic) in Central Sydney found that while the mainstream campaign focused on raising awareness about risks, appropriate environmental changes were not clearly understood by the non-English communities. The newly arrived migrants and refugees also identified barriers for environmental changes as most of these communities live in rental premises.

As some key environmental changes could not feasibly be adopted by these communities, the 'First Aid for Scalds' campaign was developed to address the lack of correct first-aid knowledge in families in the Chinese, Vietnamese, and Arabic-speaking communities.

Each target group's beliefs and practices about scalds were explored first to develop images and messages for promotion materials, that were culturally and linguistically relevant, and meaningful and effective. Information including correct and incorrect treatments was clearly demonstrated through graphic illustrations. These illustrations were designed to catch the target groups' attention and, importantly, challenged existing beliefs and practices. For example, there is a common practice in the Vietnamese community of using fish sauce as first-aid treatment on a burn. The project poster depicted the traditional 'remedy' and then introduced new information regarding this practice suggesting a more effective and therefore correct treatment to prevent serious injury. In addition, formative research was conducted to test the relevance, comprehension, and appeal of all communication materials before the promotion materials were produced and disseminated. During the development of the campaign, the target communities and their organisations were engaged to provide feedback on the communication strategies (the content of the poster, distribution channels, and the most appropriate media to promote the messages). The project team also recruited key community organisations to distribute the project materials plus training for their staff to provide scald prevention education to their clients.

The campaign message was promoted through SBS radio and relevant ethnic newspapers. These media were an effective pathway to reach the target groups. The campaign was successful in improving the knowledge (an increase from 41 per cent to 63 per cent) about correct first-aid treatment for scalds.

King, Thomas, Gatenby, Georgiou and Hua (1999) is the full article describing this intervention.

Myna Hua & Chris Rissel

CASE STUDY

2. 'Health is Gold'
An intervention to reduce tobacco use in the Vietnamese community in Sydney

In New South Wales in 1991, the smoking prevalence among Vietnamese males was found to be twice the rate of smoking among Australian-born men. It had also been reported that the Vietnamese-Australian community was less aware than the general community of the harmful effects of smoking.

The goal of the project was to reduce the prevalence of smoking among Vietnamese men living in central and south-western Sydney. Project objectives were:

1. to raise awareness of the harms of tobacco use
2. to increase the proportion of smokers who are ready to quit
3. to increase quit attempts, and
4. to decrease smoking prevalence.

A working group with representatives from a range of interested organisations, including Vietnamese community organisations, Drug and Alcohol Services, and Health Promotion Units, was established to develop and implement strategies. The project strategies included:

➤ production and distribution of culturally appropriate resources on active and passive smoking, including self-help quit-smoking booklets, posters, calendars, and stickers
➤ adaptation of a general-practitioner cessation brief intervention for smokers, and training of general practitioners, pharmacists, and health workers who provide a service to Vietnamese-speaking communities
➤ extensive coverage of tobacco control messages in the Vietnamese media, including newspaper articles, still advertisements on community television (former Channel 31 in Sydney), a quarterly newsletter, and radio programs and talkback
➤ reinforcement of project messages to community groups and at events such as Vietnamese New Year celebrations
➤ press conferences to launch specific phases of project strategies
➤ provision of a telephone tobacco cessation brief intervention in Vietnamese during World No Tobacco Day (six weeks in 2002 and 2003 as part of the NSW Health World No Tobacco Day campaign)

- promotion of smoke-free areas in restaurants
- resources (radio scripts, pamphlets, banners, posters, stickers) developed in conjunction with health workers and in consultation with the community through focus groups. Permission was granted to use television advertisements from a similar program in California (McPhee et al., 1995). Resources were distributed to the Vietnamese community through Asian groceries, Vietnamese-speaking general practitioners' surgeries, pharmacies, libraries, Vietnamese restaurants, local festivals, and Vietnamese festivals such as Vietnamese New Year and autumn festivals, and as inserts to Vietnamese newspapers. Messages were promoted through the SBS radio and Vietnamese radio stations. Banners were placed at railway stations and parking stations where many Vietnamese people lived and shopped.

The promotion of smoke-free areas in Vietnamese restaurants was gradually modified to support the implementation of the New South Wales *Smoke-free Environment Act 2000*, which banned smoking from indoor dining areas.

The effectiveness of the project was evaluated by population-based telephone surveys at pre (1993), mid-point (pooled 1995 and 1997 data), and post (2003) intervention.

In 2003, 71 per cent of respondents could recall 'Health is Gold', and 40 per cent could recall the project's main message: 'Giving up smoking will benefit the whole family'. There was an encouraging but non-significant association between recall of the project and main message and quit attempts. Between 1993 and 1997, smoking prevalence dropped from 41 per cent to 34 per cent. The smoking rate remained constant to 2003 (34 per cent). There was also a (non-significant) increase in intention to stop smoking. However, there were only limited changes in the knowledge of adverse health effects resulting from tobacco use through the life of the project.

It was concluded that the culturally and linguistically sensitive approach taken was the main reason for the initial success of the project and high level of recall of the project name and message.

The lack of continued decline in smoking prevalence may indicate a need to expand the range of strategies used over time, or that general messages about 'quit for your family' might not be strong enough. Direct and strong images of immediate harms caused by tobacco may have

Myna Hua & Chris Rissel

> been needed, accompanied by messages to quit and the extension of the telephone quit advice trial, as well as exploring appropriate cessation services with health care professionals.
>
> The unpublished full article describing this interventioncan be obtained from Sydney South West Area Health Service, Health Promotion Service, www.cs.nsw.gov.au/pophealth/ and follow the links.

Conclusion

Effective cross-cultural communication is one of the keys to providing equal access and quality health care to CALD background communities. As a health professional, it is essential to be aware of your own and your clients' cultural influences. Openness and respect are crucial for working with CALD populations, as it increases opportunities and options when developing treatment plans or population health intervention programs. To become competent in communicating with CALD communities, there are a variety of services to facilitate the learning process and to assist in communicating with the CALD populations. These include TIS, community agencies, and bilingual health professionals and websites that provide policy framework, guidelines, and on-line training.

In the process of planning a health promotion project, it is essential to be familiar with theories, principles, models and frameworks, obtain relevant data to define a health issue, conduct literature research and needs assessment, consider the concept of acculturation, and conduct formative investigation.

During the implementation phase, it is important to engage relevant multicultural health or community workers to identify potential barriers, develop links with the targeted community, and facilitate the development of appropriate resources. Testing promotional materials through focus groups for imagery, concept, comprehension, and appeal of materials is strongly recommended. The most effective and economical ways to disseminate the intervention messages are through language-specific radio, newspapers, and cable TV.

Evaluation methods used to measure outcomes of mainstream health promotion programs are generally applicable to multicultural populations. However, readers should seriously consider the cultural relevance of indicators such as literacy level, use NAATI Level III translators, use tested sampling techniques (to develop a list of traditional surnames), and employ qualified bilingual interviewers. It is also wise to plan for a realistic budget as large-scale cross-cultural health promotion programs are more costly than mainstream programs.

CRITICAL THINKING EXERCISES

1. How would you collect information to help you understand better the community you're working with?
2. What considerations are important when planning a community-based health promotion program with a multicultural migrant group?
3. How will you evaluate the effect of your program?
4. Where can you go for support or assistance when working with a multicultural population?

FURTHER READING

Milat, A.J., Carroll, T.E., & Taylor, J.J. (2005) Culturally and Linguistically Diverse Population Health Social Marketing Campaigns in Australia: A Consideration of Evidence and Related Evaluation Issues. *Health Promotion Journal of Australia*, 16(1): 20–5.

National Health and Medical Research Council (2006) *Cultural Competency in Health, A Guide for Policy, Partnerships and Participation*. NH&MRC. www.nhmrc.gov.au/publications/synopses/hp25syn.htm Access date 02/03/08

Stewart, S. (2006) Ringing in the Changes for a Culturally Competent Workforce. *Synergy, Multicultural Mental Health Australia*, 3: 8–19.

WEBPAGE RESOURCES

Centre for Culture Ethnicity and Health: www.ceh.org.au. The Centre for Culture, Ethnicity and Health specialises in assisting individuals and agencies to develop strategic and sustainable approaches to working with clients and communities from CALD backgrounds.

Community Organisations Directory: www.sesahs.nsw.gov.au/intermulticult/resources/directories/2003_dir/final/community_orgs/index.htm. This directory contains a list of key community organisations that provide services to culturally and linguistically diverse communities.

Multicultural Mental Health Australia: www.mmha.org.au. Multicultural Mental Health Australia (MMHA) provides national leadership in mental health and suicide prevention for Australians from CALD backgrounds.

Myna Hua & Chris Rissel

NSW Multicultural Health Communication Service: www.mhcs.health.nsw.gov.au. The NSW Multicultural Health Communication Service website provides over 450 on-line publications on health in a wide range of languages, and new publications are added regularly. It also posts other multilingual resources produced by other services. In addition, it outlines services to assist health professionals to communicate with non-English-speaking communities throughout New South Wales.

Quick Guide to Working with Interpreters in Mental Health Settings: www.vtpu.org.au. This website provides programs and services to assist you in working with bilingual and bi-cultural mental health clients. It provides tips from booking an interpreter to working with an interpreter in mental health settings. The guide is also applicable to other settings.

PART 5

Evaluation

Chapter 14	Frameworks of Project Evaluation	253
Chapter 15	Levels of Project Evaluation and Evaluation Study Designs	267

14

Frameworks of Project Evaluation

Margaret Dykeman
& Kathleen Cruttenden

Objectives

After reading this chapter, readers will be able to

- Recognise the significance of evaluation in health
- Integrate evaluation methods into new and existing programs
- Develop outcome indicators and use appropriate data collection methods to conduct an evaluation of a project
- Use both quantitative and qualitative processes to evaluate the evidence upon which their practice is based.

Key terms

critical theory
evaluation
evidence-informed practice
paradigms
philosophy
randomised controlled trial

Evaluation

Evaluation: action directed at collecting, analysing, interpreting, and communicating information about social programs.

The main purpose of this chapter is to build evaluation capacity among undergraduate students studying community health. First, we need to think about the need for evaluation and ask, 'What is evaluation and why is it needed?' Weiss (1998: 320) defines evaluation as 'the systematic assessment of the operation and/or the outcomes of a program or policy'. For Rossi, Lipsey and Freeman (2004: 2), evaluation is referred to as 'a social science activity directed at collecting, analyzing, interpreting and communicating information about workings and effectiveness of social programs'.

Rossi and colleagues (2004) argue that the purpose of evaluation is to aid in decision-making to determine whether programs should be continued for practical reasons, or to aid in decisions about how programs should be improved, expanded, or curtailed. Evaluation may be required to assess the utility of new programs and initiatives, to increase the effectiveness of program management and administration, and to satisfy the accountability requirements of program sponsors. Evaluations also may contribute to substantive and methodological social science knowledge (Weiss, 1998; Rossi et al., 2004). As these arguments indicate, it is evident that evaluation is critical in the social science programs associated with population health and communities, and in health promotion, the foundations of this text.

Since evaluation is a diverse and evolving discipline, many philosophies, models, and methods exist. Two prominent paradigms are the positivist and constructionist methodologies. However, scholars who are identified with evaluation argue that a broader pragmatic approach is needed to match 'concrete methods to specific questions, including the option of tactically mixing methods as needed and appropriate' (Patton, 2002: 69).

Philosophy

Philosophy: the values and principles that guide programs and policies. From an evaluation perspective, the program philosophy and features of the situation determine the method of evaluation.

As administrators, practitioners, clients, students, and researchers, we are concerned about the values and principles of underlying philosophies that guide programs and policies. From an evaluation perspective, the program philosophy and features of the situation determine the method of evaluation. Since population health, communities, and health promotion are the foundations of this text, it makes sense that we consider a philosophy with principles that guide these initiatives. The World Health Organization developed a philosophy for social justice in community health. That philosophy is Primary Health Care (PHC), with its five principles of accessibility, public participation, health promotion and prevention, intersectoral collaboration, and appropriate technology (WHO, 1986). The PHC philosophy allows evaluators to use a number of paradigms (theories/frameworks) in program and policy evaluation.

Paradigms

The *positivist paradigm* is quantitative in design and follows the scientific principles of hypothesis-testing using quantitative data to test theories (Attree, 2006). There are many quantitative models; however, the randomised controlled trial (RCT) is seen as the 'gold standard' (Sackett et al., 1985). In RTC studies, every target in the population being sampled has the same probability as any other for being in the control or experimental group (Rossi et al., 2004). Studies such as RTCs and case-control studies are frequently repeated to replicate the findings. Once sufficient quantitative studies have been done and become a 'batch of cases' evaluating the same kind of program, Weiss (1998) argues that meta-analysis may be used to evaluate the overall outcomes. The purposes of meta-analysis are threefold: to discover the overall direction of effects, to find out the conditions under which outcomes are realised, and to examine the characteristics of evaluations that have influenced the kinds of effects found in the studies.

The *constructivist paradigm* or way of thinking, as readers will discover in their theoretical and research courses, is the foundation for qualitative methodologies that identify values and experiential knowing (Denzin & Lincoln, 2005; Liamputtong & Ezzy, 2005). The paradigm is contextually based and denotes the human perception of what is real, although 'real' may not be observed in absolute terms. The Thomases' theorem that 'What is defined or perceived by people as real is real in its consequences' explains perception explicitly (Thomas & Thomas, 1928: 572). Each participant's perception is shaped by his or her culture and language. In this respect, what people perceive and experience is real to them (Guba & Lincoln, 1989; Patton, 2002; Liamputtong & Ezzy, 2005). Social researchers using constructivist philosophies seek to establish a consensus among those experiencing the perception or 'fact' 'within some value framework' (Patton, 2002: 96).

Although some argue that combining theoretical approaches constitutes pragmatic perjury (Guba & Lincoln, 1989; Denzin & Lincoln, 2005), the pragmatic paradigm is moving forward by integrating positivist (quantitative) and constructionist (qualitative) philosophies to build a complex and comprehensive

Paradigms: the different theories and frameworks in the two main methodological perspectives: positivist (quantitative), and constructivist (qualitative) paradigms.

Randomised controlled trial: a study in which people are allocated at random (by chance alone) to receive either the program of interest or not, with the latter acting as a comparison to provide a benchmark.

evaluation matrix design that utilises multiple methodologies and theories (Doane & Varcoe, 2005; Attree, 2006; Aldmeder, 2007; see also Chapter 3). The research case study which will be given later in this chapter provides an example of an evaluation that is based on a pragmatic paradigm. The use of a pragmatic paradigm necessitates the examination of the role of critical thinking in evidence-based practice and in the evaluation of the process and outcomes of programs and policies.

Critical thinking

Critical theory: a philosophy of adult learning that is the basis for critical thinking. It may use reason alone, or it may be more inclusive of diversity and include creativity, imagination, intuition, and emotional feelings.

Critical theory is a philosophy of adult learning that is the basis for critical thinking. There are a number of meanings associated with critical theory so that it is helpful to select one that addresses the process and outcomes of social evaluation. One of the criticisms of traditional critical thinking is that it supports a gender bias that uses reason alone and overlooks creativity, imagination, intuition, and emotional feelings. However, critical theory from a feminist perspective is more inclusive of diversity, is grounded in the constructivist paradigm, and represents the epistemological perspective best suited for program and policy evaluation (Thayer-Bacon, 2000). Furthermore, Brookfield (2005), in his review of critical theory, supported the position that political and ethical dimensions are integral to contemporary programs of critical thinking. In a program or policy evaluation, we show respect for the political and ethical dimensions of our identified populations by understanding and acknowledging their beliefs, experiences, and needs. Brookfield (2005: 15) states that 'in building a democratic society, we experiment, change, and discover our own and others' fallibility'. Although critical theory drives the building of the democratic society, critical thinking underlies the experimentation and changes that take place among diverse populations. Thayer-Bacon (2000: 161) views critical thinking as our best tool to reason and think clearly with others where 'knowers cannot be separated from what is known'. As you assess individuals within your population, you will realise the depth of knowledge they possess about their health issue as it exists within the context of their situation. As 'knowers', they are active participants in knowing, planning, and evaluating what will work for them. The process of critical thinking guides your analysis and integration of their knowledge with evidence-based practice for design and implementation of program evaluation. Critical thinking guides the selection of a constructivist paradigm to involve the 'knowers' in the experiential and creative processes. Actions based on critical thinking lead to programs designed to address needs or issues and to develop effective social policy. The 'knowers' also participate in the reflection and analysis of how a program or policy is meeting their needs.

Evidence-informed practice

Evaluation is one of the key components of the evidence-informed practice movement. To provide competent care, the health provider must use an evaluation process to determine if there is valid and reliable evidence to support the intended change in practice. There are a number of definitions for evidence-based practice in the literature. However, Rycroft-Malone (2006) notes that core similarities can be seen within these definitions. The core similarities noted include the recognition of the role of research, the need to use other sources of information, and the need to include individuals in the decision-making process.

Although there is controversy concerning the use of information other than research to support the evidence, Rycroft-Malone and colleagues (2004) claim that practitioners in the field depend on multiple sources of information that are based on research, the experiences of the practitioner and patient, and on the context of the local area. The belief that a broader definition of what constitutes data informs the evidence-informed process is clearly delineated by Gibbs and Gambrill (2002: 453), who suggest that:

> Evidence-based professionals pose specific answerable questions regarding decision in their practice, search electronically for the answer, critically appraise what they find, carefully consider whether findings apply to a particular client, and, together with the client, select an option to try and evaluate the results.

From Gibbs and Gambrill's discourse, there is a clear link between each phase of the process and evaluation. For instance, is the person gathering the data using credible websites? What tools are being used to decide if the findings are relevant to this particular client, and are these tools valid and reliable? Have appropriate indicators been determined to measure the results? In addition to informing practice, there is a movement at all levels to develop policies that are better informed by evidence.

Evidence-informed practice: the key component of evaluation. It is suggested that to provide competent care, the health provider must use an evaluation process to determine if there is valid and reliable evidence to support the intended change in practice.

Evidence-informed policy

In 2004, the World Health Organization held a summit in Mexico and included a round-table discussion 'Making informed policy decisions: challenges and opportunities'. Officials concluded that:

> the global community needs to improve the availability, communication, and use of the best available evidence for health policy at the global, national, and regional levels and to initiate a global fund to support these activities (WHO, 2004: 5–7).

Governments are concerned with supplying health care providers with the highest attainable standards of care, and the advice needed by individuals and communities on how to improve health and prevent disease using evidence-based care (Littlejohns & Chalkidou, 2007). Sanderson (2002: 5) notes that 'the ideal model of evidence-based policy making is predicated on the following assumptions related to: the nature of knowledge and evidence; the way in which social systems and policies work; the way in which evaluation can provide the evidence needed; the basis upon which we can identify successful or good practice; and the ways in which evaluation evidence is applied in improving policy and practice'. The intent of evaluation is to understand what is likely to work in decision-making surrounding public policies and programs.

Planning an evaluation

Planning an evaluation requires asking questions in the program or policy design phase, and how evaluation will continue throughout the life of the program or policy. Mark and colleagues (2000: 49–50) claim that there are four main purposes for conducting an evaluation. These four purposes are defined as 'assessment of merit and worth, program and organizational improvement, oversight and compliance, and knowledge development'. Although program and organisational improvement and knowledge development are fairly self-explanatory, assessment of merit and worth and oversight and compliance need further explanation. In their discussion, these authors define merit and worth as determining the value of a program or policy which they claim partially depends on whether the program 'safeguards participants' or others' rights and liberties' (Mark et al., 2000: 54). Oversight and compliance is defined by the authors as the extent to which the program will meet existing rules and regulations. The questions that need to be asked include: does the program deliver the services it was authorised to deliver, and does it enrol the participants that meet the criteria for service provision? Evaluation conducted for this purpose holds the management and staff accountable for the operation of the program.

Weiss (1998) recognises the need for ethics in evaluation. According to Weiss (1998: 320), 'intrinsic to evaluation is a set of standards that (explicitly or implicitly) define what a good program or policy looks like and what it accomplishes'. Since it is difficult to write standards for evaluation in general, the Task Force of the American Evaluation Association (2007) has developed five guiding principles for the ethical practice of evaluation. The five principles include:

- Systematic inquiry. Evaluators conduct systematic, data-based inquiries.
- Competence. Evaluators provide competent performance to stakeholders.

> Integrity/honesty. Evaluators display honesty and integrity in their own behaviour and attempt to ensure honesty and integrity in the evaluation process.
> Respect for people. Evaluators respect the security, dignity, and self-worth of respondents, program participants, clients, and other stakeholders.
> Responsibilities for general and public welfare. Evaluators articulate and take into account the diversity of general and public interests and values.

The guiding principles of the American Evaluation Association were written in 1994, and reviewed and revised in March 2007. The full text of the guiding principles was published in the *American Journal of Evaluation* (2007, 28: 129–30) and online at www.eval.org.

As Rossi and colleagues (2004) point out, the guiding principles or standards direct the ethics of evaluation, which is becoming an important element as evaluators become recognised as professionals. Evaluators and their professional associations recognise that formulated and published standards are required by professional associations to safeguard clients and their practice, stakeholders, community groups, and funding organisations.

The purposes for the evaluation are determined in the formative stage of program or policy development. In addition, during this phase the process and data needs are identified to meet the program goals and objectives.

Evaluation models

There are a number of evaluation models and a number of ways to group these models depending on which author you read. Frequently, evaluators use aspects of various models when designing their evaluation. How these elements are chosen will depend on the questions that need to be answered. Mixing model elements allows the evaluator to employ mixed methodologies also when designing evaluations to answer questions that relate to multiple aspects of the program (Weiss, 1998; Posavac & Carey, 2003). For the purpose of this text, we have chosen to discuss four models that have been used historically in health and social programs.

Four models relevant to social science program evaluation

Traditional model

In the past, evaluation was not always done systematically. It was often conducted informally by people working within an organisation with a process that served to satisfy the interests of the employer. When the standards mentioned above are not used, this model may lead to biases that favor the organisation (Posavac & Carey, 2003: 24). According to Rossi and colleagues (2004: 8), following the Second World War, federal agencies were investing heavily in social programs such as rural development, health, and nutrition. Because these commitments were so expensive the agencies were demanding 'knowledge results' from funded programs. In traditional evaluation, systematic evaluation was not built into program planning or policy design but was intended to 'increase the rationality of policymaking' (Weiss, 1998: 10).

Social sciences research model

This model was developed from the need to make evaluation more valid and reliable, and often consisted of using a control group methodology. Although it provided the rigour that was lacking in the traditional model, it frequently rules out encouraging outcomes because of the complex issues that are inherent in programming (Posavac & Carey, 2003: 25). However, Rossi and colleagues (2004) note that methodological quality has been developed and refined over the years to construct sound factual descriptions using social science techniques of systematic observation, measurement, sampling, research design, and data analysis. Such rigour in describing program performance is intended to be 'as credible and defensible as possible'.

Theory-driven evaluation

Stufflebeam (2000: 56) claims that the main purposes of theory-based program evaluation are to determine the extent to which the program of interest is theoretically sound, to understand why it is succeeding or failing, and to provide direction for program improvement. Questions for the program evaluation are derived from the guiding theory. The theory-driven model of evaluation is based on there being a set of program goals and expected outcomes of services offered by a program. The evaluation process is carried out by looking at correlations '(a) among the services and the characteristics of participants, (b) among services and immediate changes, and (c) among immediate changes and outcome variables' (Posavac & Carey, 2003: 28). This model has a better fit with program evaluation; however, in giving up the randomisation of quantitative methods, some of the rigour is lost. Currently, few social science programs are grounded in theory. Therefore, it is difficult to integrate the validation steps into the evaluation process within an acceptable time frame (Stufflebeam, 2000).

An improvement-focused model

Having provided information concerning how theories of evaluation have evolved over time to provide better information, Posavac and Carey (2003: 29) report that they have moved away from a methodology-driven evaluation process to one that is focused on program improvement. This model of evaluation seeks out the discrepancies that exist between what is actually happening and what was planned and expected to happen. These authors believe evaluations based on this model meet the needs of all stakeholders.

This model captures the elements of Thayer-Bacon's (2000) constructive critical theory and Attree's (2006: 641) proposed pragmatic paradigm that mixes methodologies to meet evaluation aims. Further, it is congruent with Weiss's (1998) need for ethics and a set of principles for use in evaluation research.

Types of evaluation

The literature discusses the types of evaluation under a number of different headings. Although there is on-going discussion about other types of evaluation, formative and summative evaluations appear to be the enduring strategies employed in evaluating programs (Scriven, 1996). Trochim (2006) suggests that the type of evaluation used will be determined by the purpose of the evaluation.

In this regard, *formative evaluation* is used when the purpose is to evaluate how the program works. For example, is the program delivered effectively for the purpose of improving the way it is offered?

In contrast, *summative evaluations* are conducted when the goal of the evaluation is to determine the output of the program (Trochim, 2006). In this case, the evaluation determines whether the goals have been met (Patton, 1994).

Wholey (1996:145) claims that formative evaluation is conducted for performance improvement while summative evaluation is needed for 'accountability, policy and budget decision-making'.

Steps in evaluation

In their text *RealWorld Evaluation* (2006: 19–20), Bamberger and colleagues discuss the methodological problems with evaluation that can affect the validity of the findings. To address these problems, these authors have developed a stepwise approach to ensure that methodological rigour is maintained. In the authors' words, these steps include:

1 planning and scoping the evaluation
2 strategies for addressing budget restraints
3 strategies for addressing time constraints

4   strategies for addressing data constraints
5   understanding and coping with political factors influencing how the evaluation is designed, implemented, disseminated, or used
6   strengthening the evaluation design and the validity of conclusions
7   helping clients [and providers] use the information.

The seven steps help to build in the credibility and accuracy of findings. Patton (2002) also discusses rigour in evaluation. He states that when you employ the criteria for quality (for example credibility, impartiality, independence of judgment), it conveys a 'sense that you are dedicated to getting as close as possible to what is really going on in whatever setting you are studying' (Patton, 2002: 93).

In research, evaluation begins with the research proposal, which establishes a framework for evaluating the process and outcomes of the study. Evaluation methods such as Program Logic (Weiss, 1998; Rossi et al., 2004) are used to evaluate research projects, particularly studies designed in phases over long periods of time.

CASE STUDY

Evaluating a housing project

In this case study, the second author (KC) is a co-investigator on the five-year Atlantic Seniors' Housing Research Alliance (ASHRA) (ashra.msvu.ca). The ASHRA study is divided into four phases involving five Atlantic Canada universities, seven researchers, and approximately 47 stakeholders, including the four provincial governments and community partners, and 23 students. The study was funded by the Social Sciences Health Research Council through a Community University Research Alliance (CURA Grant) for $1,200,000 (Canadian).

The purpose of the study is to project the housing needs for the next twenty years for seniors living in Atlantic Canada. Findings from the research component as stated in the proposal are 'to aid in informing public policy development, [and assist] community groups ... [to] increase their capacity to engage all three levels of government in implementing recommended changes'.

The four Atlantic Provinces are mainly rural, and seniors' housing policy is an issue that all three levels of government need to address. With such a comprehensive study it was critical that we include program or project evaluation as part of the study. Moreover, the funding agency requires an annual report of our progress.

Who are the evaluators associated with the ASHRA study? The Program Logic evaluation is led by an outside evaluator, community partners and stakeholders, and three of the researchers who participated in the development of the study proposal. The evaluation team uses critical thinking to maintain the integrity of the proposal and to plan for each of the four phases so that the purpose of the study, validity and reliability, are maintained. The second author, KC, of this chapter is one of the researchers on the evaluation team.

Health promotion and illness prevention, and public participation, are the philosophical principles guiding the study. The survey questionnaire is based on the twelve determinants of health that are indicators of the health promotion–illness prevention principle of primary health care (PHC). Since this is a participatory action study, key questions asked in the evaluation included:

1. How did the partnerships function? Who participated and what was their level of involvement in the project?
2. Was capacity built within academic disciplines, and government and community organisations as a result of this project?
3. Did students gain from (i) their involvement in the project, (ii) the type of training provided, (iii) students' satisfaction with their overall involvement, degree of mentoring experienced, and perceived benefits to their education, skills, and career development?
4. Was new knowledge created? Did the project process and reports lead to any change in policy? (The Principal Investigator was asked to present early findings from the survey analysis to the Canadian Senate Committee on Seniors for future policy development.) Was the research data used to develop a range of housing options within local communities and throughout the region?
5. Were stakeholder groups created in each of the four Atlantic Provinces able to work towards the creation and implementation of innovative housing options? Were the resources identified to sustain the collaborative framework of each of these groups after the project ended?

(Adapted from Atlantic Seniors' Housing Research Alliance (2004-2009) Proposal description section.)

The evaluation team has reviewed the process of confidentiality and the random selection of survey participants for the quantitative part of the study in each of the four provinces. Similarly, the evaluation team are reviewing the focus group methodology, including the participant groups and role of the community moderators, based on the methodology developed by

Krueger (1998; see also Chapter 3). The outside evaluator and students interviewed researchers, stakeholders, and community partners regarding their participation and satisfaction with the implementation of the survey and focus group research methodologies. To date, the evaluators have interviewed community partners, including focus group moderators, students performing the data analysis, and researchers, to determine whether the process was followed as outlined in the evaluation plan.

In phase three of the study, the evaluation team will review how housing models were collected and analysed in relation to data obtained from the Atlantic Seniors' survey and focus group data. In the fourth and final phase of the study, the evaluation team will analyse the process and outcomes for knowledge dissemination, including a large housing conference planned with stakeholders for May 2009 in Halifax, Nova Scotia, Canada.

Conclusion

Governments and the public recognise that evaluation has become an important part of the planning for any program or policy development. Values and principles of underlying philosophies are central to the evaluation process. The current movement in evaluation is to broaden the scope of data sources and to include community-level participation to ensure the process produces appropriate outcomes. Evaluation has evolved in the direction of pragmatic methodologies to address the needs of populations better and to inform inclusive decision-making. The reality is that evaluation is moving into the realm of a discipline that collaborates with individuals, communities, and governments to provide the evidence on which to base decisions for practice and policy-making.

CRITICAL THINKING EXERCISES

1. As part of a community group that has been asked to develop a program to meet the needs of youth who are living on the street, what steps would you take to include evaluation in the program design?

2. The World Health Organization has decreed that primary health care should be the framework for community care. In your policy evaluation, is primary health care being implemented in your practice area?

3. How does your post-secondary education address evidence-informed practice? What evidence would you use to answer the above question?

4. How would you use the *Guiding Principles for Evaluators* when choosing a research paper to guide your evidence-based practice?

5. How do you determine which websites on the internet provide valid and reliable information? Why will your instructor refuse information that you take from some websites?

FURTHER READING

Rossi, P.H., Lipsey, M.W., & Freeman, H.E. (2004) *Evaluation: A Systematic Approach*, 7th edn. Sage Publications: Thousand Oaks.

Posavac, E.J., & Carey, R.G. (2003) *Program Evaluation Methods and Case Studies*, 6th edn. Prentice Hall: Upper Saddle River.

Patton, M.Q. (2002) *Qualitative Research & Evaluation Methods*, 3rd edn. Sage Publications: Thousand Oaks.

Stufflebeam, D.L. (2000) Foundation Models for 21st Century Evaluation. In: D.L. Stufflebeam (ed.), *Evaluation Models: Viewpoints on Educational and Human Services Evaluation*, 2nd edn, 569. Kluwer Academic Publishers: Hingham, MA.

Weiss, C.H. (1998) *Evaluation*, 2nd edn. Prentice Hall: Upper Saddle River.

Renn, O, Webleer, T., Rakey, H., Dienel, P., & Johnson, B. (1993). Public Participation in Decision-making: A Three-step Procedure. *Public Sciences,* 26: 189–214.

WEBPAGE RESOURCES

Trochim, W.M. *The Research Methods Knowledge Base* (2nd edn): www.socialresearchmethods.net/kb/. These authors have introduced a new model of public participation in the policy-making process using a three-step procedure that would be of interest to students who are interested in evidence-based policy development.

American Association of Evaluation: www.eval.org. The Guiding Principles developed by the American Association of Evaluation were published in the *American Journal of Evaluation* (2007; 28: 129–130) and are available online. This document is included so that students can use it when exploring evaluation processes.

Centers for Disease Control in America: www.cdc.gov/std/program. This site is primarily aimed towards evaluating programs that deal with sexually transmitted diseases, but the information provided can be applied to most programs.

Margaret Dykeman & Kathleen Cruttenden

The W.K. Kellogg Foundation: www.wkkf.org/Pubs/Tools/Evaluation/Pub770.pdf. A downloadable handbook developed to provide the recipients of Kellogg Foundation money with information concerning how to include evaluation when developing proposals for funding to deliver services.

The W.K. Kellogg Foundation: www.wkkf.org/Pubs/Tools/Evaluation/Pub3669.pdf. This page offers a complete guide to developing logic models. The site focuses on improving current and future communities' quality of life in the United States, Latin America, the Caribbean, and southern Africa.

Enhancing Program Performance with Logic Models: www.uwex.edu/ces/lmcourse/#. This website provides an on-line course that introduces the reader to a holistic approach to planning and evaluating education and outreach programs. It provides an introduction to the process of developing a logic model and how that can enhance the evaluation process.

Atlantic Seniors' Housing Research Alliance (ASHRA): ashra.msvu.ca. This website may be used to track the process and outcomes of the four phases of the study and the policy recommendations or outcomes that will be presented at the Housing Conference planned for May 2009.

15

Levels of Project Evaluation and Evaluation Study Designs

David Dunt

Objectives

After reading this chapter, readers should be able to:

➤ Describe the features of the main types of approaches used in evaluating health promotion programs, including health promotion policy

➤ Understand the main parameters used in measuring the quality of a health promotion program

➤ Explain the role of stakeholders, particularly in promoting the utilisation of evaluation findings in relation to health promotion policy

➤ Understand the contribution of program theory and program logic in evaluating health promotion programs

➤ Identify important experimental and quasi-experimental evaluation and non-experimental study designs used in evaluating health promotion programs.

Key terms

acceptability
community trial
effectiveness
efficacy
efficiency
equity
evaluation
utilisation
experimental study design
formative evaluation
interrupted time series
non-experimental study design
outcome hierarchy
process evaluation
program cycles
program logic
matrix
program quality
program theory
quasi-experimental study design
summative evaluation

Introduction

Health program evaluation encompasses the evaluation not only of health promotion programs but also health treatments, health services, health policies, and organisational interventions (Ovretveit, 1998). Generally, an evaluation aims to assess the value or worth of a health program that is designed to produce specific changes (Hawthorne, 2000).

The topics covered in this chapter provide an overview of different approaches that are used in evaluating health promotion programs in a community. The influence of the program's objectives on the evaluation approach and the importance of evaluation on maintaining a health program are discussed. More generally, readers are consequently encouraged to think about how they might choose a particular evaluation approach for a particular specific health program, and what issues they will need to consider in selecting this choice.

The chapter also aims to illustrate how these evaluation approaches relate to research methodology in the population sciences. These include epidemiology, which can be defined as the study of the distribution, determinants, and frequency of diseases in populations (Bowling, 2002). Other disciplines that make an important contribution to the evaluation of health promotion programs include health clinical sciences, the social sciences, and health economics. Evaluation strategy and its study designs need, therefore, to be as robust and rigorous as possible.

Overview of evaluation in health promotion

Differences between evaluation study designs and traditional scientific study designs

Evaluating health programs in a community needs careful thought at an early stage. A range of factors, including key stakeholders, target population groups, policy, and health care team, can influence the process and the outcomes of the program. This makes evaluation different from traditional scientific studies. In particular, there are differences in *scope* and *context*. The health promotion evaluation has a much larger *scope*, which may include mass media campaigns, government regulations and taxes, and local community development approaches. The *context* of health program evaluation also tends to have a real-world orientation, and there may be many reasons for conducting a particular evaluation. For example, the evaluation may be conducted to ensure accountability. For local community health projects, the evaluation may occur to assess the implementation of a project with prior proven results. Health program evaluation often involves stakeholders or interest groups, and the findings of this evaluation have political and financial implications. The focus of evaluation may also be on improving programs for the future as much as making a judgment of their present value.

The context is particularly important in evaluating policy relating to health promotion. The community and decision-makers frequently have very decided views about the extent to which and in what ways governments and health services should be involved and fund health promotion. Their points of view need to be recognised and investigated by evaluators. Having a systematic evaluation of a project to show that a decision-maker's viewpoint is not correct may help remove the decision-maker's opposition to funding health promotion. The issues are frequently applied to controversial projects, for example, the introduction of a disposable container for sharp objects in a public toilet and a needle exchange program for injecting drug users.

Program cycle and evaluation strategy

According to a program cycle, evaluation may be classified into three broad strategies: *formative evaluation*, *process evaluation*, and *summative evaluation* (Scriven, 1991; Hawthorne, 2000) (see Table 15.1). The program cycle highlights that each program will go through a number of stages of planning, implementation, and measurement of the program outcomes. It involves program development, establishment, and delivery in order to achieve their effects on the population groups who are the recipients of the program.

Formative evaluation is generally conducted during the development stages of a program in order to provide feedback to program planners. The results of this formative evaluation help to review the program, if needed. *Process evaluation* involves monitoring the implementation and operation of a program in order to determine whether program activities are conducted as intended. An evaluation conducted after the completion of a program is generally classified as the *summative evaluation*.

Summative evaluation involves assessment of the effects of a program, and can be categorised as either *impact evaluation* or *outcome evaluation* (Hawthorne, 2000). *Impact evaluation* uses measures to determine the immediate or short-term effects of a particular program, such as changes in knowledge, attitudes, or behavioural intentions. These measures may be considered surrogate outputs for the actual long-term outcomes of a program. These long-term outcomes can be used to indicate the change of health status of the population, and this can be measured after the cessation of the program. In contrast, *outcome evaluation*

Program cycles: representations of the stages of the program as a circle, where completion of the program initiates a further stage of development (representing a new beginning).

Formative evaluation: the gathering of information about a program during the early stages of its existence so as to guide its future development.

Process evaluation: evaluation that focuses on how a program was implemented and operates.

Summative evaluation: evaluation that examines the effects or outcomes of program, determining their overall impact.

David Dunt

TABLE 15.1 Program cycle and evaluation strategies

Program cycle	Evaluation strategy
Planning	
Program need	*Needs analysis*
Program design	Program theory: literature review and expert/stakeholder consultation
Program development	Formative evaluation
Implementation	
Program implementation	Process evaluation
Measuring outcomes	Summative evaluation
Short-term outcomes of program	➤ Impact evaluation
Definitive outcomes of program	➤ Outcome evaluation

assesses the long term-effects of a program, such as changes in disease mortality and actual behavioural changes, rather than merely the immediate impact.

It is useful to consider here that programs often have multiple steps that are designed to have a sequence of effects. Ultimate program outcomes, such as decreased mortality from a particular illness, are thus contingent on attaining goals at different activities of the program, such as disseminating an appropriate message to a target group. This is referred to as the 'hierarchy' of outcomes of a particular program. Identifying an outcomes hierarchy is an important step in conducting an evaluation, as it identifies appropriate outcomes for evaluation at each activity of the program. This will be further discussed below.

It is noted that an evaluation encompasses very early stages of a program, including the need for a program to address a health problem in a community. An example is the severity of pain and difficulties in conducting daily activities experienced by people in the community living with arthritis, and the lack of health programs, activities, and medicines that can minimise the pain and difficulties among this population group. The conclusion that there is a gap in services is based on extensive literature review. In some situations, consultations with experts and other people with local knowledge of a health problem may be needed. It is important to note that in all evaluation strategies these literature reviews and consultations are required. The evaluators then will know what evidence exists, that the program being considered actually works, or that the program theory on which the program is based is sound.

Evaluation study design

Evaluation study designs are generally classified as one of three basic types (Scriven, 1991; Kumar, 1996; Hawthorne, 2000; Grembowski, 2001):

➤ experimental
➤ quasi-experimental, or
➤ non-experimental.

Experimental study designs

Experimental study designs are those in which the investigator has control over participants, intervention, program, and observations. They involve two or more groups, at least one of which consists of participants who receive a particular health program. This group is called an 'intervention' group, while a second group forms a control or comparison group. This 'control' group does not receive the health program or receives only a routine health program. An important feature of the experimental designs is the randomisation of participants into either the treatment or the control group. The most common form of experimental design is the *randomised controlled trial* (RCT), which involves randomisation of participants into either a treatment or a control group. There are observations or measurements of health behaviours or outcomes conducted prior to and following the intervention phase. Sometime the observations or measurements are only made following the intervention.

The Multiple Risk Factor Intervention Trial (MRFIT) was a randomised primary prevention trial to test the effect of a multifactor intervention program on mortality from coronary heart disease (CHD) in 12,866 high-risk men aged 35 to 57 years (Hennekens & Buring, 1987). These men were at high risk of developing CHD because of their current cigarette smoking, elevated blood pressure, and high blood cholesterol levels. Men were randomly assigned either to a special intervention program consisting of a stepped-care treatment for hypertension, counselling for cigarette smoking, and dietary advice for lowering blood cholesterol levels, or to their usual sources of health care in the community. After seven years of follow-up, there was a non-significant 7 per cent decrease in deaths from CHD in the stepped-care group compared with those in the usual care group. This was despite large reductions in the level of all three risk factors in the special investigation

Experimental study design: study design in which people are assigned by the researcher to an intervention group or a control group.

Non-experimental study design: study design in which people are not assigned to an intervention or control group. Sometimes called a qualitative study.

David Dunt

group. However, it transpired that a large proportion of men in the usual care group had also lowered their risk factors, presumably due to increasing awareness in the community about the three risk factors and their health effects.

From a study design viewpoint, notice how the randomised controlled trial has its starting point at the beginning of the program and not at the health outcome of the program. Information about the health outcome of the service is only obtained at some time after the delivery of the service. The crucial point of the RCT design is that the allocation to study and control groups is on a random basis.

The great advantage of randomisation is how it deals with so-called confounding factors; that is, factors related independently with the outcome and program variables. Differences in the levels of these confounding factors in the intervention and control groups in RCTs that can only occur as a result of chance are typically very small, as long as the numbers participating in the study are large enough. For any number of reasons, expected or unexpected, differences in the levels of confounding factors in the intervention and the control groups may potentially be quite large. If not measured and corrected, they may invalidate the study's results.

Quasi-experimental study designs

Quasi-experimental study design: research design that resembles an experimental design or randomised controlled trial but has no random assignment.

Quasi-experimental study designs have some features that are similar to experimental study designs. There are participants in either an intervention group or a control group. However, there is no randomisation of participants into these groups. Good quasi-experimental study designs aim to match the control group as closely as possible to the intervention group, in order to minimise differences between the two groups.

Two major quasi-experimental study designs are used in health care programs. These designs are the community trial quasi-experimental study design and an interrupted time series quasi-experimental study design. Reasons for using each design include the number of participating communities, period of the program, and resources.

Community trial quasi-experimental study design

Community trial: study in which whole communities rather than individuals are assigned to receive either the program of interest or not, with the latter acting as a comparison to provide a benchmark.

This study design requires more than two communities to compare the outcome of the program. At least one community receives a health program and the other does not. When more than two communities are participating in the program, attempts should be made to have a similar community allocated in an intervention group and a control group. The assessment of the health outcome is conducted at the commencement of the program and the end of the program. Changes in health outcome in the intervention and the control are then compared and the difference can be attributed to the introduction of the program.

Figure 15.1 shows the form of the community trial quasi-experimental study design.

FIGURE 15.1 A community trial quasi-experimental study design

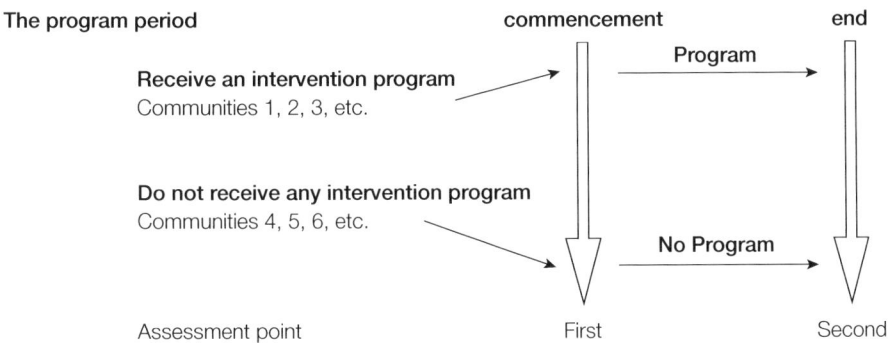

This design and the interrupted time series design are typically quasi-experimental study designs. The allocation of communities in the former case would be non-random, and random in the latter case. Both are used when an intervention is directed at a whole population, not a number of individuals. In this community trial design, a simple 'Before and After' comparison is made between the intervention and non-intervention groups. For example, fluoridation of a town's water supply system can be introduced in a number of communities while communities without fluoridated water can serve as a control group. Changes of in the percentage of children with tooth decay over a period can be used as the outcome of this community trial quasi-experimental study design.

In the community trial design, it is necessary to assume that the characteristics of the residents and other health care services relating to the health issue—in the example, tooth decay—in the intervention and control communities are similar and do not change across the study period. If this cannot be established, it is necessary to correct for these circumstances as they will be confounders of the program that influence the program's final results.

Interrupted time series trial quasi-experimental study design

In an interrupted time series design, multiple 'before and after' comparisons are made over an extended period, allowing extended comparisons to be made across time within one or more intervention communities. Sometimes, although by no means always, in an interrupted time series design, all communities receive intervention from the program for a period of time. However, there is a period in which the intervention of the program ceases temporarily. This serves as a control

Interrupted time series: study design where a single group of participants is tested repeatedly both before and after the introduction of the program.

David Dunt

within the same communities throughout the study period. Each community, in a sense, is its own control. In Figure 15.2, a program is introduced twice. The first time is between points one and two, and the second introduction is between point 3 and point 4. No program is operating in the communities between point 2 and point 3. This assumes that the characteristics of the residents and other health care services do not alter appreciably over this period of time.

Figure 15.2 illustrates the form of an interrupted time series trial quasi-experimental study design.

FIGURE 15.2 An interrupted time series trial quasi-experimental study design

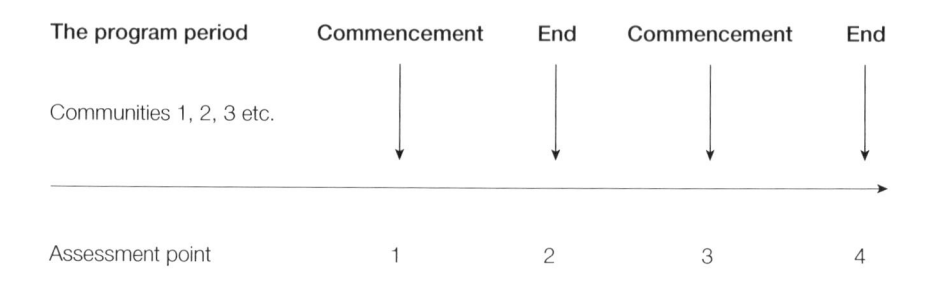

The multiple 'before and after' comparisons made over the extended time period make it possible to detect effects other than the program that may be operating during the different time periods. Changes of health outcomes at different time periods are recorded together with the introduction and withdrawal of the health program. It is assumed that, if the magnitude of an effect occurring during the period of the health program clearly exceeds the magnitude of effects occurring during the periods without the health program, it must be a program effect rather than something else. An example of a program suitable for an interrupted time series trial design is a mass media campaign to reduce accidents caused by drink driving that is aimed at a whole community or population and operates during a long holiday season.

Non-experimental study designs

Non-experimental study designs do not have the investigator's control over the participants, intervention, program, and observations (Taylor & Bogdan, 1998; Patton, 2002). Such designs are limited in their ability to establish causal links between the observed changes and a particular health program introduced to the target population group. One example of this design is observations that are conducted to gather information relating to health behaviours or outcomes of the population group at different points of the program cycle without there being any control group.

Program logic models (as described later) can be used as one form of non-experimental study design. The program logic models focus on different stages in the development, delivery, and impact of a program. Quantitative indicators may be developed to assess whether these stages have been achieved or not. It is important, however, that qualitative information be gathered at the same time to assess whether these stages have been achieved or not. Reasons for the achievement or failure will help better inform the evaluation from both summative and formative perspectives. This qualitative information will usually be obtained from interviewing the stakeholders, including users, health workers, managers, and funders, who have first-hand knowledge of the program. Observation of the stakeholders by the evaluation team members can also be used as another data collection method (see also Chapter 3).

Selection of the evaluation design

The selection of an evaluation design will depend largely on the purpose of the evaluation (Hawthorne, 2000). Where an evaluation aims to determine causality, it is generally appropriate to choose an experimental study design. In contrast, for an evaluation that aims to understand an aspect of human behaviour, an observational study design may be sufficient. In addition, it is important to consider the actual scope, context, and setting of the evaluation. While a particular design may be considered most appropriate for achieving certain aims, it may not be feasible to implement it. The barriers to using the design may include budget limitations, ethical issues, or political environments.

Restrictions on resources and time mean that the above evaluation study designs are mainly used for a summative evaluation. However, there are some common difficulties associated with the use of the RCT design in the evaluation of health programs. Other experimental and quasi-experimental designs therefore need to be considered in this summative evaluation. Study designs such as community trials and interrupted time series designs can be used to monitor a program using *quantitative* program indicators judged against explicit program *objectives* set in advance. This implies that the objectives are clearly defined and able to be measured, preferably using standardised instruments (Hawthorne, 2000).

Compared with the summative evaluations, the *formative* evaluation focuses on the design and the development of a particular program rather than the program's outcomes. This may require *qualitative* information based on the views and perceptions of stakeholders, including providers, consumers, funding bodies, and managers (see Chapter 3 for different data collection methods). These qualitative data can be used in conjunction with or in isolation from *quantitative* information, which usually are indicators of the achievement of different stages of the program cycle.

David Dunt

For the process evaluation particularly, it is important to consider indicators and measures other than disease or health outcomes. This process evaluation may be viewed as 'getting inside the black box' or knowing the factors that influence the overall outcome (Ovretveit, 1998) to determine how a program does or does not work at each level, and focus on the goals at each stage of the program's implementation. One of the evaluation frameworks, the RE-AIM evaluation framework, may be used to evaluate a complex program (Glascow et al., 2001). However, even in a relatively simple program such as child immunisations, we cannot always assume this is straightforward. There may be differences in the way parents perceive the side effects of the vaccines, media presentations of the immunisations during the program period, and level of education and support in the use of immunisation that the parents have received from health care professionals.

Program cost

Are measures of program outcomes enough to measure the summative effects of a program? It is possible that a particular health promotion program may achieve something good but that funding for the program could have been spent differently and achieved even better outcomes. Health economists call this the 'opportunity cost' of the program. To assess opportunity cost, it is important to assess the costs and effects of different projects under the same program. For this to happen, the health outcomes of different projects will need to be the same. Measurement of outcomes may be challenging if the projects or the recipients of the projects are very different. An example is a program aiming to reduce accidents by promoting the use of safety helmets in cyclists among primary-age students and an education project to reduce falls among the elderly. Health-related quality of life measures that encompass a range of population groups, regardless of the health condition, are sometimes used in this circumstance. The project cost of helping the young age group and older age group to be active members of the society may be considered. Ideally, evaluation of health promotion programs should include this sort of economic perspective.

> **Program quality**: the extent to which a program meets expectations (conforms to an ideal model).

Evaluation parameters

Donabedian (1990), in a classic paper on program quality, outlined its 'seven pillars'. These can be used in evaluating health promotion programs, as they measure the quality of the health promotion program. I discuss these in the following sections.

Efficacy

Efficacy is the ability of the science and art of a health care program to bring about improvements in health and well-being. It signifies the best that we can do, under

> **Efficacy**: the ability of the program to achieve its stated goals, objectives, and outcomes under ideal conditions.

the most favourable conditions, given condition of the society and the individual and unalterable circumstances. For a health promotion program, this would be a program conducted involving a program team and in a community where both team and community possessed ideal characteristics for its delivery.

Effectiveness
Effectiveness, in contrast to efficacy, is the improvement in health that is achieved, or can be expected to be achieved, under the ordinary circumstances of typical program teams and communities.

Effectiveness: the ability of the program to achieve its stated goals, objectives, and outcomes under normal circumstances.

Efficiency
Efficiency is simply a measure of the cost at which any given improvement in health is achieved. If two strategies of care are equally efficacious or effective, the less costly one is the more efficient.

Efficiency: the degree to which program achieves its outcomes at the lowest possible cost.

Optimality
Optimality becomes relevant when the effects of care are valued not in absolute terms, but relative to the cost of the care. This is sometimes called cost-effectiveness.

Acceptability
Acceptability of the health promotion program reflects the wishes, expectations, and values of health care clients and their families. Obviously, the clients have expectations about the effects of the program on their own health and welfare, and how these effects are attained. We can say, then, that to a large degree, acceptability depends on the program recipient's subjective valuations of effectiveness, efficiency, and optimality—but not entirely. Some new elements enter the picture, including accessibility to the program, and the attributes and amenity of the program.

Acceptability: the degree of approval of a program by the community.

Legitimacy
Legitimacy can be thought of as acceptability of the program to the community or to society at large.

Equity
Equity is the principle by which one determines what is just or fair in the distribution of a program's benefits among the members of a population. Each individual has some notion of what is equitable in access to the program and in the quality of the program that follows access. It is likely that individuals are motivated to seek what is best for them, unless they are exceptionally altruistic. However, at the societal level, the equitable distribution of access to the health promotion program

Equity: the extent to which the program is accessible to, and responsive to, the needs of all the different types of users of the program and is therefore fair to them.

David Dunt

and perceived quality of experiencing it, for different disadvantaged groups, is necessarily a matter of deliberate social policy.

Stakeholders

Why is involving the stakeholder is important? It is important to identify the stakeholders at the beginning of the program. Scriven (1991: 234) refers to a stakeholder in a program as 'one who has substantial ego, credibility, power, futures or other capital invested in the program, and thus can be held to be to some degree at risk with it' (see also Chapter 9). Stakeholders are not, therefore, just the commissioners or funders of the program.

There are a number of reasons why it is important to involve stakeholders of a program in its evaluation. The 'steering' committee with whom readers are working as an evaluator can be made up of stakeholders. Finding out the relative importance of each stakeholder, their claims on the program, and their influence can, therefore, guide the content and focus of your evaluation. In recent years, empowerment of target groups of programs has tended to reverse more traditional views of the relative power of stakeholders. Empowerment may try to bring marginal stakeholders into a steering committee.

It is often assumed that each stakeholder will hold a different point of view and that this will involve the evaluator in compromises. This may or may not be so. In fact, the key consideration is that the evaluation team is aware of each stakeholder's position, rather than making assumptions about positions. More importantly, stakeholder involvement frequently broadens the goals against which a program is evaluated.

Integrating utilisation into the evaluative process

Having stakeholders involved may help integrate long-term use of a health program into the evaluation. The study of utilisation of the evaluation comes about when people start to question the value of an expensive evaluation because the report gathers dust on the shelves despite providing a soundly based set of recommendations to rectify problems with the program. Research about utilisation has shown that utilisation should be considered from the beginning of an evaluation, and definitely not at the end. There should be no surprises for an evaluation steering committee in the last week of the evaluation. On-going meetings of the evaluators and the stakeholders throughout the evaluation should provide information as it emerges.

Evaluation utilisation: the extent to which findings and recommendations of an evaluation study are put into effect by decision-makers.

Behaviour change theory and program logic models

Another component to be considered when evaluating a health program is the underlying theory used to design it. For a health promotion program, a behaviour change theory can range from the health belief model, through the transtheoretical model of change, to the social marketing model. The evaluators need to make explicit whether the underpinning theory is to be evaluated or whether it is the program to be evaluated. The reason for this approach is to ensure that the success or failure of the program is attributed correctly. Does a program fail because its theory is unsound? Or is the program implemented poorly or incorrectly? Or is it targeted to the wrong groups?

A program theory is the set of assumptions about the manner in which the program relates to the social benefits it is expected to produce. It also determines the strategy and tactics the program has adopted to achieve its goals and objectives. Bickman (1987) describes program theory as a plausible and sensible model of how a program is supposed to work. There are more than forty theories or models that can be used (see Chapter 2). The nature of each theory can be categorised as either an impact theory or a process theory. An impact theory relates to the nature of the change in social conditions brought about by program action, and a process theory depicts the program's organisational plan and service utilisation plan (Rossi et al., 1999). For example, a smoking cessation program may be based upon the transtheoretical model of change, as described by Prochaska and colleagues (1992). In this case, the model should drive the evaluation plan. The stages of change include:

> **Program theory**: the set of assumptions about the manner in which the program relates to the social benefits it is expected to produce, and the strategy and tactics the program has adopted to achieve its goals and objectives.

- pre-contemplation: during which time the smoker is not thinking about quitting smoking
- contemplation: during which period the smoker seriously considers quitting
- preparation: preparing to quit
- action: commencing with actual cessation
- maintenance: the process of sustaining abstinence.

Then a participant may terminate smoking behaviour, or relapse into smoking behaviour.

The evaluation might determine, for example, the participant's stages of change when he or she starts and completes the program, and the frequency of relapses compared with other programs. In these deductively derived programs, the transtheoretical model of change should influence the type of evaluation questions asked.

> **Program logic**: a model that specifies the logical flow or stages of a program—its development, delivery, activities, impacts, and outcomes.

David Dunt

However, some evaluators prefer to assess the program's design, its program logic, as a fundamental step in an outcomes evaluation. Others view the derivation of a program logic as an end in itself. A program logic can be defined as a way of representing the theory behind a program's actions. It describes the assumptions or hypotheses about why the program will work and shows the presumed effects of activities or resources. The program logic is a tool that identifies the links in a chain of reasoning about 'what causes what', and links resources, activities, outputs, impact, and outcomes. Every program has a program logic. It is what happens in the program—its linkages and its causes and effects. However, it is rarely made explicit, and if it is it is usually as what should happen rather than what does happen. Every program undergoes adaptation as it is translated from policy, from the published kit, from another site, and from a plan into action. Most program logic is implicitly held knowledge, practices, and ways of doing things, approaches that are rarely challenged.

There are good reasons for constructing a program logic. In its most basic form, a program logic is inputs, processes, and outputs. A program logic model presents an overview of a program, with critical inputs, activities, and outputs identified in this evaluation context rather than a process flow chart. I will describe three techniques of program logic here as they frequently used by program evaluators: Suchman's outcomes hierarchy, Smith's 'if–then approach', and Funnell's program logic matrix.

FIGURE 15.3 Example of an evaluation using Suchman's outcomes hierarchy

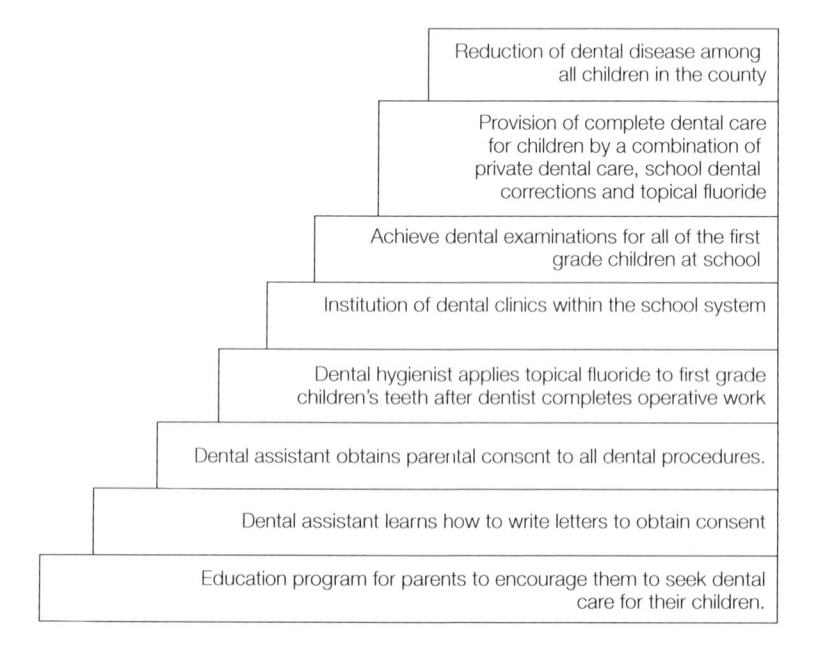

- Reduction of dental disease among all children in the county
- Provision of complete dental care for children by a combination of private dental care, school dental corrections and topical fluoride
- Achieve dental examinations for all of the first grade children at school
- Institution of dental clinics within the school system
- Dental hygienist applies topical fluoride to first grade children's teeth after dentist completes operative work
- Dental assistant obtains parental consent to all dental procedures.
- Dental assistant learns how to write letters to obtain consent
- Education program for parents to encourage them to seek dental care for their children.

Suchman's outcomes hierarchy

Suchman (1967) proposes the construction of an outcome hierarchy for a program, where the program objectives make up an ordered series, with each being dependent upon the previous one. He suggests that an evaluative effort needs to be directed at determining the degree to which each objective is met by starting with the lowest objective and moving up to the most global objective. In this approach, the program objectives are hierarchical and causally related.

Figure 15.3 is a diagram constructed from Suchman's description of a county dental health program in the USA, showing the chain of outcomes, each building upon the preceding outcome.

Outcome hierarchy: a structured set of all of the important intermediate outcomes that lead through to a final outcome within a program.

Smith's 'if–then' approach

The approach of Smith (1989) is to be favoured when causality can be attributed, or if it is to be tested in the evaluation. The following example of program logic for regular attendance at an antenatal clinic by teenage pregnant women uses Smith's 'if–then' approach (Hawthorne, 2000).

➤ If pregnant women can access information relating to pregnancy and the benefits of antenatal care then they are more likely to attend the antenatal clinic.
➤ If women increase their knowledge about pregnancy and the benefits of antenatal care then they are likely to attend the antenatal clinic.
➤ If women have little or no problem/barrier to attending the antenatal clinic, then they are likely to attend the clinic regularly.

Funnell's program logic matrix

Funnell (1997) has developed a matrix upon which program logic models can be constructed. It brings together theory and considerable practical experience, and provides some useful tools to derive and use a program logic model. The matrix is composed of a vertical flow, from output to impacts to outcomes. This 'flow' is directly comparable with Suchman's outcomes hierarchy described above. The horizontal flow records information at every stage of the vertical flow as set out in Figure 15.4.

Program logic matrix: a template used to outline explicitly the causal linkages between the components of a program.

The use of program theory and a program logic model is worth considering in all forms of evaluation of health programs. They can be applied to all evaluation study designs, experimental, quasi-experimental, or non-experimental. The use of a program logic model helps determine whether the program is successful. An example is the cell furthest to the right in Funnell's program logic matrix (Figure 15.4).

However, the application is somewhat different in the three different evaluation study designs. In a non-experimental study design, the outcome will be compared

David Dunt

FIGURE 15.4　Program logic matrix

Objectives arranged hierarchically	Success criteria	Factors affecting success within program control	Factors affecting success outside program control	Program activities and resources	Performance information relevant to success criteria: indicator data and reasons why level achieved/not achieved	Comparisons between indicator level achieved and success criteria

with the desired level of outcome, such as the percentage of program participants adopting desirable health behaviour. In an experimental or quasi-experimental study design, there may be no predetermined success level. Rather, a comparison will be made between the levels of the relevant outcome achieved in the intervention group and the levels of the relevant outcome in the control group.

CASE STUDY

Evaluation of a school-based stop-smoking program

The following case study aims to illustrate problems that can occur in the evaluation of a health program. The problems are due to inadequate consideration given to both program theory and program logic. It was the evaluation of a school-based stop-smoking program conducted in New South Wales in the 1970s. The program was well funded and aimed at early secondary school students. Much effort was spent in producing high quality curricular and kit materials to be used by both teachers and students. Project officers visited the schools chosen to be 'participants', addressing teaching staff and making the prepared material freely available. The evaluators, who were working in conjunction with the program staff, designed an impressive randomised control trial with school classes forming the unit of randomisation. The trial based on this RCT was subsequently written up, published in a prestigious, peer-refereed academic journal, and reported a null result. The program had been ineffective. There was no decrease in the proportion of students taking up smoking or increase in those who had stopped smoking.

A subsequent review of the literature revealed very few instances where school-based stop-smoking programs had been effective. Parents and peers (not schools) were much more directly linked with the take-up of smoking by these early secondary school students. In brief, the model on which the program was based, that the provision of information and clarification of values regarding smoking would influence smoking habits, had not been demonstrated to be true.

After the completion of the program, the evaluators revisited the schools to see what had happened. They then realised that the program had never been delivered in the classrooms. Acceptance of the program by the teachers was limited. Teachers, for various reasons, thought the program was not suitable. No time was allowed in the curriculum for such a program to be delivered. Teachers were unsure of their skills to deliver it, and they thought that the material did not fit in with other health materials being used in the school.

The logic on which the program was based was also defective. The program required more than anything else that the students were exposed to it, and this had not occurred. Both program managers and evaluators would have used their time much more fruitfully if they had specified the program's logic, making possible an early warning that the program was not being implemented, and checking that students were exposed to it and were responding to it, as planned. Their time would also have been even better spent to check the academic literature beforehand and find out the model on which the program was based was defective. They could have been able to predict that the program probably would be ineffective, even if it was implemented as planned.

Conclusion

In this chapter, I have described a number of the important elements used to evaluate many health programs. Evaluations can have both summative and formative dimensions. Various parameters, including acceptability, are useful in assessing the success of a program, and the program's logic needs to be specified. However, applying these elements is not straightforward. It requires planning and discussions among team members and stakeholders. If needed, evaluation experts may be called. This is because each program is different, and the precise form of these common elements will vary according to the details of each program. Nevertheless, with practice in their use, readers can feel confident that they will achieve mastery of the art and science of health program evaluation.

David Dunt

Acknowledgment

I wish to acknowledge the input of Jenni Livingston in relation to the sections on stakeholders, evaluation utilisation, and the program logic models.

CRITICAL THINKING EXERCISES

Consider a health promotion program that you know well. This may be a program that you have read about elsewhere in the book, or one with which you have had some sort of involvement.

1. What specific form would the seven evaluation parameters, discussed in this chapter, take? In other words, what actual variable would you want to measure?

2. What contribution could a program logic make to the delivery and evaluation of the program? Use Suchman's outcomes hierarchy to evaluate the program.

3. Would an experimental, quasi-experimental, or non-experimental evaluation study design be a suitable design for the evaluation of the program? If you decide that a quasi-experimental study design was suitable, explain your reasons.

FURTHER READING

Bowling, A. (2002) *Research Methods in Health: Investigating Health and Health Services*, 2nd edn. Open University Press: Buckingham.

Ovretveit, J. (1998) *Evaluating Health Interventions: An Introduction to Evaluation of Health Treatments, Services, Policies and Organisational Interventions*. Open University Press: Buckingham.

Owen, J.M., & Rogers, P.J. (1999) *Program Evaluation: Forms and Approaches*. Allen & Unwin: St Leonards.

Patton, M.Q. (1997) *Utilization Focused Evaluation: The New Century Text*. Sage Publications: Newbury Park.

Rossi, P.H., Freeman, H.E., & Lipsey, M.W. (1999) *Evaluation: A Systematic Approach*, 6th edn. Sage Publications: Thousand Oaks.

WEBPAGE RESOURCES

Evaluation of a Health Promotion Program (Community Trial Design): www.ajph.org/cgi/content/abstract/88/8/1193?ijkey=67ab9165156f831595316dac8b878858a4f27f40&keytype2=tf_ipsecsha. Forster, J.L., Murray, D.M., Wolfson, M., Blaine, T.M., Wagenaar, A.C., & Hennrikus, D.J. (1998) The Effects of Community Policies to Reduce Youth Access to Tobacco, *American Journal of Public Health,* 88: 1193–8. This is a good example of an evaluation of a health promotion program using a community trial design.

Evaluation of a Health Promotion Program (Interrupted Time Series Design): www.ajph.org/cgi/reprint/91/2/292.pdf. Palmgreen, P., Donohew, L., Lorch, E.P., Hoyle, R.H., & Stephenson, M.T. (2001) Television Campaigns and Adolescent Marijuana Use: Tests of Sensation Seeking Targeting, *American Journal of Public Health*, 91: 292–6. This is a good example of an evaluation of a health promotion program using an interrupted time-series design.

Evaluation of a Health Promotion Programme (Randomised Control Trial Design): www.bmj.com/cgi/content/full/311/7001/363. Gourlay, S.G., Forbes, A., Marriner, T., Pethica, D. & McNeil, J.J.(1995) Double Blind Trial of Repeated Treatment with Transdermal Nicotine for Relapsed Smokers, *British Medical Journal,* 31: 363–6. This is a good example of an evaluation of a health promotion program using a randomised controlled trial design.

Transcript of an Evaluation Workshop on Planning and Constructing Performance-based Evaluations: www.ed.uiuc.edu/sped/tri/evalwkshp.htm. This sets out Joseph Wholey's approach to the use of logic models in program planning. He is a seminal figure in program evaluation and the website is strongly recommended.

David Dunt

Appendix 1

Selected theories, models, and frameworks used in health promotion

Focus on the individual

Theories and models that attempt to explain health behaviour and health behaviour change by focusing on the individual include:

- Health belief model
- Theory of reasoned action
- Theory of planned behaviour
- Transtheoretical model of change
- Social learning theory
- Coping theory
- Learned helplessness theory.

Focus on groups

Theories and models that attempt to explain health behaviour and health behaviour change by focusing on a group, including interpersonal influence on health, include:

- Reference group based social influence theory
- Social support and social network
- Natural helper model.

Focus on the community

Theories and models that attempt to explain health behaviour and health behaviour change by focusing on a community include:

- Ecological models
- Social marketing theory
- Diffusion of innovation theory.

Other important models

Other models and theories are used for multilevel collaborative planning or evaluation of a program in a community include:

- PRECEDE–PROCEED planning model to apply health behaviour theories
- RE-AIM evaluation framework
- The planned approach to community health (PATCH model)
- The community health improvement process (CHIP model)
- Mobilising for action through planning and partnership (MAPP model)
- The theory of gender and power
- Pender's health promotion model.

SOURCES

Bartholomew, L.K., Parcel, G.S., Kok, G., & Gottlieb, N.H. (eds) (2006) *Planning Health Promotion Programs*. Wiley: San Francisco.

DiClemente, R.A., Crosby, R.A., & Kegler, M.C. (eds) (2002) *Emerging Theories in Health Promotion Practice and Research: Strategies for Improving Public Health*. Wiley: San Francisco.

Glanz, K., Rimer, B.K., & Lewis, F.M. (eds) (2002) *Health Behaviour and Health Education: Theory, Research and Practice.* Wiley: San Francisco.

Huff, R.M., & Kline, M.V. (eds) (1999) *Promoting Health in Multicultural Populations: A Handbook for Practitioners*. Sage Publications: Thousand Oaks.

Appendix 2

Example of project planning and protocol

This appendix illustrates part of the planning done in Townsville in 1990 as part of a multicentre survey of pigmented naevi, commonly known as moles, in children at primary and secondary schools. Sun exposure increases the number of naevi. They are not cancers, but their number is correlated with the risk of malignant melanoma.

Letter to Director of Education in Queensland state government

May 30, 1989

Director General of Education
Dept. of Education
P.O. Box 33
North Quay QLD 4001

Dear Sir,

Melanoma is steadily increasing in all Australian states and in New Zealand. The strongest risk factor for melanoma is the number of melanocytic naevi ('moles') on the skin. There is also good evidence that sun exposure in childhood is related to the subsequent risk of melanoma. Naevi are acquired mainly in childhood, and although both naevi and melanoma are broadly related to ambient levels of ultraviolet radiation, the types of sun exposure that increase their risk are not understood. Depletion of ozone in the atmosphere will increase ambient ultraviolet radiation and consequent skin cancer and melanoma.

A programme for collaborative study of the development of skin naevi in school children has been proposed by the Sydney Melanoma Unit, the Alfred Hospital in Melbourne, the Anton Breinl Centre for Tropical Health and Medicine, Townsville, and the Queensland Institute of Medical Research. We propose to survey naevi in children at different ages in several geographical locations in Australia. These locations will be selected on the basis of what is already known about variation in ultraviolet radiation. We propose to compare and relate naevus counts to variation in environmental ultraviolet radiation and information on past sun exposure. The long term goal is the prevention of skin cancer from sun exposure in childhood.

We propose to collect information on type of skin, hair colour, and previous patterns of sun exposure by a questionnaire sent to parents when asking for their permission for a child to participate. Naevi will be assessed by inspection of the skin by dermatologists or doctors with special training. All areas of the skin will be inspected except for the scalp, bra, and underpants areas. In each geographical area we would like to include 100 children in each of the age groups 6, 9, 12 and 15 years. It is hoped to re-examine as many of the same children as possible after 3 years. During this time, they will be periodically requested to complete a simple chart recording the time they spend in the sun.

To obtain the sample of children it will be necessary to approach a number of schools in representative areas in Queensland for permission to examine a group of children of each appropriate age. Once selected, permission will be sought from the parents before any contact is made with a selected child.

This letter is to request permission from the Department of Education to approach heads of appropriate schools in Queensland. The investigators in this project in Queensland are Professor H. Peach and myself. I would be pleased to come to the Department to discuss details of the project with appropriate departmental personnel, and/or provide a more detailed protocol. We would value departmental assistance in selection of appropriate schools for study.

I look forward to your favourable response to this request.
Yours faithfully,

Robert MacLennan MB BS, FRACP
Senior Principal Research Fellow

Letter to schools to gain participation in the project

(ALFRED BREINL CENTRE LETTERHEAD)

Date

Name and address of the Principal

Dear (recipient)

This letter is in follow-up to our recent telephone conversation. I would like to thank you for allowing our research team to conduct our study at your school in late May of this year.

As indicated, I represent a group of skin cancer research doctors from Queensland, New South Wales, and Victoria. The research aims to study factors that influence the frequency and cause of common moles on the skin.

Learning more about what causes moles is important because moles sometimes turn into malignant melanoma (a type of skin cancer) in later life. Most moles form between about 5 and 15 years of age, so we must study children if we are to understand the causes of moles. Knowing what causes moles may help us to prevent melanomas.

Dr MacLennan from the Queensland Institute of Medical Research will be in Townsville on April 24 and 26, and we hope to visit you then and discuss details of the proposed study, which has been approved by the Departments of Education in Queensland, New South Wales, and Victoria. We will discuss how your school might assist us in obtaining informed consent from parents and children before proceeding. We would need an area in your school to examine the students. During the survey we will measure a child's height, weight, count the moles on his or her skin, and take a photograph of the back. The mole counts will be carried out by the same dermatologist and medical doctors with special training as in Sydney and Melbourne. The boys will be examined in underpants or swim shorts and the girls in panties and a bra (if worn) in addition to a hospital gown. Girls and boys will be seen at different times in private surroundings. Elsewhere mothers have volunteered to spend half a day acting as chaperones and generally assisting the study.

We estimate that it will take approximately 30 minutes per student to perform the examination. Although this survey places an additional load on the school, the success of our study in Melbourne in March 1990 suggests that the amount of disruption will be minimal. We will, of course, do our best to lighten the load, and we do believe that the study will be worthwhile.

We are most grateful that you are willing to assist the study in your school. It was chosen on the basis that your students come from a predominantly stable population of Australian-born individuals. We estimate that we would be at each school for about 2–3 days.

Information sheet for participants and their parents

(ALFRED BREINL CENTRE LETTERHEAD)

In Association with the Queensland Institute of Medical Research

Melanoma, Moles and Sunlight—The Australian Schools Study

Malignant melanoma is a form of skin cancer that develops from moles. The number of Australians who are getting melanoma each year is doubling with the passing of every ten years. On average melanoma will affect at least one person on every street in

Australia (2% of the Australian population) and even more in Queensland. This rate is higher than in any other country in the world. Melanoma affects relatively younger people than other forms of cancer and is already the major cause of cancer death among young Australian adults. The prevention of deaths from melanoma is a major challenge to the Australian population and, particularly, to Australian health care providers.

Recent evidence has shown that the most important risk factor for melanoma is the number of moles on a person's skin. This knowledge has focused attention on moles as a vital piece in the melanoma jigsaw. Yet, we still have a lot to learn about moles and the factors that cause them.

The aim of this study is to discover when moles develop, how they are distributed over the body surface, and whether they are caused by sunlight. To find the answers to these questions we are studying school children in Melbourne, Sydney, and Townsville. The study is being conducted by the Monash University Department of Medicine, Alfred Hospital; the Sydney Melanoma Unit; and by the Queensland Institute of Medical Research and James Cook University with assistance from the Queensland Cancer Fund. The study has been approved by the Queensland Department of Education.

Each student will bring home a questionnaire with questions relating to lifestyle factors, including sun exposure. The help of parents will be necessary to complete these forms. Parents will also be asked to sign a consent form for their child to have his or her skin examined for moles. The examinations will be conducted by doctors with special expertise in skin examination. Measurements of height and weight will be made and a photograph will be taken of the moles on the back of each student. The examination will take about 10 minutes. Students will be required to undress only as far as their underwear or swim briefs, and a hospital gown will be provided. Every effort will be made to preserve the privacy of each child during the examination, and mothers will be requested to volunteer to spend half a day as chaperones. The results of the questionnaire and examination will be kept strictly confidential.

If your child is found to have a serious skin problem we will let you know and recommend appropriate referral.

The results of this survey will provide vital information related to the causes of moles and melanoma skin cancer. The reliability of our results depends on obtaining accurate information and on the involvement of every student. We therefore urge you to help us if you possibly can.

Principal Investigators

Professor Hedley Peach	James Cook University, Townsville
Professor Robert MacLennan	Queensland Institute of Medical Research, Brisbane
Dr Jason Rivers	Sydney Melanoma Unit, Royal Prince Alfred Hospital

Dr John Kelly	Alfred Hospital, Melbourne
Dr Anne Lewis	Alfred Hospital, Melbourne
Dr Bruce Tait	Alfred Hospital, Melbourne

Excerpt from plan of action: Proposed time schedule for Townsville Mole Survey

Dates were planned from the last activity to the first activity of the project:

Wed May 30	end skin examination study
Mon May 21	begin skin examination study
Mon May 14	return of consent forms and questionnaires
Mon May 9	consent forms must be in the hands of the students (aged 6, 9, 12)
Fri May 4	forms must be in the schools and in the mail to parents of 15 year olds
Wed May 2	preparation of packages for parents—collating of forms and applications of labels

All forms must be printed (from QIMR). Envelopes should be addressed 'Please return to Main School Office.'

Package to include:

1 information sheet on Breinl Centre letterhead (attached). In addition should include a request to help, why important, call for chaperones, deadlines, locations for return
2 consent form
3 letter from Principal (call for chaperones to leave phone number)
4 questionnaire and limited mole assessment to be completed by parent
5 request that forms be returned by May 14 at the latest.

Tue Apr 24–26	visit principals and teachers of primary and high schools.

Then/later: At designated schools, meet with principals, discuss program for promoting the study, see layout of examination area.

Speak with school teachers at a staff meeting (20 minute presentation concerning background to study, details of study, request their help in distributing forms to students and in collection).

Speak to students: in each age group at each school.

Offer to speak to parents during one evening at a central locale (after questionnaires have been distributed).

Excerpts from Project Manual (Townsville Mole Survey 1990)

- *Form #* Class lists with DOB (and phone numbers).
- Prior to study we need to know the numbers of eligible students in each age group.
- Specific names and addresses on envelopes. Must be marked 'Return to main school office by (date)'.
- *Form #* Teachers to keep a list of eligible students approached in each class.
- *Form #* List of organised volunteers: On initial information sheet of principal's letter. Time, where to report, to whom.
- *Form #* For 15 year olds stamped return-addressed envelopes for parents to return to the school.
- *Form #* Outline of Information.
- Talks to principals and teachers; students in class; parents in evening. Jason Rivers to loan slides on melanoma incidence and naevi as risk factor.
- *Form #* Instructions for taking a sample of children.

    We aim to recruit 100 children aged 6, 9, 12, 15 at time of survey. Thus a child who is 6 or 9 by May 20 will be eligible. Response rates of 80–90% were achieved at these ages in Melbourne. Because of the lower response rates at 12 (60%) and 15 (35%) we broadened the age to children who were or would be 12 or 15 at any time during the survey, between March 1 and June 30, 1990. Thus we included some children who were not quite 12 or 15 at the time of the examination, and others who have just turned 13 and 16. If this seems too complicated we could use the same criteria as for 6 and 9, if there are sufficient numbers in the school. In Melbourne we did not achieve the sample size for age 15—only 60 were seen. The sample was probably biased, and an instrument is now being produced to assess this—all parents will be asked to mark their child's moles on charts of the back and upper arms. The instrument will be validated among those who consent to have their child examined. Since consent varied inversely with the age of a child, we do not think there will be a difference in how accurately parents count naevi in those who consent compared with those who do not consent to the examination. The instrument will have full colour printing, and is likely to be ready only for Townsville.

    School selection: Aim for sufficient eligible children in each age group to examine 100. If more than 100 respond, all will be examined.

    High Schools: Identifying 'ring leaders', to emphasise that privacy is maintained.

- *Form #* Condition and equipment for examination of the skin.

Privacy and Modesty: Boys may prefer to wear swim briefs to underpants, and girls bikinis. All will be given a hospital gown to wear, and only the part being examined will be uncovered at any one time. In Melbourne, for undressing private cubicles were constructed from plastic clothes line and opaque black plastic sheeting held on by clothes pegs. This system is easily portable. For examinations, 4 cubicles would be desirable using this system, or preferably movable hospital screens.

Chaperones: mothers in each school in Melbourne volunteered as chaperones and generally to assist for half a day each.

Equipment: bathroom scales, examination lamps, gowns 40–50, reflectometer, angle-poise lamps (from QIMR) with clamps for attaching to tables; small tables for examiners, with chairs for child, examiner, and chaperone/scribe.

Schedule A. Questionnaires: At least 600.

➤ *Form #.* Return of questionnaires: each day teachers should find out how many returned, also encourage students to return them by due date.

Nurse/assistant to measure height, weight, skin reflectance.

Compliance: Emphasise that compliance is a potential problem (teachers must assume some responsibility).

Slides for talks

Initially by Bob MacLennan to teachers, and by Simone Harrison to classes and parent meeting: study background, methodology, aims, roles: what teachers must do to help, parents. Set of slides to be provided by April 24.

Appendix 3

Applications of PRECEDE–PROCEED

TABLE A3.1 PRECEDE–PROCEED applied to child pedestrian injuries

Rationale/needs assessment	Program goal and objectives
Statement on severity/type of health issue: Child pedestrian injury Target group: Based on this information the primary target groups were identified as 6–9-year-old children, their parents and teachers. The secondary target groups were identified as city officials, school administrators, legislators, police, road safety advisory committee members, and drivers.	Goal: By the end of the program there will be a 10% reduction in pedestrian injuries among 6–9 year olds in the intervention communities

Identify behavioural and environmental risk/protective factors, contributing factors and their corresponding measurable objectives		Strategies to achieve the objectives
Risk/protective factor Child behaviour The behavioural assessment identified two main risk factors for the children's road-related behaviours: ▲ Inappropriate road crossing behaviour; and ▲ Children failing to seek help to cross roads. **Contributing Factor (predisposing, enabling, or reinforcing)** Predisposing factors related directly to child pedestrians included: ▲ lack of knowledge about safe road crossing behaviour, and ▲ a perception of low risk of injury associated with crossing busy roads. Enabling factors for these children included: ▲ inability to identify safer road crossing places; ▲ undeveloped road crossing skills; ▲ lack of social skills required to ask people to assist them cross roads; and ▲ insufficient road safety education in the schools. Reinforcing factors were: ▲ parents allowing their children to cross roads unaccompanied;	**Objectives** ▲ Reduce % of children crossing at busy roads ▲ Increase % of children crossing at safer times ▲ Improve % of children crossing road using appropriate behaviour ▲ Increase % of children getting help to cross roads **Sub-objectives** Increase in % of children who indicate ▲ sound knowledge about road crossing behaviour ▲ understanding of injury associated with crossing busy roads ▲ ability to identify safe road crossing places ▲ good road crossing skills ▲ confidence and skills to ask for assistance ▲ positive family role modelling about road safety	Road crossing curriculum for Grades 2,3,4 students Home education component aimed at parents. Review of school policies Improve signage, paint curbs and increase number of crossing attendants Create action/experience/modelling school pedestrian safety education program Provide teacher training and follow up support to ensure implementation of the school, pedestrian safety education program

Appendix 3

Risk/protective factor	Objectives	
Parent behaviour	▲ Increase % of parents supervising children at road crossing	Parent pedestrian safety education program
▲ Parents failing to supervise children at road crossing	▲ Increase % of parents teaching children appropriate road-crossing procedures	Community education and media
▲ Parents failing to teach their children appropriate road crossing procedures	▲ Increase in % of parents modelling appropriate road crossing behaviour	
▲ Parents failing to model appropriate road-crossing behaviors.	**Sub-objectives**	
Contributing factor (predisposing, enabling, or reinforcing):	Increase in % of parents who indicate sound knowledge about road crossing behaviour	
▲ parents' perceptions that that their children have adequate abilities to cross roads safely, while alone.	▲ realistic perceptions about child road-crossing skills development and capacity	

Risk/protective factor	Objectives	
Environmental—traffic	▲ Reduce residential traffic volume by %	School Road Safety Committees to advocate for improved traffic management around schools; reduction of speed limits to 40kmh, reduction or obstacles/parking alternatives)
▲ high volume of traffic on residential streets;	▲ Reduce average speed of vehicles by %	
▲ speed of vehicles too fast on residential streets	**Sub-objectives**	Community education campaign/programs
Contributing factors	▲ Reduce posted residential speed limit to 40 km per hour around schools	
▲ Posted residential speed limits too high	▲ Change road design to discourage speeding	
▲ Road design in residential areas encourages speeding and high traffic volume	▲ Increase police enforcement	
▲ Perception of drivers they will not be caught by police of cause injury	▲ Increase in % of drivers who report accurate understanding of child road crossing capabilities	
▲ Drivers overestimate child road crossing capabilities		
Environmental–structural	▲ Reduce impact of roadside obstacles including parked cars and structures	
▲ Roadside obstacles obscuring children		

This is an example of a small project focused only on those young people from X culture who access a specific service.

Health issue and target group	Goals and objectives
Health issue or concern: Low confidence and skills in condoms use amongst sexually active adolescents from X culture Potential target group: Young people accessing specific youth program	**Goal** Within 12 months 70% of young people accessing X outreach services report self-confidence, skills, and access to use condoms should they choose to be sexually active. (This project was part of a broader program to reduce STIs and unplanned pregnancy)

Identify behavioural and environmental risk/protective factors, contributing factors and their corresponding measurable objectives		
Risk factor Lack of access to information and skills development that is culturally appropriate and relevant	**Contributing factors** ▲ Inability to reconcile cultural background and condom use ▲ Low knowledge about how to use a condom ▲ Low skills and confidence to negotiate the use of condoms	60% of young people report abstinence or safe sex (condom use) is consistent with their culture 90% of young people can list key steps in using a condom 80% of young people report an increase in their skills and confidence to use condoms
Risk factor Lack of access to condoms to practice with and be familiar	**Contributing factors** ▲ Cost barriers to purchasing condoms ▲ Low confidence in accessing condoms ▲ Fear of community assumptions if found with condoms	80% of young people can name three places they could access condoms within their budget 80% of young people report they are able to access condoms discretely and confidently 70% of young people report that they feel people who they look up to would support them accessing of condoms
		Strategies ▲ Conduct interactive workshops, designed with and for young people, that deals with skills, role-playing negotiation, and discussion about community and cultural issues. ▲ Develop and distribute with relevant supportive community members and young people a youth-focused media resource about condom use and options for where condoms can be accessed. ▲ Implement policy in relevant services that increase access to free condoms for young people ▲ Recruit and train local community leaders and youth role models to encourage and support the normalisation of condom access and use

Glossary

Aboriginal Community Controlled Health Service: a primary health care service that is initiated and operated by the local Aboriginal community to deliver holistic, comprehensive, and culturally appropriate health care to the community.

Aboriginal health: the physical well-being of an individual in conjunction with the social, emotional, and cultural well-being of the whole community so that each individual is able to achieve his or her full potential as a human being, thereby bringing about the total well-being of the community. It is a whole-of-life view and includes the cyclical concept of life–death–life.

Acceptability: the degree of approval of a program by the community.

Acculturation: a process through which migrants and their children acquire the values, behavioural norms, and attitudes of the host society.

Active partnership: partners having an equal role in decision-making.

Advocacy: action directed at changing the policies, positions, or programs of government or any other institution. It is one of the principal means by which environmental change can be achieved.

Amenability: how successful a public health intervention will be.

Attitudes: feelings of respect or familiarity, affection or hostility, rights or obligations by which people feel bound and which will manifest themselves in certain patterns of behaviour.

Attributed influentials: people in informal leadership positions, such as religious leaders and health care professionals.

Capacity domains: areas of influence that enable a community to organise and mobilise itself better towards increasing its assets and attributes.

Communication: the production and exchange of information and meaning by use of signs and symbols.

Community: a group of people with a common identity or perspective, occupying space during a given period of time, and functioning through a social system to meet its needs within a social environment. It can include geographic, professional, cultural, racial, religious, or socio-economic status.

Community capacity building: increasing the assets and attributes of a community through improvements in skills, knowledge, and competencies.

Community development: a process of organising or supporting community groups in identifying their priority health issues, and planning and acting upon their strategies for social action and change, thereby gaining increased self-reliance and decision-making power as a result of their experiences (Labonte, 1993).

Community engagement: the ability to establish a meaningful contact, conversation, or discussion with individuals and groups with the aim of maximising their participation and decision-making in issues that are of concern to them. Engagement involves strategies that assist communities to understand and use their strengths as the basis for change, and forms the critical initial steps towards effective community development and empowerment.

Community trial: a study in which whole communities rather than individuals are assigned to receive either the program of interest or not, with the latter acting as a comparison to provide a benchmark.

Consultation: the process of referring to others for information to seek their opinion; can vary in level of involvement from basic consideration to active engagement.

Critical theory: a philosophy of adult learning that is the basis for critical thinking. It may use reason alone, or it may be more inclusive of diversity and include creativity, imagination, intuition, and emotional feelings.

Cross-cultural: pertaining to or involving different cultures or comparison between them.

Culture is a learned, non-random, systematic behaviour that is transmitted from person to person and from generation to generation.

Deontologicalism: an ethical approach that seeks a set action irrespective of consequences, most often used in law and legislation; ends do not justify the means.

Determinant of health: the range of personal, social, economic, and environmental factors that determine the health status of individuals or populations. The factors that influence health are multiple and interactive.

Displaced persons: people forced to leave their homes because of conflict, natural disasters, or trauma. Internally displaced persons remain within their regional or national boundaries, externally displaced persons (refugees) move across national and international boundaries.

Economic dominants: people of wealth within a community.

Ecosystem: the integrated natural life-support system for humans and all other life forms. Environmental damage beyond the ability of the planet's ecosystems to recover results in climate change, natural disasters, and altered disease patterns.

Effectiveness: the ability of the program to achieve its stated goals, objectives, and outcomes under normal circumstances.

Efficacy: the ability of the program to achieve its stated goals, objectives, and outcomes under ideal conditions.

Efficiency: the degree to which program achieves its outcomes at the lowest possible cost.

Empowerment: a process whereby individuals and groups of people become stronger and more confident in controlling or exerting influence over the issues affecting their lives. This involves the ability of people to assert and claim their legitimate rights in any given situation, and their capacity to accept and willingly discharge responsibilities towards themselves, others, and society. It entails special responsibility of a wider society to work consciously towards creating social environments and relationships that bring out the best in people.

Enabling (facilitating) factors: factors that facilitate or hinder the desired behavioural or environmental changes, such as availability of and access to health resources and personal health-related skills.

Equity: the extent to which the program is accessible to, and responsive to, the needs of all the different types of users of the program and is therefore fair to them.

Equity in health: the aim not of eliminating all health differences so that everyone has the same level of health, but rather reducing or eliminating those differences that result from factors that are considered to be both avoidable and unfair. Equity is, therefore, concerned with creating equal opportunities for health and with bringing health differentials down to the lowest levels possible.

Essential public health services: ten core processes used in public health to promote health and prevent disease. These are to monitor health status to identify and solve community health problems, diagnose and investigate health problems and health hazards in the community, inform, educate, and empower people about health issues, mobilise community partnerships and take action to identify and solve health problems, develop policies and plans that support individual and community health efforts, enforce laws and regulations that protect health and ensure safety, link people to needed personal health services and assure the provision of health care when otherwise unavailable, assure a competent public and personal health care workforce, evaluate effectiveness, accessibility, and quality of personal and population-based health services, and research for new insights and innovative solutions to health problems.

Evaluation: a social science activity directed at collecting, analysing, interpreting, and communicating information about the workings and effectiveness of social programs.

Evaluation utilisation: the extent to which findings and recommendations of an evaluation study are put into effect by decision-makers.

Evidence-informed practice: the key component of evaluation. It is suggested that to provide competent care, the health provider must use an evaluation process to determine if there is valid and reliable evidence to support the intended change in practice.

Experimental study design: study design in which people are assigned by the researcher to either an intervention group or a control group.

Formative evaluation: the gathering of information about a program during the early stages of its existence so as to guide its future development.

Gap analysis: an assessment identifying differences between a current state of public health delivery and an optimal desired level.

Global burden of disease: the gap between current health and an ideal health status in countries of the world where individuals live a normal lifespan free of illness and disease. Populations of impoverished countries carry a greater burden of disease than wealthy countries.

Goals (or aims) of a program: the broad, long-term, quantifiable outcomes of a program of which a planned project is a part.

Health: a state of complete physical, mental, and social well-being and not merely the absence of disease or infirmity.

Health education: an educational process concerned with providing a combination of approaches to lifestyle change that can assist individuals, families, and communities in making informed decisions on matters that affect the restoration, achievement, and maintenance of health.

Health promotion: a combination of educational, organisational, economic, and political actions, designed with genuine consumer participation, to enable individuals, groups, and whole communities to increase control over, and to improve, their health through knowledge, attitudinal, behavioural, social, and environmental changes. It is any combination of educational, political, regulatory, and organisational supports for actions and conditions of living conducive to the health of individuals, groups, or communities. It also can be defined as the process of enabling people to increase control over their lives and health.

Human resources: the people who are required in order to plan for, undertake, and evaluate the project.

Impact: in MAPP, a short-term measurable change in areas such as knowledge, attitudes, and behaviour.

Indigenous Australians: people of Aboriginal or Torres Strait Islander descent who identify as Aboriginal or Torres Strait Islander and are accepted as such by the community with which they are associated.

Interrupted time series: a study design where a single group of participants is tested repeatedly both before and after the introduction of the program.

Key informants: important individuals or organisations that provide valuable data, information, and context towards a public health assessment.

KSAs: knowledge, skills, attitudes. Although knowledge and skills are separate from actual performance, they are important steps towards building competence.

Likert scale: a graphic scale intended to quantify the level of agreement or disagreement with a question or issue, typically numbered 3, 5, or 7.

MAPP: an abbreviation of Mobilising Action through Planning and Partnership, a process developed by the CDC for planning in public health and available on-line.

Measurement: the collection and comparison of information.

Mentoring: taking an interest in, coaching, and supporting another person in his or her career.

Mixed method: both quantitative and qualitative methods used in needs assessment.

Model: a subclass of a theory that provides a plan for investigating or addressing a phenomenon. It does not attempt to explain the processes underlying learning, but only to represent them. It also provides the vehicle for applying the theories.

Non-experimental study design: a study design in which people are not assigned to an intervention or control group. Sometimes called a qualitative study.

Needs assessment: a systematic means for researchers to be able to identify the unmet health and health care needs of a target group, as well as to make changes to meet those unmet needs.

Objectives of a project: specific, usually short-term outcomes. They are stated in a concise paragraph that specifies the population (community) in which the project is to be implemented, and the scope and extent of the observations and/or interventions.

Optimality: cost-effectiveness; it is relevant when the effects of care are valued not in absolute terms, but relative to the cost of the care.

Outcome: a change of health status of an individual, group, or population that can be directly attributed to a public health intervention; outcomes in MAPP are long-term measurable changes in areas such as mortality, morbidity, and disability.

Outcome hierarchy: a structured set of all of the important intermediate outcomes that lead through to a final outcome within a program.

Paradigms: the different theories and framework in the two main methodological perspectives: positivist (quantitative) and constructivist (qualitative) paradigms.

Participatory learning action (PLA): a collaborative approach towards collecting information in ways convenient and useful to the target population, characterised by engagement in a non-directive manner.

Philosophy: the system of values and principles that guides a programs and policy. From an evaluation perspective, the program philosophy and features of the situation determine the method of evaluation.

Plan of action: the proposed chronology of the various stages of a project. It may be a part of the project manual.

Policy: a program of action adopted by government, or the set of principles on which it is based. Policies come in many forms and can be represented by a government document that states action intent, a piece of legislation, budget allocations, or promises made by ministers.

Population health: health groups, families, and communities. Populations may be defined through locality, biological criteria such as age and gender, social criteria such as socio-economic status, or cultural criteria.

Power: the ability to affect change rather than the power to exploit or dominate others. Differentiation is made between 'power over', whereby individuals, groups, or institutions assume the right to make decisions for others, versus 'power with', which involves a commitment to self-determination or capacity of people to determine their own affairs.

Predisposing (motivating) factors: knowledge, beliefs, values, and attitudes that facilitate or hinder motivation for change.

Prescribed influentials: people formally designated to positions of authority, such as mayors, sheriffs, chiefs.

Prevalence: a measurement of how widespread a condition or disease is among a population.

Process evaluation: evaluation that focuses on how a program was implemented and operates.

Process objectives: in MAPP, a short-term assessment of the level of professional practice.

Program cycles: representation of the stages of the program as a circle, where completion of the program initiates a further stage of development (representing a new beginning).

Program logic: the logical flow or stages of a program—its development, delivery, activities, impacts, and outcomes.

Program logic matrix: a template used to outline explicitly the causal linkages between the components of a program.

Program quality: the extent to which a program meets expectations (conforms to an ideal model).

Program theory: the set of assumptions about the manner in which the program relates to the social benefits it is expected to produce, and the strategy and tactics the program has adopted to achieve its goals and objectives.

Project manual: a management tool for various phases of a project. It has all the detail needed for planning the project, and for the collection and analysis of data. It includes correspondence and decisions (such as changes to procedures) made throughout the project and forms a permanent record of its implementation.

Project protocol: the rationale of the project, specific objectives, the procedures that it will follow, ethics review application, plans for data analysis, and plans for reporting.

Protective factors: those factors that produce resilience to, or reduce the probability of, the development of a disorder, disease, or specific cause of death (adapted from Spence, 1996).

Public health: the art and science of preventing disease, promoting health, and prolonging life through the organised efforts of society.

Qualitative methods: research methods employed when researchers wish to understand the health needs of their target group rather than wanting to know about the prevalence of illness and diseases. Qualitative methods are employed to obtain in-depth information about people's perceptions, feelings, and experiences, and do not rely on numbers.

Quantitative methods: research methods that rely on standardised research tools such as surveys. They are used to gain information that can be counted (for example, how many people make use of an alternative medical system).

Quasi-experimental study design: a research design that resembles an experimental design or randomised controlled trial but has no random assignment.

Randomised controlled trial: a study in which people are allocated at random (by chance alone) to receive either the program of interest or not, with the latter acting as a comparison to provide a benchmark.

Reinforcing (maintaining or rewarding) factors: rewards or incentives for the continuation or maintenance of behaviours. Social support, peer influences from other significant people such as parents, teachers, and health professionals, are examples of reinforcing factors. They also include tangible or imagined rewards, social benefits, and physical benefits, along with mass media messages.

Risk factors: those characteristics, variables, or hazards that, if present for a given individual, will increase the probability that they will develop a disorder, disease, or specific cause of death.

Social integration: is defined as the existence of social ties.

Social network: refers to the web of social relationships that surround individuals. The provision of social support is one of the important functions of social relationships.

Stakeholders: those groups and organisations having an interest or stake in a program; the people who will be affected by a project, or who will have an impact on the success of a project.

Summative evaluation: examinination of the effects or outcomes of program, determining their overall impact.

Sustainability: the continuation of activities related to the project after the project team has officially concluded its input.

SWOT analysis: an abbreviation of Strengths and Weaknesses (internal to organisation), and Opportunities and Threats (external to organisation), plotted to assess strategic positioning.

Theory: an integrated set of propositions that serves as an explanation for a phenomenon. It is introduced after a phenomenon has already revealed a systematic set of uniformities. It is a systematic arrangement of fundamental principles that provide a basis for explaining certain happenings of life.

Utilitarianism: an ethical approach commonly used in public health that seeks maximum benefit for the greatest number of people; the needs of the many outweigh the needs of the few.

Value: a conception of the desirable, which may be explicit or implicit, distinctive of an individual or characteristic of a group, that influences the selection from viable modes, means and ends of action.

Vulnerable target group: people who face particular social vulnerability. These include children, unemployed people, homeless people, drug-addicted people, sex workers, refugees, and ethnic and religious minority groups.

Zoonotic diseases: diseases shared by infectious agents that can be transmitted between, or are shared by, animals and humans.

References

Chapter 1

Abel, T., Ritchie, J., Jacoby, E.R., Amuyunzu-Nyamongo, M., & Sivarajah, N. (2007) *Assets for Health and Development: Creating Supportive Environments*. Panel Discussion, 13 June 2007, 19th International Union for Health Promotion and Education (IUHPE) World Conference on Health Promotion & Health Education, 10–15 June 2007. IUHPE: Vancouver.

Association of Schools of Public Health (2007) *What is Public Health?* Association of Schools of Public Health: Washington DC. www.asph.org/document.cfm?page=300 Access date: 5/102007.

Australian Bureau of Statistics (ABS) (2006a) *Injury in Australia: A Snapshot, 2004–05* (ABS cat. no. 4825.0.55.001). www.abs.gov.au/ausstats/abs@.nsf/mf/4825.0.55.001 Access date: 12/08 2007.

Australian Bureau of Statistics (2006b) *Health of Older People in Australia: A Snapshot, 2004–2005* (ABS cat. no. 4833.0.55.001). www.abs.gov.au/ausstats/abs@.nsf/mf/4833.0.55.001 Access date: 24/07/2005.

Australian Bureau of Statistics (2007a) *Census of Population and Housing: Media Releases and Fact Sheets, 2006* (ABS cat. no. 2914.0.00.002–2006). www.abs.gov.au/ausstats/abs@.nsf/7d12b0f6763c78caca257061001cc588/ Access date: 24/07/2007.

Australian Bureau of Statistics (2007b) *Causes of Deaths, Australia, 2005* (ABS cat. no. 3303.0.) Access www.abs.gov.au/ausstats/abs@.nsf/mf/3303.0 Access date: 24/07/2005.

Australian Institute of Health and Welfare (AIHW) (1994) *Australia's Health 1994*. Australian Institute of Health and Welfare: Canberra.

Australian Institute of Health and Welfare (1998) *Australia's Health 1998*. Australian Institute of Health and Welfare: Canberra.

Australian Institute of Health and Welfare (2000) *Australia's Health 2000*. Australian Institute of Health and Welfare: Canberra.

Australian Institute of Health and Welfare (2003) *BreastScreen Australia Monitoring Report 2000–2001* (AIHW cat. no. CAN 20). Cancer series no. 25. Australian Institute of Health and Welfare: Canberra.

Australian Institute of Health and Welfare. (2006) *Australia's Health 2006* (AIHW cat. no. AUS 73). Australian Institute of Health and Welfare: Canberra.

Baum, F. (2008) *The New Public Health: An Australian Perspective*. Oxford University Press: Melbourne.

Beaglehole, R., & Bonita, R. (eds) (2004) *Public Health at the Crossroads: Achievements and Prospects*. Cambridge University Press: Cambridge.

Bell, M. (1995) *Internal Migration in Australia, 1986–91: Overview Report*. AGPS: Canberra.

Berkman, L.F., & Kawachi, I. (eds) (2000) *Social Epidemiology*. Oxford University Press: New York.

Bosch, F.X., Manos, M.M., Muñoz, N., Sherman, M., Jansen, A.M., Peto, J., Schiffman, M.H., Moreno, V., Kurman, R., Shan, K.V., & International Biological Study on Cervical Cancer (IBSCC) Study Group (1995) Prevalence of Human Papillomavirus in Cervical Cancer: A Worldwide Perspective. *Journal of the National Cancer Institute*, 87(11): 796–802.

Christchurch Community Mapping Project (2004) *Christchurch Community Mapping Project: Part 4, Social Connectedness*. www.library.christchurch.org.nz/CommunityMapping/Report/socialconnectedness.pdf Access date: 10/05/2007.

Cohen, D.A., Mason, K., Margolis, L.H., Eng, E., & Henriquez-Roldan, C. (2003) Neighborhood Physical Conditions and Health. *American Journal of Public Health*, 93(3): 467–71.

Committee for Inquiry into the Future Development of the Public Health Function (1988) *Public Health in England*. HMSO, Cmnd 289: London.

Department of Communities (2004) *Cross Government Project to Reduce Social Isolation of Older People* (Summary Report for Demonstration Project Funding Round). Department of Communities: Brisbane.

Department of Health and Ageing (2003) *What is Q Fever? The National Q Fever Management Program*. www.immunise.health.gov.au/internet/immunise/publishing.nsf/Content/q-fever-man Access date: 4/10/2007.

Department of Health and Ageing (2007) *Population Health*. www.aihw.gov.au/pophealth/index.cfm Access date: 4/07/2007.

Draper, G., Turrell, G., & Oldenburg, B. (2004) *Health Inequality in Australia: Mortality*. Health Inequality Monitoring No. 1 (AIHW cat. no. PHE 55). Queensland University of Technology and Australian Institute of Health and Welfare: Canberra.

Duckett, S.J. (2007) *The Australian Health Care System*. Oxford University Press: Melbourne.

Egger, G., Spark, R., Lawson, J., & Donovan, R. (1999) *Health Promotion Strategies and Methods*. McGraw-Hill: Sydney.

Fitzpatrick, M. (2001) *The Tyranny of Health: Doctors and the Regulation of Lifestyle.* Routledge: London.

Fuller, J., Edwards, J., Procter, N., & Moss, J. (2002) Mental Health in Rural and Remote Australia. In D. Wilkinson, & I. Blue (eds), *The New Rural Health*, 171–87. Oxford University Press: Melbourne.

Garrard, J., Lewis, B., Keleher, H., Tunny, N., Burke, L., & Harper, S. (2004) *Planning for Healthy Communities: Reducing the Risk of Cardiovascular Disease and Type 2 Diabetes through Healthier Environments and Lifestyles*, 1–123. Department of Human Services (Victoria): Melbourne.

Gent, V.M. (2004) *The Impact of Fly-in/fly-out Work on Well-being and Work–life Satisfaction.* Honours Thesis. Department of Psychology, Murdoch University: Perth.

Germov, J. (2005a) Theorising Health: Major Theoretical Perspectives in Health Sociology. In: J. Germov (ed.), *Second Opinion: An Introduction to Health Sociology*, 28–50. Oxford University Press: Melbourne.

Germov, J. (2005b) Imagining Health Problems as Social Issues. In: J. Germov (ed.), *Second Opinion: An Introduction to Health Sociology*, 3–27. Oxford University Press: Melbourne.

Ginzberg, E. (1999) US Health Care: A Look Ahead to 2025. *Annual Review of Public Health*, 20: 55–66.

Glover, J., & Tennant, S. (1999) *A Social Health Atlas of Australia, Volume 4: Queensland.* Public Health Information Development Unit: Canberra.

Hermeston, W.A. (2005) Telling You Our Story: How Apology and Action Relate to Health and Social Problems in Aboriginal and Torres Strait Islander Communities. *Medical Journal of Australia*, 183(9): 479–81.

Higgs, Z.R., & Gustafson, D.D. (1985) *Community as a Client: Assessment and Diagnosis.* F.A. Davis: Philadelphia.

Hodgens, H. (2005) *How Does the Built Environment Affect Your Health?—Planning for Changes.* Report on HSV Public Lecture given by Stephanie Knox, Social and Strategic Planner, 28 April, Balwyn Library. home.vicnet.net.au/~humanist/whatsnew/meetings/lectures/april2005lecture.html Access date: 3/10/2007.

Huff, R.M., & Kline, M.V. (1999) *Promoting Health in Multicultural Populations: A Handbook for Practitioners.* Sage Publications: Thousand Oaks.

Hugo, G. (2002) Australia's Changing Non-metropolitan Population. In: D. Wilkinson & I. Blue (eds), *The New Rural Health*, 12–43. Oxford University Press: Melbourne.

International Wellbeing Group (2006) *Personal Wellbeing Index*, 4th edn. Australian Centre on Quality of Life, Deakin University: Melbourne. www.deakin.edu.au/research/acqol/instruments/wellbeing_index.htm Access date: 27/05/2007.

Jirojwong, S., & Manderson, L. (1999) Physical Health, Life Styles and Preventive Health Behaviours: What are Implications for Health Care for Immigrants? In:

P. Liamputtong Rice (ed.), *Living in a New Country: Understanding Migrants' Health*, 79–102. Ausmed Publications: Melbourne.

Jirojwong, S., & Manderson L. (2002) Physical Health and Preventive Health Behaviours among Thai Women in Urban Australia. *Health Care for Women International*, 23: 197–206.

Jirojwong, S., Prior, J., & Wowan/Dululu Community Volunteer Group (2005) Chronic Illnesses in Queensland Rural and Remote Communities Using Two Sampling Units. *Southeast Asian Journal of Tropical Medicine & Public Health*, 36(5): 1275–82.

Jones, K. (2003) *Health and Human Behaviour*. Oxford University Press: Melbourne.

Kelaher M., Gillespie A., Allotey P., Manderson L., Potts H., Sheldrake M., & Young M. (1998) *The Impact of Culture and Ethnicity on Cervical Screening in Queensland: Final Report* (manuscript). Tropical Health Program, Australian Centre for International and Tropical Health and Nutrition, University of Queensland: Brisbane.

Keleher, H. (2007) Population Health Issues in Australia. In: W. St John, & H. Keleher (eds), *Community Nursing Practice: Theory, Skills and Issues*, 39–58. Allen & Unwin: Crows Nest.

Kickbusch, I. (2003) The Contribution of the World Health Organization to the New Public Health and Health Promotion. *American Journal of Public Health*, 93(3): 383–7.

Kindig, D., & Stoddart, G. (2003) What is Population Health? *American Journal of Public Health*, 93(3): 380–2.

Kleinman, A. (1980) *Patients and Healers in the Context of Culture*. University of California Press: Berkeley.

Korda, R.J., Butler, J.R.G., Clements, M.S., & Kunitz, S.J. (2007) Differential Impacts of Health Care in Australia: Trend Analysis of Socioeconomic Inequalities in Avoidable Mortality. *International Journal of Epidemiology*, 36(1): 157–65.

Kwok, C., & Sullivan, G. (2007) The Concepts of Health and Preventive Health Practices of Chinese Australian Women in Relation to Cancer Screening. *Journal of Transcultural Nursing*, 18(2): 118–26.

Landrine, H., & Klonoff, E.A. (1992) Culture and Health-related Schemas: A Review and Proposal for Interdisciplinary Integration. *Health Psychology*, 11: 267–76.

Le Fanu, J. (1999) *The Rise and Fall of Modern Medicine*. Abacus: London.

Liamputtong, P., Lin, V., & Bagley, P. (2003) Living in a Different Place at a Different Time: Health Policy and Australian Ethnic Communities. In: P. Liamputtong & H. Gardner (eds), *Health, Social Change and Communities*, 257–81. Oxford University Press: Melbourne.

Liamputtong Rice, P. (1999) Multiculturalism and the Health of Immigrants: What Public Health Issues Do Immigrants Face when They Move to a New Country?

In: P. Liamputtong Rice (ed.), *Living in a New Country: Understanding Migrants' Health*, 1–21. Ausmed Publications: Melbourne.

MacLennan, R., Green, A., Martin, N., & McLeod, R. (1992) Increasing Incidence of Cutaneous Melanoma in Queensland. *Journal of the National Cancer Institute*, 84: 1427–32.

MacLennan, R., Kelly, J., & Martin, N.G. (1999) Melanocytic Naevi in Eastern Australia: Latitude Is Important but Most Variation Is within Cities. *Australasian Journal of Dermatology*, 40(3): 167.

Marmot, M., & Syme, S. (1976) Acculturation and Coronary Heart Disease in Japanese-Americans. *American Journal of Epidemiology*, 14: 225–47.

McDermott, L., Russell, A., & Dobson, A. (2002) *Cigarette Smoking among Women in Australia*. Commonwealth Department of Health and Ageing: Canberra.

McQueen, D., Nutbeam, D., Hawe, P., Speller, V., Waters, E., & Mercer, S. (2007) *Health Promotion Effectiveness*. Panel Discussion, 11 June 2007, 19th International Union for Health Promotion and Education (IUHPE) World Conference on Health Promotion & Health Education, 10–15 June 2007. IUHPE: Vancouver.

Milio, N. (1983) Commentary: Next Steps in Community Health Policy: Matching Rhetoric and Reality. *Community Health Studies*, 7(2): 185–92.

Modeste, N.N., & Tamayose, T.S. (2004) *Dictionary of Public Health Promotion and Education: Terms and Concepts*. Jossey-Bass: San Francisco.

Mohsin M., Bauman A.E., & Jalaludin, B. (2006) The Influence of Antenatal and Maternal Factors on Stillbirths and Neonatal Deaths in New South Wales, Australia. *Journal of Biosocial Science*, 38(5): 643–57.

National Health and Medical Research Council (2007) *Index of /Publications/Synopses*. www.nhmrc.gov.au/publications/synopses/ Access date: 4/10/2007.

Rissel C., Lesjak M., & Ward J. (1998) Cardiovascular Risk Factors among Arabic-speaking Patients Attending Arabic-speaking General Practitioners in Sydney, Australia: Opportunities for Intervention. *Ethnicity & Health*, 3(3): 213–22.

Rootman, I., Frank, J., Matlin, S., Martinez, R., & Mittelmark, M. (2007) *Knowledge Translation: Linking Research and Policy*. Panel Discussion, 12 June 2007, 19th International Union for Health Promotion and Education (IUHPE) World Conference on Health Promotion & Health Education, 10–15 June 2007. IUHPE: Vancouver.

Ross, N.A. (2004) *What Have We Learned Studying Income Inequality and Population Health?* Department of Geography, McGill University: Ontario.

Schwartz, S., Susser, E., & Susser, M. (1999) A Future for Epidemiology. *Annual Review of Public Health*, 20: 15–33.

Syme, S., Hyman, M., & Enterline, P. (1965) Cultural Mobility and the Occurrence of Coronary Heart Disease. *Journal of Health and Human Behaviour*, 6: 178–89.

Turrell, G., Oldenberg, B., McGuffog, I., & Dent, R. (1999) *Socioeconomic Determinants of Health: Towards a National Program and a Policy and Intervention Agenda.* Queensland University of Technology, School of Public Health, Ausinfo: Canberra.

Vindigni, D.R., Parkinson, L., Blunden, S., Perkins, J., Rivett, D.A., & Walker, B.F. (2004) *Aboriginal Health in Aboriginal Hands: Development, Delivery and Evaluation of a Training Programme for Aboriginal Health Workers to Promote Musculoskeletal Health of Indigenous People Living in Rural Community (Rural and Remote Health, 281).* www.rrh.org.au. Access date: 4/10/2007.

Wahlqvist, M.L. (2002) Asian Migration to Australia: Food and Health Consequences. *Asia Pacific Journal of Clinical Nutrition,* 11 (Suppl. 3): S562–8.

Wilkinson, R., & Marmot, M. (eds) (2003) *Social Determinants of Health: The Solid Facts,* 2nd edn. World Health Organization: Geneva.

World Health Organization (WHO) (1946) *Preamble to the Constitution of the World Health Organization.* As adopted by the International Health Conference, New York, 19–22 June 1946, and entered into force on 1948. World Health Organization: Geneva.

World Health Organization (1978) *Alma-Ata 1978: Primary Health Care.* World Health Organization: Geneva.

World Health Organization (1986) *Ottawa Charter for Health Promotion.* World Health Organization: Geneva.

World Health Organization (1998) *Draft Amendments to the Constitution of the World Health Organization.* Executive Board 101st Session, 19–27 January 1998 (EB101/1998/REC/2, Summary Record). World Health Organization: Geneva.

World Health Organization (1999) *Health 21: The Health for All Policy Framework for the WHO European Region.* World Health Organization Regional Office for Europe: Copenhagen.

World Health Organization (2004) *The World Health Report 2003: Shaping the Future.* World Health Organization: Geneva. www.who.int/whr/2003/en/Annex4-en.pdf Access date: 4/10/2007.

Chapter 2

Alliance for Healthy Cities (2007) *Alliance for Healthy Cities.* www.alliance-healthycities.com/ Access date: 6/11/07.

Ashton, J. (1992a) The Origin of Healthy Cities. In: J. Ashton (ed.), *Healthy Cities,* 1–14. Open University Press: Milton Keynes.

Ashton, J. (1992b) Preface and Acknowledgements. In: J. Ashton (ed.), *Healthy Cities,* xiii–xiv. Open University Press: Milton Keynes.

Australian Institute of Health and Welfare (AIHW) (2002) *Older Australia at a Glance 2002,* AIHW Cat. No. AGE 25. Australian Institute of Health and Welfare & Department of Health and Ageing: Canberra.

Australian Institute of Health and Welfare (AIHW) (2005) *Australia's Welfare 2005*, AIHW cat. no. AUS65. Australian Institute of Health and Welfare: Canberra.

Australian Institute of Health and Welfare (2004a) *Longitudinal Studies of Ageing: Implications for Future Studies*, AIHW cat. no. 42. Australian Institute of Health and Welfare: Canberra.

Australian Institute of Health and Welfare (2004b) Diversity among Older Australians in Capital Cities 1996–2011. *Bulletin* issue 18.

Australian Institute of Health and Welfare (2006) *Australia's Health 2006*, AIHW cat. no. AUS 73. Australian Institute of Health and Welfare: Canberra.

Baibach, E.W., Rothschild, M.L., Novelli, W.D. (2002) Social Marketing, In: K. Glanz, B.K. Rimer & F.M. Lewis (eds), *Health Behavior and Health Education: Theory, Research and Practice*, 437–461. Wiley: San Francisco.

Bartholomew, L.K., Parcel, G.S., Kok, G., & Gottlieb, N.H. (eds) (2006) *Planning Health Promotion Programs*. Wiley: San Francisco.

Berkman, L.F., & Kawachi, I. (eds) (2000) *Social Epidemiology*. Oxford University Press: New York.

Bronfenbrenner, U. (1979) *The Ecology of Human Development*. Harvard University Press: Cambridge, Massachusetts.

Catford, J. (2007) Ottawa 1986: The Fulcrum of Global Health Development. *Promotion & Education*, Supplement 2: 6.

Chen, L.C., Kleinman, A., & Ware, N.C. (eds) (1992) *Advancing Health in Developing Countries: The Role of Social Research*. Auburn House: New York.

Cummins, R.A., & Hughes, J. (2007) *Special Report: The Wellbeing of Australians—Carer Health and Wellbeing*. Australian Centre on Quality of Life, Deakin University: Melbourne. www.deakin.edu.au/research/acqol/index_wellbeing/index.htm Access date: 4/11/07.

Department of Health and Ageing (2006) *Australian Better Health Initiative: Promoting Good Health, Prevention and Early Intervention*. www.aodgp.gov.au/internet/wcms/publishing.nsf/content/feb2006coag03.htm Access date: 22/4/07.

Department of Health and Ageing (2007) *Health Priorities*. www.health.gov.au/internet/wcms/publishing.nsf/Content/pq-ncds Access date: 10/10/07.

Department of Health & Human Services (USA) (2005) *A Systematic Approach to Health Improvement, Healthy People 2010*. www.healthypeople.gov/document/html/uih/uih_2htm Access date: 29/10/07.

Department of Health and Social Security (United Kingdom) (1976) Prevention and Health: Everybody's Business. Discussion document: HMSO. Cited in M. Fitzpatrick (2001) *The Tyranny of Health: Doctors and the Regulation of Lifestyle*. Routledge: London.

Department of Human Services, Victoria (2002) *Health Promoting Health Services—Hume Region 2002 Forum*. www.Health.vic.gov.au/healthpromotion/environ_settings/hume_reg2002_forum.htm Access date: 6/11/07.

Duckett, S.J. (2007) *The Australian Health Care System*. Oxford University Press: Melbourne.

Finnegan, J.R., & Viswanath, K. (2002) Communication Theory and Health Behaviour Change: The Media Studies Framework. In: K. Glanz, B.K. Rimer, & F.M. Lewis (eds), *Health Behavior and Health Education: Theory, Research and Practice*, 361–88. Wiley: San Francisco.

Flauhault, D., & Roemer, M.I. (1986) *Leadership for Primary Health Care, Public Health Papers 82*. World Health Organization: Geneva.

Frankish, C.J., Lovato, C.Y., & Shannon, W.J. (1999) Models, Theories, and Principles of Health Promotion with Multicultural Populations. In: R.M. Huff, & M.V. Kline (eds), *Promoting Health in Multicultural Populations: A Handbook for Practitioners*, 41–72. Sage Publications: Thousand Oaks.

Germov, J. (2005) Theorising Health: Major Theoretical Perspectives in Health Sociology. In: J. Germov (ed.), *Second Opinion: An Introduction to Health Sociology*, 28–50. Oxford University Press: Melbourne.

Goldstein, G. (1992) Foreword. In: J. Ashton (ed.), *Healthy Cities*, xi–xii. Open University Press: Milton Keynes.

Gottschalk, J., & Baker, S.S. (2004) Primary Health Care. In: E.T. Anderson, & J. McFarlane (eds), *Community as Partner: Theory and Practice in Nursing*, 3–27. Lippincott Williams & Wilkins: Philadelphia.

Harpham, T., Burton, S., & Blue, I. (2001) Healthy City Projects in Developing Countries: The First Evaluation. *Health Promotion International*, 16(2): 111–25.

Heaney, C.A., & Israel, B.A. (2002) Social Network and Social Support. In: K. Glanz, B.K. Rimer, & F.M. Lewis (eds), *Health Behavior and Health Education: Theory, Research and Practice*, 185–209. Wiley: San Francisco.

Hills, M., & McQueen, D.V. (2007) At Issue: Two Decades of the Ottawa Charter. *Promotion and Education*, Supplement 2: 5.

Hodge, A.M., English, D.R., O'Dea, K., & Giles, G. (2004) Increased Diabetes Incidence in Greek and Italian Migrants to Australia: How Much can be Explained by Known Risk Factors? *Diabetes Care*, 27(10): 2330–4.

Kaplan, L. (1992) Healthy Cities in Australia. In: J. Ashton (ed.), *Healthy Cities*, 57–63. Open University Press: Milton Keynes.

Kegler, M.C., Crosby, R.A., & DiClemente, R.J. (2002) Reflections on Emerging Theories in Health Promotion Practice. In: R.J. DiClemente, R.A. Crosby, & M.C. Kegler (eds), *Emerging Theories in Health Promotion Practice and Research: Strategies for Improving Public Health*, 386–96. Wiley: San Francisco.

Kickbusch, I. (2007) The Move towards a New Public Health. *Promotion and Education*, Supplement 2: 9.

Lalonde, M. (1974) *A New Perspective on the Health of Canadians.* Ministry of Supply and Services: Ottawa.

Le Fanu, J. (1999) *The Rise and Fall of Modern Medicine.* Abacus: London.

Malcolm, L. (1994) Primary Health Care and the Hospital: Incompatible Organizational Concepts? *Social Science & Medicine*, 39: 455–8.

Marmot, M., & Wilkinson, R.G. (eds) (1999) *Social Determinants of Health.* Oxford University Press: New York.

McDermott, L., Russell, A., & Dobson, A. (2002) *Cigarette Smoking among Women in Australia.* Department of Health and Ageing: Canberra.

McKeown, T. (1979) *The Role of Medicine: Dream, Mirage or Nemesis.* Blackwell: Oxford.

McLeroy, K.R., Bibeau, D., Steckler, A., & Glanz, K. (1988) An Ecological Perspective on Health Promotion Programs. *Health Education Quarterly*, 15: 351–77.

Mir, N.S. (1998) Health Promotion in South East Asia. *Health Millions*, 24(4): 10–11.

Modeste, N.N., & Tamayose, T.S. (2004) *Dictionary of Public Health Promotion and Education: Terms and Concepts.* Jossey-Bass: San Francisco.

Montaño, D.E. Kasprzyk, D. (2002) The Theory of Reasoned Action and the Theory of Planned Behavior. In: K. Glanz, B.K. Rimer, & F.M. Lewis (eds), *Health Behavior and Health Education: Theory, Research and Practice*, 67–98. Wiley: San Francisco.

Moodie, R., & Hulme, A. (eds) (2004) *Hands on Health Promotion.* IP Communications: East Hawthorn.

National Public Health Partnership (2002) *Report: The Role of Local Government in Public Health Regulation.* National Public Health Partnership: South Melbourne.

Owen, N., Fotheringham, M.J., & Marcus, B.H. (2002) Communication Technology and Health Behavior Change. In: K. Glanz, B.K. Rimer, & F.M. Lewis (eds), *Health Behavior and Health Education: Theory, Research and Practice*, 510–29. Wiley: San Francisco.

Pender, N. (1996) Health Promotion in Nursing Practice. Cited in F.A. Maurer, & C.M. Smith (eds), *Community/Public Health Nursing Practice: Health for Families and Populations.* Elsevier Saunders: St Louis.

Prochaska, J.O., Redding, C.A., & Evers, K.E. (2002) The Transtheoretical Model and Stages of Change. In: K. Glanz, B.K. Rimer, & F.M. Lewis (eds), *Health Behavior and Health Education: Theory, Research and Practice*, 99–120. Wiley: San Francisco.

Richard, L., Potvin, L., Kishchuk, N., Prlic, H., & Green, L.W. (1996) Assessment of the Integration of the Ecological Approach in Health Promotion Programs. *American Journal of Health Promotion*, 10(4): 318–28.

Rockhampton—60 and Better Program (2007) *Rockhampton—60 and Better.* www.60betterrok.org.au/index.htm Access date: 6/11/07.

Rosenstock, I.M. (1974) The Health Belief Model and Preventive Health Behaviour. *Health Education Monographs*, 2(4): 354–86.

Rothschild, M.L. (1999) Carrots, Sticks, and Promises: A Conceptual Framework for the Management of Public Health and Social Issue Behaviours. *Journal of Marketing*, 63: 24–37.

Sallis, J.F., & Owen, N. (2002) Ecological Model of Health Behavior. In: K. Glanz, B.K. Rimer, & F.M. Lewis (eds), *Health Behavior and Health Education: Theory, Research and Practice*, 462–84. Wiley: San Francisco.

Sheykhi, M.T. (2007) Ageing and Quality of Life in Asia and Europe: A Comparative Sociological Appraisal. In: H. Mollenkopf, & A. Walker (eds), *Quality of Life in Old Age: International and Multi-Disciplinary Perspectives*, 167–78. Springer: Dordrecht.

University of the Third Age, Adelaide, Inc. (2007) *The Growth of U3A's in Australia.* www.adelaideu3a.mx.com.au/U3AGrowth.html Access date: 6/11/07.

Tsouros, A.D., Dowding, G., Thompson, J., & Dooris, M. (eds) (1998) *Health Promoting Universities: Concept, Experience and Framework for Action.* World Health Organization Regional Office for Europe: Copenhagen.

Tsuji, I., Minami, Y., Fukao, A., Hisamichi, S., Asano, H., & Sato, M. (1995) Active Life Expectancy among Elderly Japanese. *Journal of Gerontology*, 50(3): M173–6.

Turrell, G., Oldenburg, B., McGufog, I., & Dent, R. (1999) *Socioeconomic Determinants of Health: Towards a National Research Program and Policy an Intervention Agenda.* Queensland University of Technology, School of Public Health, Ausinfo: Canberra.

Wass, A. (2000) *Promoting Health: The Primary Health Care Approach.* Harcourt Saunders: Sydney.

World Health Organization (WHO) (1978) *Alma-Ata 1978: Primary Health Care.* World Health Organization: Geneva.

World Health Organization (1986) *Ottawa Charter for Health Promotion.* World Health Organization: Geneva.

World Health Organization (1999a) *Health21: Health for All in the 21st century: An Introduction.* World Health Organization Regional Office for Europe: Copenhagen.

World Health Organization (1999b) *Health21: The Health for All Policy Framework for the WHO European Region.* World Health Organization Regional Office for Europe: Copenhagen.

World Health Organization (2007) *Health Promoting Hospitals.* www.euro.who.int/healthpromohosp Access date: 23/10/07.

Chapter 3

Anderson, D.G., & Hatton, D.C. (2000) Accessing Vulnerable Populations for Research. *Western Journal of Nursing Research*, 22(2): 244–51.

Barbour, R. (2007) *Doing Focus Groups*. Sage Publications: London.

Beebe, J. (2001) *Rapid Assessment Process: An Introduction*. AltaMira Press: Walnut Creek.

Benoit, C., Jansson, M., Millar, A., & Phillips, R. (2005) Community–Academic Research on Hard-to-Reach Populations: Benefits and Challenges. *Qualitative Health Research*, 15(2): 263–82.

Berkowitz, S. (1996). Using Qualitative and Mixed Method Approaches. In: R. Reviere, S. Berkowitz, C.C. Carter, & C.G. Ferguson (eds), *Needs Assessment: A Creative and Practical Guide for Social Scientists*, 53–70. Taylor & Francis: Washington DC.

Birman, D. (2005) Ethical Issues in Research with Immigrants and Refugees. In: J.E. Trimble, & C.B. Fisher (eds), *Handbook of Ethical Research with Ethnocultural Populations and Communities*, 155–77. Sage Publications: Thousand Oaks.

Bosworth, T.W. (1999) *Community Health Needs Assessment: The Healthcare Professional's Guide to Evaluating the Needs in Your Defined Market*. McGraw-Hill: New York.

Bowie, C., Richardson, A., & Sykes, W. (1995) Consulting the Public About Health Care. *British Medical Journal*, 311: 1155–8.

Bradshaw, J. (1972) The Concept of Social Need. *New Society*, 30: 640–3.

Bradshaw, J. (1994) The Conceptualization and Measurement of Need: A Social Policy Perspective. In: J. Popay & G. Williams (eds), *Researching the People's Health*, 45–57. Routledge: London.

Brooks, C., Poudrier, J., & Thomas-MacLean, R. (in press). Creating Collaborative Visions with Aboriginal Women: A Photovoice Project. In Liamputtong, P. (ed.), *Doing Cross-Cultural Research: Ethnical and Methodological Considerations*. Springer: Dordrecht.

Colucci, E. (2007). 'Focus Groups Can Be Fun': The Use of Activity-Oriented Questions in Focus Group Discussions. *Qualitative Health Research*, 17(10): 1422–33.

Delbecq, A.L., Van de Ven, A.H., & Gustafson, D.H. (1975) *Group Techniques for Program Planning: A Guide to Nominal Group and Delphi Processes*. Scott-Foreman: Glenview.

Denzin, N.K. (1970) *The Research Act: A Theoretical Introduction to Sociological Methods*. Prentice-Hall: Englewood Cliffs.

Duffield, C. (1993) The Delphi Technique: A Comparison of Results Obtained Using Two Expert Panels. *International Journal of Nursing Studies*, 30: 227–37.

Eng, E., & Blanchard, L. (1990) Action-Oriented Community Diagnosis: A Health Education Tool. *International Journal of Community Health Education*, 11(2): 93–100.

Fitch, C., Rhodes, T., Hope, V., Stimson, G.V., & Renton, A. (2002) The Role of Rapid Assessment Methods in Drug Use Epidemiology. *Bulletin on Narcotics*, LIV(1 & 2): 61–72.

Gilmore, G.D., & Campbell, M.D. (1996). *Needs Assessment Strategies for Health Education and Health Promotion*. Brown & Benchmark: Dubuque.

Gilmore, G.D., Campbell, M.D., & Becker, B.L. (1989). *Needs Assessment Strategies for Health Education and Health Promotion*. Brown & Benchmark: Dubuque.

Goldman, K.D., & Schmalz, K.J. (2001) Focus on Focus Groups! *Health Promotion Practice*, 2(1): 14–15.

Hesse-Biber, S.N., & Leavy, L.P. (2005) *The Practice of Qualitative Research*. Sage Publications: Thousand Oaks.

Hodges, B.C., & Videto, D.M. (2005) *Assessment and Planning in Health Programs*. Jones and Bartlett, Boston.

Jackson, C.A., Pitkin, K & Kington, R. (1998) *Evidence-based Decision-making for Community Health Programs*. RAND Corporation: Santa Monica.

Jirojwong, S., Prior, J., & Wowan/Dululu Community Volunteer Group (2005) Chronic Illnesses in Queensland Rural and Remote Communities Using Two Sampling Units. *Southeast Asian Journal of Tropical Medicine & Public Health*, 36(5), 1275–82.

Johnson, J. M. (2002) In-Depth Interviewing. In: J.F. Gubrium & J.A. Holstein (eds), *Handbook of Interview Research: Context & Method*, 103–19. Sage Publications: Thousand Oaks.

Jordan, J., Dowswell, T., Harrison, S., Lilford, R.J. & Mort, M. (1996). Whose Priorities? Listening to Patients and Professionals. In: J. Wright (ed.), *Health Needs Assessment in Practice*, 60–69. BMJ Books: London.

Joseph, J.G., Emmons, C.A., Kessler, R.C., Wortman, C.B., O'Brien, K., Hockev, W.T., & Schaefer, C. (1984) Coping with the Threat of AIDS: An Approach to Psychosocial Assessment. *American Psychologist*, 39:1297–302.

Kellehear, A. (1993) *The Unobtrusive Researcher: A Guide to Methods*. Allen & Unwin: Sydney.

Khan, M.E., & Manderson, L. (1992) Focus Groups in Tropical Diseases Research. *Health Policy and Planning*, 7(1): 56–66.

Kitzinger, J. (1994) Focus Groups: Method or Madness? In: M. Boulton (ed.), *Challenge and Innovation: Methodological Advances in Social Research on HIV/AIDS*, 159–75. Taylor & Francis: London.

Kitzinger, J. (1995) Qualitative Research: Introducing Focus Groups. *British Medical Journal* 311: 299–302.

Krueger, R.A., & Casey, M.A. (2000) *Focus Groups*, 3rd edn. Sage Publications: Thousand Oaks.

Lenaghan, J., New, B., & Mitchell, E. (1996) Setting Priorities: Is There a Role for Citizens' Juries? *British Medical Journal*, 312: 1591–3.

Liamputtong, P. (2007) *Researching the Vulnerable: A Guide to Sensitive Research Methods*. Sage Publications: London.

Liamputtong, P., & Ezzy, D. (2005) *Qualitative Research Methods*, 2nd edn. Oxford University Press: Melbourne.

Liamputtong Rice, P. (1995) Health Research and Ethnic Communities: Reflections on Practices. In: D. Colquhoun, & A. Kellehear (eds), *Health Research in Practice*, vol. 2: *Personal Experiences, Public Issues*, 50–61. Chapman and Hall: London.

Madriz, E.L. (1998) Using Focus Groups with Lower Socioeconomic Status Latina Women. *Qualitative Inquiry*, 4(1): 114–29.

Manderson, L. (1998) Applying Medical Anthropology in the Context of Infectious Disease. *Tropical Medicine and International Health*, 3(12): 1020–7.

Marie Stopes International Australia (2005) *Photovoice: Sexual health through the eyes of Indigenous Youth*. Marie Stopes International Australia: Melbourne.

Ministry of Health, New Zealand (2000) *Health Needs Assessment for New Zealand: An Overview and Guide*. Ministry of Health: New Zealand. www.moh.govt.nz Access date: 11/6/2007.

Ministry of Public Works and Government Services Canada (2000) *Community Health Needs Assessment: A Guide for First Nations and Inuit Health Authorities*. Health Canada: Ottawa.

Minkler, M., & Wallerstein, N. (eds) (2003) *Community-Based Participatory Research in Health*. Jossey-Bass: San Francisco.

Morgan, D.L. (1988) *Focus Group as Qualitative Research*. Sage Publications: Newbury Park.

Murray, S., & Graham, C. (1995) Practice Based Health Needs Assessment: Use of Four Methods in a Small Neighbourhood. *British Medical Journal*, 310: 1443–8.

Needle, R.H., Trotter, R.T., Singer, M., Bates, C., Page, B., Metzger, D., & Marcelin, L.H. (2003) Rapid Assessment of the HIV/AIDS Crisis in Racial and Ethnic Communities: An Approach for Timely Community Interventions. *American Journal of Public Health*, 93(6): 970–9.

Nicholson, P., & Burr, J. (2003) What is 'Normal' About Women's Hetero Sexual Desire and Orgasm?: A Report of An In-Depth Interview Study. *Social Science and Medicine*, 57: 1735–45.

Ong, B.N., & Humphris, G. (1994) Prioritizing Needs with Communities: Rapid Appraisal Methodologies in Health. In: J. Popay & G. Williams (eds), *Researching the People's Health*, 58–82. Routledge: London.

Payne, J. (1999) *Researching Health Needs*. Sage Publications: London.

Pelto, P.J., Bentley, M.E., Bhattacharyya, K., & Jensen, J.L. (1998) *Rapid Assessment Procedures (RAP): Ethnographic Methods to Investigate Women's Health*. International Nutrition Foundation (INF): Boston.

Petersen, D.J., & Alexander, G.R. (2001) *Needs Assessment in Public Health: A Practical Guide for Students and Professionals*. Kluwer Academic/Plenum Publishers: New York.

Piper, D., & Krolik, P. (1991) *A Needs Assessment: St Ives*. Health Promotion Unit, Hornsby Ku-ring-gai Hospital: Hornsby.

Quest, T., & Marco, C.A. (2003) Ethics Seminars: Vulnerable Populations in Emergency Medicine Research. *Academic Emergency Medicine*, 10(11): 1294–8.

Reviere, R., Berkowitz, S., Carter, C.C., & Ferguson, C.G. (1996) *Needs Assessment: A Creative and Practical Guide for Social Scientists*. Taylor & Francis: Washington DC.

Robinson, J., & Elkan, R. (1996). *Health Needs Assessment: Theory and Practice*. Churchill Livingstone: New York.

Sanderowitz, J., Hainsworth, G., & Solter, C. (2003) *A Rapid Assessment of Youth Friendly Reproductive Health Services*. Pathfinder International: Watertown.

Schoenberg, N.E., Hopenhayn, C., Christian, A., Knight, E.A., & Rubio, A. (2005) An In-Depth and Updated Perspective on Determinants of Cervical Cancer Screening among Central Appalachian Women. *Woman & Health*, 42(2): 89–105.

Schweitzer, R., & Steel, Z. (in press) Researching Refugees: Methodological and Ethical Considerations. In Liamputtong, P. (ed.), *Doing Cross-Cultural Research: Ethnical and Methodological Considerations*. Springer: Dordrecht.

Scrimshaw, N.V., & Gleason, G.R. (1992) *Rapid Assessment Procedures: Qualitative Methodologies for Planning and Evaluation of Health Related Programs*. International Nutrition Foundation: Boston.

Sharpe, P.A., Greany, M.L., Lee, P.R., & Royce, S.W. (2000) Assets-Oriented Community Assessment. *Public Health Reports*, 113: 205–11.

Simons-Morton, B., Green, L., & Gottleib, N. (1995) *Introduction to Health Education and Health Promotion*, 2nd edn. Waveland: Prospect Heights.

Stewart, D.W., & Shamdasani, P.N. (1990) *Focus Groups: Theory and Practice*. Sage Publications: Newbury Park.

Stimson, G.V., Fitch, C., Rhodes, T., & Ball, A. (1999) Rapid Assessment and Response: Methods for Developing Public Health Responses to Drug Problems. *Drug and Alcohol Review*, 18: 317–25.

Thompson, N.J., & McClintock, H.O. (1998) *Demonstrating Your Program's Worth: A Primer on Evaluation for Programs to Prevent Unintentional Injury*. Centers for Disease Control and Prevention, National Center for Injury Prevention and Control: Atlanta.

Umaña-Taylor, A.J., & Bámaca, M.Y. (2004) Conducting Focus Groups with Latino Populations: Lessons from the Field. *Family Relations*, 53: 261–72.

Wang, C.C. (1999) Photovoice: A Participatory Action Research Strategy Applied to Women's Health. *Journal of Women's Health*, 8(2): 185–92.

Wang, C. & Burris, M.A. (1994) Empowerment through Photo Novella: Portraits of Participation. *Health Education Quarterly*, 21(2): 171–86.

Winslow, W., Honein, W., & Elzubeir, M.A. (2002) Seeking Emirati Women's Voices: The Use of Focus Groups with an Arab Population. *Qualitative Health Research*, 12(4): 566–75.

World Health Organization (WHO) (1978) *Alma-Ata 1978: Primary Health Care*. World Health Organization: Geneva.

World Health Organization (1985) *Targets for Health for All*. World Health Organization Regional Office for Europe: Copenhagen.

World Health Organization (1986) *The Ottawa Charter for Health Promotion*. World Health Organization: Geneva.

World Health Organization (2000) *Reproductive Health during Conflict and Displacement: A Guide for Program Managers*. World Health Organization: Geneva.

Wright, J., Williams, R., & Wilkinson, J. (1998). The Development and Importance of Health Needs Assessment. In : J. Wright (ed.), *Health Needs Assessment in Practice*, 1–11. BMJ Books: London.

Ziglio, E. (1996) The Delphi Method and Its Contribution to Decision-Making. In: M. Adler & E. Ziglio (eds), *Gazing into the Oracle: The Delphi Method and its Application to Social Policy and Public Health*, 3–33. Jessica Kingsley: London.

Chapter 4

Anonymous (2006) A Broader Understanding of Indigenous Health. *Australian Nursing Journal*, 14(4): 25.

Australian Bureau of Statistics (ABS) & Australian Institute of Health and Welfare (AIHW) (2003) *The Health and Welfare of Australia's Aboriginal and Torres Strait Islander Peoples, 2003*. (ABS cat. no. 4704.0, AIHW cat. no. IHW11). Australian Bureau of Statistics: Canberra.

Australian Bureau of Statistics & Australian Institute of Health and Welfare (2005) *The Health and Welfare of Australia's Aboriginal and Torres Strait Islander Peoples, 2005*. (ABS cat. no. 4704.0, AIHW cat. no. IHW14). Australian Bureau of Statistics: Canberra.

Australian Bureau of Statistics (2007) *Population Distribution, Aboriginal and Torres Strait Islander Australians, 2006*. www.abs.gov.au/AUSSTATS/abs@.nsf/Lookup/4705.0 Main+Features12006?OpenDocument Access date: 20/10/2007.

Australian Government Culture and Recreation Portal (2007a) *Australian Indigenous Cultural Heritage. Australian Government: Australia*. www.cultureandrecreation.gov.au/articles/indigenous/ Access date: 5/11/2007.

Australian Government Culture and Recreation Portal (2007b) *European Discovery and the Colonisation of Australia.* www.cultureandrecreation.gov.au/articles/australianhistory/ Access date: 4/10/2007.

Australian Indigenous Health *Infonet* (2007) *Mortality.* www.healthinfonet.ecu.edu.au/html/html_overviews/overviews_our_mortality.htm Access date: 5/11/2007.

Australian Indigenous Health Promotion Network (2006) *Australian Indigenous Health Promotion Network Workshop: Working Towards an Indigenous Model of Health Promotion.* Australian Indigenous Health Promotion Network: Sydney.

Australian Institute of Health and Welfare (AIHW) (2003) *National Health Data Dictionary.* Australian Institute of Health and Welfare: Canberra.

Brough M., Bond C., & Hunt J. (2004) Strong in the City: Towards a Strengths Based Approach in Indigenous Health Promotion. *Health Promotion Journal of Australia*, 15(3): 215–20.

Campbell, D., Wunungmurra, P., & Nyomba, H. (2007) Starting where the People Are: Lessons on Community Development from a Remote Aboriginal Australian Setting. *Community Development Journal,* 42(2): 151–66.

Collaborative Centre for Aboriginal Health Promotion (2006) www.ccahp.org.au/ Access 13/3/08.

Davis, B., McGrath, N., Knight, S., Davis, S., Norval, M., Freelander, G., & Hudson L. (2004) Aminina Nud Mulumuluna ('You gotta look after yourself'): Evaluation of the Use of Traditional Art in Health Promotion for Aboriginal People in the Kimberley Region of Western Australia. *Australian Psychologist*, 39(2): 107–13.

Gray, D., Sputore, B., & Walker, J. (1998) Evaluation of an Aboriginal Health Promotion Program: A Case Study from Karalundi. *Health Promotion Journal of Australia,* 8(1): 24–8.

Gray, D., Saggers, S., Sputore, B., & Bourbon, D. (2000) What Works? A Review of Evaluated Alcohol Misuse Interventions among Aboriginal Australians. *Addiction*, 95(1): 11–22.

Human Rights and Equal Opportunity Commission (2006) *Social Justice Report.* www.hreoc.gov.au/Social_Justice/sj_report/index.html#2006. Access date: 10/09/07.

Human Rights and Equal Opportunity Commission (1997) *Bringing Them Home, the Stolen Children Report.* www.hreoc.gov.au/Social_Justice/bth_report/. Access date: 10/09/2007.

Hurst, S., & Nader, P. (2006) Building Community Involvement in Cross-cultural Indigenous Health Programs. *International Journal for Quality in Health Care*, 18(4): 294–8.

Ivers, R. (2003) A Review of Tobacco Interventions for Indigenous Australians. *Australian and New Zealand Journal of Public Health*, 27(3): 294–9.

Jackson, N., & Waters, E. (2005) For the Guidelines for Systematic Reviews in Health Promotion and Public Health Taskforce: Criteria for the Systematic Review of Health Promotion and Public Health Interventions. *Health Promotion International*, 20(4): 367–74.

Johnston, F., Beecham, R., Dalgleish, P., MalpraBurr, T., & Gamarania, G. (1998) The Maningrida 'Be Smoke Free' Project. *Health Promotion Journal of Australia*, 8(1): 12–17.

Kelly, K, & Lenthall, S. (1997) *An Introduction to Recent Aboriginal and Torres Strait Islander History in Queensland*. Rural Health Training Centre, Queensland Health: Queensland.

Laverack, G., & Labonte, R., (2000) A Planning Framework for Community Empowerment Goals within Health Promotion. *Health Policy and Planning*, 15(3): 255–62.

Manne, R. (2007) Pearson's Gamble, Stanner's Dream: The Past and Future of Remote Australia. *The Monthly* No. 26, August 2007.

Marmot, M. (2005) Social Determinants of Health Inequalities. *Lancet*, 365(9464): 1099–104.

Marmot, M. (2006) Harveian Oration: Health in an unequal world. *Lancet*, 368(9552): 2081–95.

McLennan, V., & Khavarpour, F. (2004) Culturally Appropriate Health Promotion: Its Meaning and Application in Aboriginal Communities. *Health Promotion Journal of Australia*, 15(3): 237–9.

Mikhailovich, K., Morrison, P., & Arabena, K. (2007) Evaluating Australian Indigenous Community Health Promotion Initiatives: A Selective Review. *Rural and Remote Health 7* (online), No. 746. Available from: www.rrh.org.au.

Mitchell, J. (2007) History. In: Carson, B., Dunbar, T., Chenhall, R., & Bailie, R., (eds), *Social Determinants of Indigenous Health*, 41–64. Allen & Unwin: Crows Nest.

National Aboriginal Community Controlled Health Organisation (2006) *About NACCHO*. www.naccho.org.au Access date: 2/3/2007.

National Aboriginal Health Strategy Working Party (1989). *National Health Strategy*. Department of Aboriginal Affairs: Canberra.

National Health and Medical Research Council (NH&MRC) (1995) *Health Australia: Promoting Health in Australia*. Discussion Paper. National Health and Medical Research Council: Canberra.

National Health and Medical Research Council (1997) *Promoting the Health of Aboriginal and Torres Strait Islander Communities: Case Studies and Principles of Good Practice*. National Health and Medical Research Council: Canberra.

National Health and Medical Research Council (2002) *The NH&MRC Road Map: A Strategic Framework for Improving Aboriginal and Torres Strait Islander Health Through*

Research. www.nhmrc.gov.au/publications/synopses/_files/r28.pdf Access date: 20/10/2007.

NSW Health (2002) *Principles for Better Practice in Aboriginal Health Promotion: The Sydney Consensus Statement.* NSW Health: North Sydney.

Office of Indigenous Policy Coordination (2007) Survey of Outstation Resource Centres in the Northern Territory. *The Australian,* 10 August, p. 7.

Oldenburg, B., McGuffog, I. & Turrell, G. (2000). Socioeconomic Determinants of Health in Australia: Policy Responses and Intervention Options. *Medical Journal of Australia,* 172: 489–92.

Pearson, N. (2000). *Our Right to Take Responsibility.* Noel Pearson and Associates: Cairns.

Pearson, N. (2006) *Arthur Mills Oration: Our Vision for the Future of Cape York Peninsula,* 7 May. Congress of the Royal Australasian College of Physicians: Cairns.

Poelina, A., & Perdrisat, I. (2004) *A Report of the Derby, West Kimberley Project: Working with Adolescents to Prevent Domestic Violence.* Attorney-General's Department: Canberra.

Potvin, L., Cargo, M., McComber, A., Delormier, T., & Macaulay, A. (2003) Implementing Participatory Intervention and Research in Communities: Lessons from the Kahnawake Schools Diabetes Prevention Project in Canada. *Social Science & Medicine,* 56(6): 1295–305.

Ring, I., & Wenitong, M. (2007) Interventions to Halt Child Abuse in Aboriginal Communities. *Medical Journal of Australia,* 187(4): 204–5.

Rose, G. (1992) *Strategy of Preventive Medicine.* Oxford University Press: Oxford.

Saggers, S., & Gray, D. (2007) Defining What We Mean. In: Carson, B., Dunbar, T., Chenhall, R., and Bailie, R. (eds), *Social Determinants of Indigenous Health,* 1–20. Allen & Unwin: Crows Nest.

Sanson-Fisher, R., Campbell, E., Perkins, J., Blunden, S., & Davis, B. (2006) Indigenous Health Research: A Critical Review of Outputs over Time. *Medical Journal of Australia,* 184(10): 502–5.

Shannon, C., Canuto C., Young. E., Craig, D., Schluter, P., Kenny, G., & McClure, R. (2001) Injury Prevention in Indigenous Communities: Results of a Two-year Community Development Project. *Health Promotion Journal of Australia,* 12(3): 233–7.

Steering Committee for the Review of Government Service Provision (2005) *Overcoming Indigenous Disadvantage: Key Indicators 2005.* Productivity Commission: Canberra.

Steering Committee for the Review of Government Service Provision (2007) *Overcoming Indigenous Disadvantage: Key Indicators 2007.* Productivity Commission: Canberra.

Swerrisen, H., Duckett S.J., Daly, J., Bergen, K., Marshall, S., Borthwick, C., & Crisp, B.R. (2001) Health Promotion and Evaluation: A Programmatic Approach. *Health Promotion Journal of Australia,* 11(1 Suppl): 1–28.

Tsey, K., Patterson, D., Whiteside, M., Baird, L., & Baird, B. (2002) Indigenous Men Taking their Rightful Place in Society? A Participatory Action Research Process with Yarrabah Men's Health Group. *Australian Journal of Rural Health*, 10(6): 278–84.

Tsey, K., Patterson, D., Whiteside, M., Baird, L., Baird, B, & Tsey, K.A. (2004a) A Micro Analysis of a Participatory Action Research Process with a Rural Aboriginal Men's Health Group. *Australian Journal of Primary Health,* 10(1): 64–71.

Tsey, K., Wenitong, M., McCalman, J., Baird, L., Patterson, D., Baird, B., Whiteside, M., Fagan, R., Cadet-James, Y., & Wilson, A. (2004b) A Participatory Action Research Process with a Rural Indigenous Men's Group: Monitoring and Reinforcing Change. *Australian Journal of Primary Health*, 10(3): 130–6.

Turrell, G., Oldenburg, B., McGuffog, I., Dent, R. (1999) *Socio-economic Determinants of Health: Towards a National Research Program and a Policy and Intervention Agenda*. Queensland University of Technology, School of Public Health, AusInfo: Canberra.

United Nations (1986) *Study of the Problem of Discrimination*. Addenda 1–4. UN Sub-Commission on Prevention of Discrimination and Protection of Minorities. United Nations: New York.

Wallerstein, N. (1992) Powerlessness, Empowerment and Health: Implications for Health Promotion Programs. *American Journal of Health Promotion*, 6(3): 197–205.

Wallerstein, N. (2006) *What is the Evidence on Effectiveness of Empowerment to Improve Health?* Health Evidence Network Report. WHO Regional Office for Europe: Copenhagen. www.euro.who.int/Document/E88086.pdf Access date: 1/2/2006.

Whitehead, M. (1985) *The Concepts and Principles of Equity and Health*. WHO Regional Office for Europe: Copenhagen.

Wilson, T., Condon, J., & Barnes, T. (2007) Northern Territory Indigenous Life Expectancy Improvements, 1967–2004. *Australian and New Zealand Journal of Public Health*, 31(2): 184–8.

Winch, J. (1999) Aboriginal Youth. *New Doctor*, 70: 22–4.

World Health Organization (WHO) (1986) *The Ottawa Charter for Health Promotion*. World Health Organization: Geneva.

Chapter 5

Allotey, P., & Zwi, A. (2007) Population Movements. In: I. Kawachi & S. Wamala (eds), *Globalization and Health*, 1st edn, 340. Oxford University Press: Oxford.

Baum, F. (1999) *The New Public Health: An Australian Perspective*, Oxford University Press: Melbourne.

Bertolote, J., Fleischmann, A., Butchart, A., & Besbelli, N. (2006) Suicide, Suicide Attempts and Pesticides: A Major Hidden Public Health Problem. *Bulletin of the World Health Organization*, 84(4): 260.

Corvalán, C., Hales, S., & McMichael, M. (2005) *Ecosystems and Human Well-Being: Health Synthesis: A Report of the Millenium Ecosystem Assessment.* World Health Organization: Geneva.

Department of Foreign Affairs and Trade (2007). www.dfat.gov.au/ Access date: 26/07/2007.

Environmental Protection Agency (US) (1972) *DDT Ban Takes Effect.* www.epa.gov/history/topics/ddt/01.htm. Access date 24/9/2007.

Frumkin, H. (2003) Agent Orange and Cancer: An Overview for Clinicians. *CA: A Cancer Journal for Clinicians,* 53(4): 245–55.

Goldsworthy, D. (2005) *The Physical and Psycho-Social Consequences of Allergic Responses Attributed to Parthenium Hysterophorus Linn in a Rural Community of Central Queensland.* Paper presented at the Queensland Health and Medical Scientific Meeting. Brisbane.

Hagopian, A., Thompson, M., Fordyce, M., Johnson, K., & Hart, L. (2004) The Migration of Physicians from Sub-Saharan Africa to the United States of America: Measures of the African Brain Drain. *Human Resources for Health,* 2(17). www.human-resources-health.com/content/2/1/17 Access date: 30/11/2007.

Hall, J., & Taylor, R. (2003) Health for All Beyond 2000: The Demise of the Alma-Ata Declaration and Primary Health Care in Developing Countries. *The Medical Journal of Australia,* 178(1). www.mja.com.au/public/issues/178_01_060103/hal10723_fm.html Access date: 16/05/2007.

Hollingsworth, T., Ferguson, N., & Anderson, R. (2007) Frequent Travellers and the Rate of Spread of Disease. *Emerging Infectious Diseases,* 13: 1288–94.

Kawachi, I., & Wamala, S. (2007) *Globalization and Health.* Oxford University Press: New York.

King, L. (2007) The Convergence of Animal and Human Health. Paper presented at the the 2007 Annual Conference on Antimicrobial Resistance, Bethesda, MD.

Kramárová, E., Kogevinas, M., Anh, C.T., Cau, H.D., Dai, L.C., Stellman, S.D., & Parkin, D.M. (1998) Exposure to Agent Orange and Occurrence of Soft-Tissue Sarcomas or Non-Hodgkin Lymphomas: An Ongoing Study in Vietnam. *Environmental Health Perspectives,* April 1998, 106(Suppl. 2): 671–8. www.pubmedcentral.nih.gov:80/articlerender.fcgi?artid=1533419 Access date: 15/3/08.

Lloyd, M. (2003) *The Passport: The History of Man's Most Travelled Document.* Stroud: Sutton.

Macdowall, W., Bonell, C., & Davies, M. (2006) *Health Promotion Practice,* 1st edn. Open University Press: Maidenhead.

MacPherson, W.D., Gushulak, B.D., & Macdonald, L. (2007) Health and Foreign Policy: Influences of Migration and Population Mobility. *Bulletin of the World Health Organization,* 85(3): 200–6.

McCarthy, J., Canziani, O., Leary, N., Dokken, D., & White, K. (2001) *Climate Change 2001: Impacts, Adaptation and Vulnerability.* Intergovernmental Panel on Climate Change. Cambridge University Press: Cambridge.

McMichael, A.J., & Butler, C.D. (2005) *Emerging Health Issues: The Widening Challenge for Population Health Promotion.* 6th Global Conference on Health Promotion: Bangkok.

McMichael, J., Woodruffe, R.E., & Hales, S. (2006) Climate Change and Human Health: Present and Future Risks. *Lancet*, 367: 859–69.

Miller, J., Boyd, H., Cookson, S., Parise, M., Gonzaga, P., Addiss, D., Wilson, M., Nguyen-Dinh, P., Wahlquist, S., Weld, T., Wainwright, R., Gushlak, B., & Cetron, M. (2000) Malaria, Intestinal Parasites and Schistosomiasis among Barawan Somali Refugees Resettling to the United States: A Strategy to Reduce Morbidity and Decrease the Risk of Imported Infections. *American Journal of Tropical Medicine and Hygiene*, 62(1): 115–21.

Moser, M.R., Bender, T.R., Margolis, H.S., Noble, G.R., Kend, A.P., & Ritter, D.G. (1979) An Outbreak of Influenza aboard a Commercial Airliner. *American Journal of Epidemiology*, 110(1): 1–6.

Newton, S. Personal communication, cited in US Department of Health and Human Services Environmental Health Policy Committee Risk Communication and Education Subcommittee, *An Ensemble of Definitions of Environmental Health*, 20 November 1998. http://www.health.gov:80/environment/DefinitionsofEnv Health/ehdef2.htm Access date: 15/3/08.

Olsen, S., Chang, H., Cheung, T., & Tang, A.E.A. (2003) Transmission of the Severe Acute Respiratory Syndrome on Aircraft. *New England Journal of Medicine*, 349(25): 2416.

O'Neill, K., & Meert, J. (2007) *Putting People and Health Needs on the Map.* World Health Organization: Geneva.

Parashar, U., Alexander, M., & Glass, R. (2006). *Prevention of Rotavirus Gastroeneteritis among Infants and Children.* Division of Viral Diseases, National Center for Immunization and Respiratory Diseases: Atlanta.

Paz, J., McGeehin, M., Bernard, S., Ebi, K., Epstein, P., Gramsbsch, A., Gubbler, D., Reiter, P., Romieu, I., Rose, J., Samet, J., & Trtanj, J. (2000). The Potential Health Impacts of Climate Variability and Change for the United States: Executive Summary of the Report of the Health Sector of the US National Assessment. *Environmental Health Perspectives,* 108(4): 367–76.

Prüss-Üstűn, A., & Corvalán, C. (2006) *Preventing Disease through Healthy Environments: Towards an Estimate of the Environmental Burden of Disease.* World Health Organization: Geneva.

Purdy, K., Hay, J., Botteman, M., & Ward, J. (2004) Evaluation of Strategies for Use of Acellular Pertussis Vaccine in Adolescents and Adults: A Cost Benefit Analysis. *Clinical Infectious Diseases,* 39(1): 20–8.

Queensland Health (2007) *Travel Health.* access.health.qld.gov.au/hid/HealthConsumer Information/TravelHealth/index.asp. Access date: 12/07/2007.

Radosavljevic, V., & Jakovljevic, B. (2007) Bio-Terrorism: Types of Epidemics, New Epidemiological Paradigm and Levels of Prevention. *Public Health,* (121): 549–57.

Schnur, A. (2006) SARS in China: Prelude to Pandemic? *Journal of the American Medical Association,* 295: 1712–13.

Select Committee of Sciences and Technology (2000) *Fifth Report—Air Travel and Health.* House of Lords: London.

Travel Information Association (2006) *Travel through the Generations.* Travel Information Association: Sacramento.

Ugalde, A., Selva-Sutter, E., Castillo, C., Paz, C., & Canas, S. (2000) The Health Costs of War: Can They be Measured? Lessons from El Salvador (Conflict and Health). *British Medical Journal,* 321: 7254.

United Nations High Commission for Refugees (2006) *The State of the World's Refugees: Human Displacement in the New Millennium.* Oxford University Press: Oxford.

World Health Organization (WHO) (2005a) *Fifty-ninth World Health Assembly, Resolution WHA59.2: Application of the International Health Regulations.* World Health Organization: Geneva.

World Health Organization (2005b) *Combating Emerging Infectious Diseases in the South-East Asia Region.* World Health Organization: New Delhi.

World Health Organization (2007a) *International Travel and Health,* World Health Organization: Geneva. www.who.int/ith/en Access date: 20/03/07.

World Health Organization (2007b) *World Health Statistics 2007.* World Health Organization: Geneva.

World Health Organization (1978) *Alma-Ata 1978: Primary Health Care.* World Health Organization: Geneva.

World Health Organization (2006) *Weekly Epidemiological Record.* No. 38, 22 September 2006: 358. www.who.int/wer. Access date: 12/08/2007.

Whyatt, R., Camann, D., Kinney, P., & Perera, F. (2002) Residential Pesticide Use during Pregnancy among a Cohort of Urban Minority Women. *Environmental Health,* 110(5): 507–14.

Chapter 6

Adair, J.E. (2005). *The Handbook of Management and Leadership.* Thorogood: London.

Ayler, A.A., Mayer, J., Rafii, R., Housemann, R., Brownson, R., & King, A.C. (1999) Key Informant Surveys as a Tool to Implement and Evaluate Physical Activity Interventions in the Community. *Health Education Research,* 14(2): 289–98.

Bagley, P., Lin, V., Sainsbury, P., Wise, M., Keating, T., & Roger, K. (2007) In What Ways Does the Mandatory Nature of Victoria's Municipal Public Health Planning

Framework Impact on the Planning Process and Outcomes? *Australia and New Zealand Health Policy*, 4(4). www.pubmedcentral.nih.gov/articlerender.fcgi?artid=1851012 Access date: 15/11/2007.

Barrett, K., Greene, R., & Mariani, M. (2004) A Case of Neglect: Why Health Care Is Getting Worse, Even Though Medicine Is Getting Better. *Congressional Quarterly*. www.governing.com/gpp/2004/intro.htm Access date: 15/11/2007.

Bayron, H. (2006) Philippines Medical Brain Drain Leaves Public Health System in Crisis. *VOA News*, 3 May. www.voanews.com/english/archive/2006-05/2006-05-03-voa38.cfm Access date: 15/11/2007.

Berkowitz, B. (2004) Rural Public Health Service Delivery: Promising New Directions. *American Journal of Public Health*, 94(10):1678–81.

Brand, M., Kerby, D., Elledge, B., Johnson, D., & Olga, M. (2006) A Model for Assessing Public Health Emergency Preparedness Competencies and Evaluating Training Based on the Local Preparedness Plan. *Journal of Homeland Security and Emergency Management*, 3(2): 1–19.

Bundred, P.E. & Levitt, C. (2000) Medical Migration: Who Are the Real Losers? *Lancet*, 356(9225): 245–6.

Calhoun, J.G., Rowney, R., Eng, E., & Hoffman, Y. (2005) Competency Mapping and Analysis for Public Health Preparedness Training Initiatives. *Public Health Reports*, 120(S1): 91–9.

Castelloe, P., Watson, T., & White, C. (2002) Participatory Change: An Integrative Approach to Community Practice. *Journal of Community Practice*, 10(4): 7–31.

Center for Health Policy Columbia University School of Nursing & Association of Teachers of Preventive Medicine (2004) *Competency to Curriculum Toolkit: Developing Curricula for Public Health Workers*. www.nursing.hs.columbia.edu/research/ResCenters/chphsr/pdf/toolkit.pdf Access date: 1511/2007.

Chauvin, S.W., Anderson, A.C., & Bowdish, B.E. (2001) Assessing the Professional Development Needs of Public Health Professionals. *Journal of Public Health Management Practice*, 7(4): 23–37.

Corso, L.C., Wiesner, P.J., Halverson, P.K., & Brown, C.K. (2000) Using the Essential Services as a Foundation for Performance Measurement and Assessment of Local Public Health Systems. *Journal of Public Health Management and Practice*, 6(5): 1–18.

Dessel, A., Rogge, M.E., & Garlington, S.B. (2006) Using Intergroup Dialogue to Promote Social Justice and Change. *Social Work*, 51(4): 303–15.

Dougherty, D., & Drumheller, K. (2006) Sensemaking and Emotions in Organizations: Accounting for Emotions in a Rational(ized) Context. *Communication Studies*, 57(2): 215–38.

Dunabin, J., & Levitt, L. (2003) Rural Origins and Rural Medical Exposure: Their Impact on the Rural and Remote Medical Workforce in Australia. *Rural and Remote Health*, 3(1): 212–38.

Dutton, G. (1998) One Workforce, Many Languages. *Management Review*, 87(11): 42–7.

Ellis, I., & Kelly, K. (2005) Health Infrastructure in Very Remote Areas: An Analysis of the CRANA Bush Crisis Line Database. *Australian Journal of Rural Health*, 13(1): 1–2.

Ha-Redeye, O. (2006) *A Bioethical Model for Emergency Medical Response*. 3rd Annual Canadian Risk and Hazards Network Symposium, 11–13 October 2006. Université du Québec à Montréal: Montreal.

Hays, R., Veitch, C., Franklin, L., & Crossland, L. (1998) Methodological Issues in Medical Workforce Analysis: Implications for Regional Australia. *Australian Journal of Rural Health*, 6: 32–5.

Kälvemark, S., Höglund, A.T., Hansson, M.G., Westerholm, P., & Arnetz, B. (2004) Living with Conflicts: Ethical Dilemmas and Moral Distress in the Health Care System. *Social Science and Medicine*, 58(6):1075–84.

Loveridge, K. (2006) Profile of an RN(NP) in Primary Health Care. *SRNA Newsbulletin*, Summer, 8(3): 20.

Kennedy, V.C., & Moore, F.I. (2001) A Systems Approach to Public Health Workforce Development. *Journal of Public Health Management Practice*, 7(4): 17–22.

Kuruvilla, S., & Joseph, A. (1999) Identifying Disability: Comparing House-to-house Survey and Rapid Rural Appraisal. *Health Policy and Planning*, 14(2): 182–90.

Maggie, M., Convery, I., Baxter, J., & Bailey, C. (2005) Psychosocial Effects of the 2001 UK Foot and Mouth Disease Epidemic in a Rural Population: Qualitative Diary Based Study. *British Medical Journal*, 331(7527): 1234–7.

Napoles-Springer, A.M., Santoyo, J., Houston, K., Perez-Stable, E.J., & Stewart, A.L. (2005) Patients' Perceptions of Cultural Factors Affecting the Quality of their Medical Encounters. *Health Expectations*, 8(1): 4–17.

National Association of County & City Health Officials (2008) *Mobilizing for Action through Planning and Partnerships (MAPP)* www.naccho.org/topics/infrastructure/MAPP.cfm Access date: 6/3/2008.

Nelligan, P., Grinspun, D., Jonas-Simpson, C., McConnell, H., Peter, E., Pilkington, B., Balfour, J., Connolly, L., Reid-Haughian, C., & Sherry, K. (2002) Client-Centred Care: Making the Ideal Real. *Hospital Quarterly*, 5(4): 70–6.

Pang, T., Lansang, M.A., & Haines, A. (2002) Brain Drain and Health Professionals. *British Medical Journal*, 324: 499–500. www.bmj.com/cgi/content/full/324/7336/499 Access date: 15/11/2007.

Pellegrino, E.D. (1994) Patient and Physician Autonomy: Conflicting Rights and Obligations in the Physician–Patient Relationship. *Journal of Contemporary Health Law & Policy*, 10: 47–68.

Potter, M.A., Barron, G., & Cioffi, J.P. (2003) A Model for Public Health Workforce Development Using the National Public Health Performance Standards Program. *Journal of Public Health Management and Practice*, 9(3): 199–207.

Reischl, T.M., & Buss, A.N. (2005) Responsive Evaluation of Comptency-based Public Health Preparedness Training Programs. *Journal of Public Health Management and Practice*, 11(6): S100–5.

Robinson, G., d'Abbs, P., Togni, S., & Bailie, R. (2003) Aboriginal Participation in Health Service Delivery: Coordinated Care Trials in the Northern Territory of Australia. *International Journal of Healthcare Technology & Management*, 5(1/2): 45.

Telleen, S., & Simpson, H. (2006) *Identifying Evidence-based Resources in Public Health*, Skills Building Session, 5 March 2006, Association of Maternal and Child Health Programs Annual Conference. http://nnlm.gov/ner/training/material/ebph2006_class.ppt Access date: 17/3/08.

Schofield, D.J., Page, S.L., Lyle, D.M., & Walker, T.J. (2006) Ageing of the Baby Boomer Generation: How Demographic Change Will Impact on City and Rural GP and Nursing Workforce. *Rural and Remote Health*, 6 (online): 604. www.rrh.org.au/articles/subviewnew.asp?ArticleID=604 Access date: 14/11/2007.

Slack, M.K., Cummings, D.M., Borrego, M.E., Fuller, K., & Cook, S. (2002) Strategies Used by Interdisciplinary Rural Health Training Programs to Assure Community Responsiveness and Recruit Practitioners. *Journal of Interprofessional Care*, 16(2): 129–38.

Department of Health and Human Services (US) (1997) T*he Public Health Workforce: An Agenda For The 21st Century*. www.health.gov/phfunctions/pubhlth.pdf Access date: 17/11/2007.

Victorian Government Health Information (2006) *Municipal Public Health Planning Framework—Environments for Health*. Department of Public Health, State Government of Victoria. www.health.vic.gov.au/localgov/mphpfr/index.htm Access date: 17/11/2007.

Wakefield, M.A., Wilson, D.H. (1986). Community Organisation for Health Promotion. *Community Health Studies*, 10(4): 444–51.

World Health Organization (WHO) (1999) *Community Participation in Local Health and Sustainable Development: A Working Document on Approaches and Techniques*. European Sustainable Development and Health Series 4. www.health.vic.gov.au/localgov/downloads/who_book4.pdf Access date: 17/11/2007.

Zapf, M.K. (1993) Remote Practice and Culture Shock: Social Workers Moving to Isolated Northern Regions. *Social Work*, 38(6): 694–704.

Chapter 7

Bailey, D.M. (1997) *Research for the Health Professional: A Practical Guide*. Davis: Philadelphia.

Bonita, R., Beaglehole, R., & Kjellström, T. (2006) *Basic Epidemiology*, 2nd edn. World Health Organization: Geneva.

Centeno, C., Arnillas, P., Hernansanz, S., Flores, L.A., Gómez, M., & López-Lara, F. (2000) The Reality of Palliative Care in Spain. *Palliative Medicine*, 14: 387–94.

Freeman, D. (1983) *Margaret Mead and Samoa: The Making and Unmaking of an Anthropological Myth*. Harvard University Press: Boston.

Geitgey, D.A., & Metz, E.M. (1969) A Brief Guide to Designing Research Proposals. *Nursing Research*, 18: 339–44.

Hill, A.B. (1962) *Statistical Methods in Clinical and Preventive Medicine*. Livingstone: Edinburgh.

Liamputtong, P., & Ezzy, D. (2005) *Qualitative Research Methods*, 2nd edn. Oxford University Press: Melbourne.

Marshall, B.J., & Warren, J.R. (1984) Unidentified Curved Bacilli in the Stomach of Patients with Gastritis and Peptic Ulceration. *Lancet*, 1: 1311–15.

Medawar, P.B. (1967) *The Art of the Soluble*. Methuen: London.

Chapter 8

Baum, F. (2008) *The New Public Health*. Oxford University Press: Melbourne.

Department of Health & Ageing (2001) *National Alcohol Strategy: A Plan for Action 2001–2003/04*. Ministerial Council and Drug Strategy, Commonwealth of Australia: Canberra.

Cross, D., Hall, M., & Howat, P. (2003) Using Theory to Guide Practice in Children's Pedestrian Safety Education. *American Journal of Health Education*, 34(5): S42–S47.

Green, L.W., & Kreuter, M.W. (1999) *Health Promotion Planning: An Educational and Ecological Approach*. Mayfield: Mountain View.

Green, L.W., & Kreuter, M.W. (2005) *Health Program Planning: An Educational and Ecological Approach*, 4th edn. McGraw-Hill: New York.

Hawe, P., Degeling, D., & Hall, J. (1990) *Evaluating Health Promotion: A Health Workers Guide*. MacLennan & Petty: Sydney.

Howat, P., Jones, S., Hall, M., Cross, D., & Stevenson, M. (1997) Adaptation of the PRECEDE–PROCEED Framework for Planning a Child Pedestrian Injury Prevention Program. *Injury Prevention*, 3: 282–7.

Howat, P., Maycock, B., Cross, D., Collins, J., Jackson, L., & Burns, S. (2003) Towards a More Unified Definition of Health Promotion. *Health Promotion Journal of Australia*, 14(2): 82–5.

Hubley, J. (2004) *Communicating Health: An Action Guide to Health Education and Health Promotion*. Macmillan: Oxford.

Iredell, H., Howat, P., Shaw, T., James, R., & Granich, J. (2004) Introductory Postcards: Do They Increase Response Rate in a Telephone Survey of Older Persons? *Health Education Research: Theory and Practice*, 19(2): 1–6.

Liamputtong, P. (2006) *Health Research in Cyberspace: Methodological, Practical and Personal Issues*. Nova Science: New York.

Mrazek, P.J., & Haggerty. R.J. (1994) *Reducing Risks for Mental Disorders: Frontiers for Preventive Intervention Research*. National Academy Press: Washington DC.

Naidoo, J., & Wills, J. (2000) *Health Promotion: Foundations for Practice*. Harcourt: London.

O'Connor-Fleming, M., & Parker, E. (eds) (2001) *Health Promotion: Principles and Practice in the Australian Context*, 2nd edn. Allen & Unwin: Crows Nest.

Poland, B.D., Green, L.W., & Rootman, I. (2000) Reflections on Settings for Health Promotion. In: B.D. Poland, L.W. Green, & I. Rootman (eds), *Settings for Health Promotion: Linking Theory and Practice*, 341–51. Sage Publications: Thousand Oaks.

Spence, S.H. (1996). A Case for Prevention. In P. Cotton & H. Jackson (eds), *Early Intervention and Prevention in Mental Health*, 1–19. Australian Psychological Society: Melbourne.

Stevenson, M., Jamrozik, K., & Spittle, J. (1995) A Case-Control Study of Traffic Risk Factors and Child Pedestrian Injuries. *International Journal of Epidemiology*, 24(5): 957–64.

Stevenson, M., Iredell, H., Howat, P., Cross, D., & Hall, M. (1999) Measuring Community/Environmental Interventions: The Child Pedestrian Injury Prevention Project. *Injury Prevention*, 5: 26–30.

Chapter 9

Degeling, P.J., Maxwell, S., Iedema, R., & Hunter, D.J. (2004) Making Clinical Governance Work. *British Medical Journal*, 329: 679–81.

Dwyer, J., Stanton, P., & Thiessen, V. (2004) *Project Management in Health and Community Services*. Allen & Unwin: Crows Nest.

Jirojwong, S., & Savage P. (2003) *The Evaluation of the Community Development Health Strategy 'Owning Our Health Project'*, Report submitted to Wowan/Dululu Community Volunteer Group Inc., Central Queensland University: Rockhampton.

Kouzes, J.M., & Posner, B.Z. (2002) *The Leadership Challenge*, 3rd edn. Jossey-Bass: San Francisco.

Lee, J.-W. (2006) *Working Together for Health: The World Health Report 2006*. World Health Organization: Geneva.

Macfarlane, S., Racelis, M., & Muli-Musiime, F. (2000) Public Health in Developing Countries. *Lancet*, 356: 841–6.

McIntosh, J., & McCormack, D. (2001) Partnerships Identified within Primary Health Literature. *International Journal of Nursing Studies*, 38: 547–55.

McMurray, A. (2007) *Community Health and Wellness: A Sociological Approach*, 3rd edn. Mosby Elsevier: Sydney.

Murray, W.E., & Storey, D. (2003) Political Conflict in Postcolonial Oceania. *Asia Pacific Viewpoint*, 44(3): 213–24.

New Zealand Nurses Organisation (1995) Cultural Safety in Nursing Education: In: *Policy and Standards on Nursing Education*. New Zealand Nurses Organisation: Wellington.

O'Connor-Fleming, M.L., & Parker, E. (eds) (2001) *Health Promotion: Principles and Practice in the Australian Context,* 2nd edn. Allen & Unwin: Crows Nest.

Postlen-Slattery, D., & Foley, K. (2006) Meeting Staff Socialization and Educational Needs for Team Building. In: B.S. Marquis & C.J. Huston (eds), *Leadership Roles and Management Functions in Nursing*, 5th edn, 386–415. Lippincott Williams & Wilkins: Philadelphia.

Scally, G., & Donaldson, L.J. (1998) Clinical Governance and the Drive for Quality Improvement in the New NHS in England. *British Medical Journal*, 317: 61–5.

Smeltzer, C.H. (2006) Career Development. In: B.S. Marquis & C.J. Huston (eds), *Leadership Roles and Management Functions in Nursing*, 5th edn, 245–68. Lippincott Williams & Wilkins: Philadelphia.

Stewart, L. (2006) The Nurse as Consultant. *Royal College of Nursing Australia Connections*, 1: 17–18.

Stewart, L., Hanson, J., & Usher, K. (2006a) Evidence-based Management in Clinical Governance. *Collegian*, 13(4): 12–15.

Stewart, L., Usher, K., Nadakuitavuki, R., & Tollefson, J. (2006b) Developing the Future Nurse Leaders of Fiji. *Australian Journal of Advanced Nursing*, 23(4): 47–51.

Talbot, L., & Verrinder, G. (2005) *Promoting Health: The Primary Health Care Approach*, 3rd edn. Elsevier Churchill Livingstone: Sydney.

Vanu Som, C. (2007) Exploring the Human Resource Implications of Clinical Governance. *Health Policy*, 80: 291–6.

Vincent, C. (2001) *Clinical Risk Management: Enhancing Patient Safety*. BMJ Books: London.

Chapter 10

Chapman, S., & Wakefield, M. (2001) Tobacco Control Advocacy in Australia: Reflections on 30 Years of Progress. *Health Education Behaviour*, 28: 274–89.

Colebatch, H. (1998) *Policy*. Open University Press: Buckingham.

Cowal, S. (2000) *Inequalities in Health: Reflecting Back, Stepping Forward*. Health Promotion Conference, 29 October–1 November, Melbourne.

Gladwell, M. (2000) *The Tipping Point: How Little Things Can Make a Big Difference*. Time Warner: London.

Hawe, P., & Stickney, E.K. (1997) Developing the Effectiveness of an Intersectoral Food Policy Coalition through Formative Evaluation. *Health Education Research*, 12(2): 213–25.

Heyman, S.J. (2000) Health and Social Policy. In: L. Berkman & I. Kawachi (eds), *Social Epidemiology*, 368–82. Oxford University Press: Oxford.

Institute of Medicine (1999) Leading Health Indicators for Healthy People 2010: Second Interim Report. National Academy Press: Washington DC.

Kar, S.B. (2000) *Empowerment of Women for Health and Welfare Systems Development*. Background Paper of International Meeting on Women and Health, 5–7 April, Awaji Island. WHO Kobe Centre: Kobe.

Penrith City Council (2001) *The Penrith Food Project*. www.penrithcity.nsw.gov.au/index.asp?id=360. Access date: 23/03/2007.

Penrith Food Project (1998) *Strategic Intent*. Penrith City Council: Sydney.

Public Interest Advocacy Centre (1996) *Working the System: A Guide for Citizens, Consumers and Committees*. Pluto Press: Sydney.

Wallack, L., & Dorfman, L. (1996) Media Advocacy: A Strategy for Advancing Policy and Promoting Health. *Health Education Quarterly*, 23(3): 293–317.

Wallack, L. (1994) Media Advocacy: A Strategy for Empowering People and Communities. *Journal of Public Health Policy*, 15(4): 420–36.

World Health Organization (WHO) (1986) *Ottawa Charter for Health Promotion*. World Health Organization: Geneva.

World Health Organization (1999) *TB Advocacy: A Practical Guide*. WHO Global Tuberculosis Programme: Geneva.

Yeatman, H. (2003) Food and Nutrition Policy at the Local Level: Key Actors that Influence the Policy Development Process. *Critical Public Health*, 13(2): 125–38.

Chapter 11

Bjaras, G., Haglund, B.J.A., & Rifkin, S. (1991) A New Approach to Community Participation Evaluation. *Health Promotion International*, 6(3): 1999–2206.

Bopp, M., Germann, K., Bopp, J., Littlejohns, L.B., & Smith, N. (2000) *Assessing Community Capacity for Change*. Four Worlds Development: Calgary.

Constantino-David, K. (1995) Community Organising in the Philippines: The Experience of Development NGOs. In: G. Craig & M. Mayo (eds), *A Reader in Participation and Development*, 154–67. Zed Books: London.

Freire, P. (1973) *Education for Critical Consciousness*. Seabury Press: New York.

Gibbon, M., Labonte, R., & Laverack, G. (2002) Evaluating Community Capacity. *Health and Social Care in the Community*, 10(6): 485–91.

Goodman, R., Speers, M., McLeroy, K., Fawcett, S., Kegler, M., Parker, E., Rathgeb Smith, S., Sterling, T., & Wallerstein, N. (1998) Identifying and Defining the Dimensions of Community Capacity to Provide a Base for Measurement. *Health Education and Behaviour*, 25(3): 258–78.

Jones, A., & Laverack, G. (2003) *Building Capable Communities within a Sustainable Livelihoods Approach: Experiences from Central Asia.* www.livelihoods.org/lessons/kyrgyz_SLLPC. Access date: 12/01/2007.

Kumpfer, K., Turner, C., Hopkins, R., & Librett, J. (1993) Leadership and Team Effectiveness in Community Coalitions for the Prevention of Alcohol and Other Drug Abuse. *Health Education Research: Theory and Practice*, 8(3): 359–74.

Labonte, R., & Laverack, G. (2001a) Capacity Building in Health Promotion, Part 1: For Whom? And for What Purpose? *Critical Public Health*, 11(2): 111–27.

Labonte, R., & Laverack, G (2001b) Capacity Building in Health Promotion, Part 2: Whose Use? And with What Measure? *Critical Public Health*, 11(2): 129–38.

Laverack, G. (1999) *Addressing the Contradiction between Discourse and Practice in Health Promotion.* Unpublished PhD Thesis. Deakin University: Melbourne.

Laverack, G. (2000) *Health and Housing Repair in a Rural Community in the Northern Territory of Australia.* Territory Health Services, Operations North: Darwin.

Laverack, G. (2001) An Identification and Interpretation of the Organizational Aspects of Community Empowerment. *Community Development Journal*, 36(2): 40–52.

Laverack, G. (2003) Building Capable Communities: Experiences in a Rural Fijian Context. *Health Promotion International*, 18(2): 99–106.

Laverack, G. (2004) *Health Promotion Practice: Power and Empowerment.* Sage Publications: London.

Laverack, G. (2005) *Public Health: Power, Empowerment & Professional Practice.* Palgrave Macmillan: London.

Laverack, G. (2007a) Building the Capacity of Fijian Communities to Improve Health. Paper submitted to *Journal of Community Health and Clinical Medicine for the Pacific.*

Laverack, G. (2007b) *Health Promotion Practice: Building Empowered Communities.* Open University Press: London.

O'Connor, M., & Parker, E. (1995) *Health Promotion: Principles and Practice in the Australian Context.* Allen & Unwin: St Leonards.

Rifkin, S.B., Muller, F., & Bichmann, W. (1988) Primary Health Care: On Measuring Participation. *Social Science & Medicine*, 9: 931–40.

Rifkin, S.B. (1990) *Community Participation in Maternal and Child Health/Family Planning Programmes.* World Health Organization: Geneva.

Roughan, J.J. (1986) *Village Organization for Development.* Unpublished PhD Dissertation, Department of Political Science, University of Hawaii: Honolulu.

Sustainable Livelihoods for Livestock Producing Communities Project (SLLPC) (2004) *Monitoring and Evaluation Report for December. Sustainable Livelihoods for Livestock Producing Communities.* SLLPC: Bishkek.

Wang, C., Yi, W.K., Tao, Z.W., & Carvano, K. (1998) Photovoice as a Participatory Health Promotion Strategy. *Health Promotion International*, 13(1): 75–86.

World Health Organization (WHO) (1986) *Ottawa Charter for Health Promotion*. World Health Organization: Geneva.

Chapter 12

Anderson, I. (2003) Aboriginal Australians, Governments, and Participation in Health Systems. In: P. Liamputtong & H. Gardner (eds), *Health, Social Change & Communities*, 224–40. Oxford University Press: Melbourne.

Apunipima Cape York Health Council (2006) *Family Wellbeing Facilitators Manual*, Apunipima Cape York Health Council: Cairns.

Behrendt, L. (2003) *Achieving Social Justice*. Federation Press: Annandale.

Boffa, J., George, C., & Tsey, K. (1994) Sex, Alcohol and Violence: A Community Collaborative Action against Strip Tease Shows. *Australian Journal of Public Health*, 18(4): 359–65.

Bruner, J. (1990) *Acts of Meaning*. Harvard University Press: Cambridge, Massachusetts.

Campbell, D., Pyett, P., McCarthy, L., Whiteside, M., & Tsey, K. (2007) Community Development and Empowerment: A Review of Interventions to Improve Aboriginal Health. In: I. Anderson, F. Baum & M. Bentley (eds), *Beyond Bandaids: Exploring the Underlying Social Determinants of Aboriginal Health*, 165–80. Papers from the Social Determinants of Aboriginal Health Workshop, Adelaide, July 2004, Cooperative Research Centre for Aboriginal Health: Darwin.

Campfens, H. (1997) *Community Development around the World: Practice, Theory, Research, Training*. University of Toronto Press: Toronto.

Cape York Institute (2007) From Hand Out to Hand Up. *Cape York Welfare Reform Project*. Cape York Institute: Cairns.

Couzos, S., & Murray, R. (eds) (2003) *Aboriginal Primary Health Care: An Evidence-Based Approach*, 2nd edn. Oxford University Press: Melbourne.

Flyvbjerg, B. (2001) *Making Social Science Matter: Why Social Inquiry Fails and How It Can Succeed Again*. Cambridge University Press: Cambridge.

Ife, J. (2002) *Community Development: Community-Based Alternatives in an Age of Globalisation*. Pearson Education Australia: Frenchs Forest.

Labonte, R. (1993) Community Development and Partnerships. *Canadian Journal of Public Health*, 84: 237–40.

Laverack, G., & Wallerstein, N. (2001) Measuring Community Empowerment: A Fresh Look at Organizational Domains. *Health Promotion International*, 16(2): 179–85.

McCashen, W. (1998). *Our Job Is to Bring Hope*. Handout. St Luke's Innovative Resources: Bendigo.

National Aboriginal Community Controlled Health Organisation (NACCHO) (2006). www.naccho.org.au Access date: 02/03/2008.

Pearson, N. (2000) *Our Right to Take Responsibility*. Noel Pearson Associates: Cairns.

Pearson, N. (2001) *Outline of a Grog and Drugs (and Therefore Violence) Strategy*. Cape York Institute for Policy and Development: Cairns.

Rissel, C. (1994) Empowerment: The Holy Grail of Health Promotion? *Health Promotion International*, 9(1): 39–47.

Scrimgeour, D. (1997) *Community Control of Aboriginal Health Services in the Northern Territory*. Territory Health Services: Darwin.

Short, S., & Tsey, K. (1992) The Economic Rationalisation of Health Policy in Ghana and Australia: A Cross-National Public Policy Analysis. In: *Primary Health Care: Development and Diversity, An International Conference Proceedings*, 103–12, November 1992. University of Sydney Press: Sydney.

Syme, L. (1998) Social and Economic Disparities in Health: Thoughts about Intervention. *Milbank Quarterly*, 76: 493–502.

Tsey, K. (1994a) Black Health: The Third World Myth. *Alice Springs News*, No. 11, 12 May 1994, 1.

Tsey, K. (1994b) Aboriginal Health: How Others Cope. *Alice Springs News*, No. 12, 19 May 1994, 2.

Tsey, K. (1994c) How British Ambition Shaped Two Different Black Destinies: Colonialism and Indigenous Health in Ghana and Australia. *Alice Springs News*, No. 13, 26 May 1994, 2.

Tsey, K. (1994d) Health and Independence: How Effective is Indigenous Self Determination in Ghana and Australia? *Alice Springs News*, No. 14, 3 April 1994, 2.

Tsey, K. (1996) Aboriginal Health Workers: Agents of Change? *Australian and New Zealand Journal of Public Health*, 20(3): 227–9.

Tsey, K. (1997a) Traditional Medicine in Ghana: A Public Policy Analysis. *Social Science and Medicine*, 45(7): 1065–74.

Tsey, K. (1997b) Aboriginal Self-Determination, Education and Health: Towards a More Radical Attitude towards Aboriginal Education. *Australian and New Zealand Journal of Public Health*, 21(1): 77–83.

Tsey, K. (2000) An Innovative Family Support Program By and For Indigenous Australians: Reflections in Evaluation Practice. *Journal of Family Studies*, 6(2): 302–8.

Tsey, K., & Every, A. (2000) Evaluating Aboriginal Empowerment Programs: The Case of Family WellBeing. *Australian and New Zealand Journal of Public Health* 24(5): 509–14.

Tsey, K., Patterson, D., Whiteside, M., Baird, L., & Baird, B. (2002) Indigenous Men Taking their Rightful Place in Society? A Participatory Action Research Process

With Yarrabah Men's Health Group. *Australian Journal of Rural Health*, 10(6): 278–84.

Tsey, K., Travers, H., Gibson, T., Whiteside, M., Cadet-James, Y., Haswell-Elkins, M., McCalman, J., & Wilson, A. (2005a) The Role of Empowerment through Life Skills Development in Building Comprehensive Primary Health Care Systems in Indigenous Australia. *Australian Journal of Primary Care*, 11(2): 16–25.

Tsey, K., Wenitong, M.., McCalman, J., Baird, L., Patterson, D., Baird, B., Whiteside, M., Fagan, R., Cadet-James, Y., Wilson, A. (2004) A Participatory Action Research Process with a Rural Indigenous Men's Group: Monitoring and Reinforcing Change. *Australian Journal of Primary Health*, 10(3): 130–6.

Tsey, K., Whiteside, M., Daly, B., Deemal, A., Gibson, T., Cadet-James, Y., Wilson, A., Santhanam, R., & Haswell, M. (2005b) Adapting the Family Wellbeing Empowerment Program to the Needs of Remote Indigenous School Children. *Australian and New Zealand Journal of Public Health*, 29(2): 112–16.

Tsey, K., Whiteside, M., Deemal, A., & Gibson, T. (2003) Social Determinants of Health, the 'Control Factor', and the Family Wellbeing Empowerment Program. *Australasian Psychiatry*, 11(Suppl.), S34–S39.

Turrell, G., Oldenburg, B., McGuffog, I., & Dent, R. (1999) *Socio-Economic Determinants of Health: Towards a National Research Program and Policy and Intervention Agenda*. Queensland University of Technology, Ausinfo: Canberra.

Wallerstein, N. (1992) Powerlessness, Empowerment, and Health: Implications for Health Promotion Programs. *American Journal of Health Promotion*, 6: 197–205.

Wallerstein, N. (2006) *What Is the Evidence on Effectiveness of Empowerment to Improve Health?* Copenhagen, WHO Regional Office for Europe (Health Evidence network report. www.euro.who.int/Document/E88086.pdf Access date: 01/02/06.

Whiteside, M., Tsey, K., McCalman, J., Cadet-James, Y., & Wilson, A. (2006) Empowerment as a Framework for Indigenous Workforce Development and Organisational Change. *Australian Social Work*, 59(4): 422–34.

Chapter 13

Australian Bureau of Statistics (ABS) (2001) *Basic Community Profile* (ABS cat. no. 2001.0). Australian Bureau of Statistics: Canberra.

Department of Immigration and Multicultural Affairs (DIMA) (1998) *Responding to Diversity: Progress in Implementing the Charter of Public Service in a Culturally Diverse Society, Access and Equity Annual Report*. DIMA: Canberra.

Cortes, D.E., Rogler, L.H., & Malgady, R.G. (1994) Biculturality among Puerto Rican Adults in the United States. *American Journal of Community Psychology*, 22: 707–21.

DeFleur, M.L., Kearney, P., & Plax, T.G. (1992) *Fundamentals of Human Communication*. Mayfield: Mountain View.

Grbich, C. (2004) Qualitative Research Design. In: V. Minichiello, G. Sullivan, K. Greenwood & R. Axford (eds), *Handbook of Research Methods for Nursing and Health Sciences*, chapter 7. Pearson Education Australia: Sydney.

Huff, R.M., & Kline, M.V. (1999) *Promoting Health in Multicultural Populations: A Handbook for Practitioners*. Sage Publications: Thousand Oaks.

Jochelson, T., Hua, M., & Rissel, C. (2003) Knowledge, Attitudes and Behaviours of Caregivers Regarding Children's Exposure to Environmental Tobacco Smoke among Arabic and Vietnamese-Speaking Communities in Sydney, Australia. *Ethnicity and Health*, 8(4): 339–51.

Khavarpour, F., & Rissel, C. (1997) Mental Health Status of Iranian Migrants in Sydney. *Australian and New Zealand Journal of Psychiatry*, 31(6): 828–34.

King, L., Thomas, M., Gatenby, K., Georgiou, A., & Hua, M. (1999) 'First Aid for Scalds' Campaign: Reaching Sydney's Chinese, Vietnamese, and Arabic Speaking Communities. *Injury Prevention*, 5: 104–8.

McPhee, J., Jenkins, C.N.H., Wong, C., Fordham, D., Lai, K.Q., Bird, J.A., & Moskowitz, J.M. (1995) Smoking Cessation Intervention among Vietnamese Americans: A Controlled Trial. *Tobacco Control*, 4 (suppl. 1): S16–S24.

Nutbeam, D., & Harris, E. (2004) *Theory in a Nutshell: A Practical Guide to Health Promotion Theories*, 2nd edn. McGraw-Hill: Sydney.

O'Connor, C., Wen, L.M., Rissel, C., & Shaw, M. (2007) Sexual Behaviour and Risk in Vietnamese Men Living in Metropolitan Sydney. *Sexually Transmitted Infections*, 83(2): 147–50.

Pauwels, A. (1995) *Cross-Cultural Communication in the Health Sciences: Communicating with Migrant Patients*. Macmillan Education Australia: Melbourne.

Rissel, C. (1997) The Development and Application of a Scale of Acculturation. *Australian and New Zealand Journal of Public Health*, 21(6): 606–13.

Rissel, C., McLellan, L., & Bauman, A. (2000a) Factors Associated with Delayed Tobacco Uptake among Vietnamese and Arabic Youth in Sydney, NSW. *Australian and New Zealand Journal of Public Health*, 24(1): 22–8.

Rissel, C., McLellan, L., & Bauman, A. (2000b) Social Factors Associated with Ethnic Differences in Alcohol and Marijuana Use by Vietnamese-, Arabic- and English-Speaking Youth in Sydney, Australia. *Journal of Paediatrics and Child Health*, 36(2): 145–52.

Chapter 14

Aldmeder, R. (2007) Pragmatism and Philosophy of Science: A Critical Survey. *International Studies in the Philosophy of Science*, 21(2): 171–95.

American Evaluation Association (2007) Guiding Principles for Evaluators. *American Journal of Evaluation*, 28: 129–30.

Atlantic Seniors' Housing Research Alliance (2004–2009) *Projecting the Housing Needs of Aging Atlantic Canadians.* In progress.

Attree, M. (2006) Evaluating Healthcare Education: Issues and Methods. *Nurse Education Today,* 26: 640–6.

Bamberger, M., Rugh, J., & Mabry, L. (2006) *Realworld Evaluation: Working under Budget, Time, Data and Political Restraints.* Sage Publications: Thousand Oaks.

Brookfield, S. (2005) *Power of Critical Theory for Adult Learning and Teaching.* McGraw-Hill: Berkshire.

Denzin, N.K., & Lincoln, Y.S. (2005) Introduction: The Discipline and Practice of Qualitative Research. In: N.K. Denzin & Y.S. Lincoln, *Handbook of Qualitative Research,* 3rd edn, 1–32. Sage Publications: Thousand Oaks.

Doane, G.H., & Varcoe, C. (2005) Toward Compassionate Action: Pragmatism and the Inseparability of Theory/Practice. *Advances in Nursing Science,* 28(1), 81–90.

Gibbs, L., & Gambrill, E. (2002) Evidence-based Practice: Counterarguments to Objections. *Research on Social Work Practice,* 12: 452–76.

Guba, G., & Lincoln, Y.S. (1989) *Fourth Generation Evaluation.* Sage Publications: Thousand Oaks.

Krueger, R.A. (1998) Moderating Focus Groups. In: D. Morgan & R.A. Krueger, *Focus Group Kit.* Sage Publications: Thousand Oaks.

Liamputtong, P., & Ezzy, D. (2005) *Qualitative Research Methods,* 2nd edn. Oxford University Press: Melbourne.

Littlejohns, P., Chalkidou, K. (2006) Evidence for Health Policy. *Journal of Research in Nursing,* 11: 110–17.

Mark, M.M., Henry, G.T., & Julnes, G. (2000) *Evaluation.* Jossey-Bass: San Francisco.

Patton, M.Q. (1994) Developmental Evaluation. *Evaluation Practice,* 15(3): 311–19.

Patton, M.Q. (2002) *Qualitative Research & Evaluation Methods,* 3rd edn. Sage Publications: Thousand Oaks.

Posavac, E.J., & Carey, R.G. (2003) *Program Evaluation Methods and Case Studies,* 6th edn. Prentice Hall: Upper Saddle River.

Rossi, P.H., Lipsey, M.W., & Freeman, H.E. (2004) *Evaluation: A Systematic Approach,* 7th edn. Sage Publications: Thousand Oaks.

Rycroft-Malone, J. (2006) The Politics of the Evidence-Based Practice Movements: Legacies and Current Challenges. *Journal of Research in Nursing,* 11: 95–108.

Rycroft-Malone, J., Seers, K., Titchen, A., Harvey, G., Kitson, A., & McCormack, B. (2004) What Counts as Evidence in Evidence-Based Practice? *Journal of Advanced Nursing,* 47(1): 81–90.

Sackett, D.L., Haynes, R.B., & Tugwell, P. (1985) *Clinical Epidemiology: A Basic Science for Clinical Medicine.* Little, Brown: Boston.

Sanderson, I. (2002) Evaluation, Policy Learning and Evidence-based Policy Making. *Public Administration*, 80: 1–22.

Scriven, M. (1996) Types of Evaluation and Types of Evaluator. *Evaluation Practice*, 17: 151–62.

Stufflebeam, D.L. (2000) Foundation Models for 21st Century Evaluation. In: D.L. Stufflebeam (ed.), *Evaluation Models: Viewpoints on Educational and Human Services Evaluation,* 2nd edn, 569. Kluwer Academic Publishers: Hingham, MA.

Thayer-Bacon, B. (2000) *Transforming Critical Thinking Constructively*. Teachers College Press, Columbia University: New York.

Thomas, W.I., & Thomas, D.S. (1928) *The Child in America: Behavior Problems and Programs*. Knopf: New York.

Trochim, W.M. *The Research Methods Knowledge Base*, 2nd edn. www.socialresearchmethods.net/kb/ Access date: 20/10/06.

Weiss, C.H. (1998) *Evaluation*, 2nd edn. Prentice Hall: Upper Saddle River.

Wholey, J.S. (1996) Formative and Summative Evaluation: Related Issues in Performance Measurement. *American Journal of Evaluation*, 17: 145.

World Health Organization (WHO) (1986) *Ottawa Charter for Health Promotion*. World Health Organization: Geneva.

World Health Organization (2004) *Report from the Ministerial Summit on Health Research*, 5–7. Mexico City. www.who.int/rpc/summit/documents/summit_report_final2.pdf Access date: 13/11/07.

Chapter 15

Bickman, L. (ed.) (1987) Using Program Theory in Evaluation. *New Directions for Program Evaluation*, 33: 1–116.

Bowling, A. (2002) *Research Methods in Health: Investigating Health and Health Services*, 2nd edn. Open University Press: Buckingham.

Donabedian, A. (1990) The Seven Pillars of Quality. *Archives of Pathology & Laboratory Medicine*, 114: 1115–18.

Funnell, S. (1997) Program Logic: An Adaptable Tool for Designing and Evaluating Programs. *Evaluation News and Comment*, 6(1): 5–17.

Glasgow, R.E., McKay, H.G., Piette, J.D., Reynolds, K.D. (2001) The RE-AIM Framework for Evaluating Interventions: What Can it Tell us about Approaches to Chronic Illness Management? *Patient Education and Counseling*, 44: 119–27.

Grembowski, D. (2001) *The Practice of Health Program Evaluation*. Sage Publications: Thousand Oaks.

Hawthorne, G. (2000) *Introduction to Health Program Evaluation*. Program Evaluation Unit, Centre for Health Program Evaluation: Melbourne.

Hennekens, C.H., & Buring, J.E. (1987) *Epidemiology in Medicine*. Little, Brown: Boston.

Kumar, R. (1996) *Research Methodology: A Step-by-Step Guide for Beginners*. Longman Australia: Melbourne.

Ovretveit, J. (1998) *Evaluating Health Interventions: An Introduction to Evaluation of Health Treatments, Services, Policies and Organisational Interventions*. Open University Press: Buckingham.

Patton, M.Q. (2002) *Qualitative Research and Evaluation Methods*. Sage Publications: Thousand Oaks.

Prochaska, J.O., DiClemente, C.C., & Norcross, J.C. (1992) In Search of How People Change. *American Psychologist*, 47: 1102–14.

Rossi, P.H., Freeman, H.E., & Lipsey, M.W. (1999) *Evaluation: A Systematic Approach*, 6th edn. Sage Publications: Thousand Oaks.

Scriven, M. (1991) *Evaluation Thesaurus*, 4th edn. Sage Publications: Newbury Park.

Smith, M.F. (1989) *Evaluability Assessment: A Practical Approach*. Kluwer Academic Publishers: Norwell.

Suchman, E.A. (1967) *Evaluative Research: Principles and Practice in Public Service and Social Action Programs*. Russell Sage Foundation: New York.

Taylor, S.J., & Bogdan, R. (1998) *Introduction to Qualitative Research Methods*. Wiley: Indianapolis.

Index

Aboriginal and Torres Strait Islander people   8, 21–2, 23
Aboriginal community (NT), building community capacity   209–12
Aboriginal Community Controlled Health Services (ACCHS)   16, 73, 220
Aboriginal Education Development Branch (AEDB)   222
Aboriginal health   71
   see also Indigenous Australians
acceptability   277
acculturation   240–1
active partnership   163
advocacy
   approach   183
   assessing climate for change   180–1
   campaigns   182–3
   and coalition building   187–8
   definition   174
   health   175–6, 187, 188–90
   key concepts   174–5
   lobbying and government relations   183–5
   media   185–7
   messages, targeting and framing   182
   planning   174, 179–83
   policy advocacy for health   176–9
   for policy change   174
   success factors   188–90
   toolkit   183–9
Agent Orange   100
Alma-Ata Declaration   27, 29, 163
amenability   111
American Evaluation Association   259
attitudes   241
attributed influentials   110
Australian Better Health Initiatives   29, 32, 34

Australian Indigenous Health Promotion Network   79
Australian Institute of Health and Welfare (AIHW)   9, 10, 11, 12, 74, 75, 82
avian influenza   94, 96

baby boomers   105
Beaglehole, R.   15
behaviour change theory   279–82
Better Health Commission   29
behaviour change theories, group level   37–9
   diffusion of innovation   38–9
   social networks   38
   social support   38
behaviour change theories, individual level   36–7
   health belief model (HBM)   36
   theory of reasoned action   36–7
   transtheoretical model (TTM) of change   37
behaviour change theories, population level   39–41
   communication and media   39–40
   ecological model of health behaviour   40–1
   social marketing   39
behavioural factors and epidemiological assessment   140
Bichmann, W.   205
Bickman, L.   279
bilingual data collection   244
bioethical analysis guidelines   113
bioethical model for decision-making   112
Bjaras, G.   205
Bonita, R.   15
bovine spongiform encephalopathy (BSE)   96
Bradshaw, Jonathan   47
Brough, M.   81
budgetary planning   244

345

built environment   19
Butler, C.D.   97

Campbell, M.D.   85, 216
cancer   11
Carey, R.G.   260
Centers for Disease Control and Prevention (CDC)   106, 107, 119, 265
Charter of the Public Service in Culturally Diverse Society   235
Child Pedestrian Injury Prevention Project (CPIPP)   138, 139, 140, 144–7, 148
climate change   31, 93, 99–102
coalition building and health advocacy   187–8
communication
    cross-cultural   234–5, 238, 248
    and media   39–40
communities and population health   17–23
community capacity
    Aboriginal community (NT)   209–12
    building   201–4, 212
    critical consciousness   199
    definition   196
    domains   196–7, 203
    in Fiji   207–8
    links to other organisations/people   200
    local leadership   196
    measuring   201–4, 212
    organisational structures   198–9
    outside agents   200
    problem-assessment capacity   199
    resource mobilisation   199–200
    stakeholder control over program management   201
    stakeholder participation   197
    strategic plan development   204
    visual representation   205–6
community development and empowerment   216–28
    approaches   219–20
    definition   216
    evaluating   224–7
    Indigenous Australian communities   220–1
    monitoring   224–7
    principles   219–20
    strategies   219–20
community empowerment   226–7
community engagement   216

community health   56, 67, 71, 106–7, 157, 160, 167, 254, 268, 286–7
Community Health Program   13, 16, 29
community trial   272
community-based methods, needs assessment   61–2
community-based services   236–7
Competency to Curriculum Toolkit   108, 119
competing interest groups   109–11
Constantino-David, Karina   198
constructivist paradigm   255
critical consciousness   199
critical thinking   256
cross-cultural
    communication   234–5, 238, 248
    competency training   238–9
    population-based health promotion program   239–44
cultural characteristics and health   21–2
cultural diversity   238
culturally and linguistically diverse (CALD) backgrounds   234, 235–9
culturally inclusive health assessment   237–9
culture   9

data collection   46, 48, 50, 51, 52, 125
    checklist   130–1
    monitoring   130
    schedules   129
death rates   11, 19–20
decision-making
    bioethical model   112
    government   183
deep vein thrombosis   94
DeFleur, M.L.   234
Delphi method   54–5, 59
demographics and health   19–20, 240
deontologicalism   111
developing countries
    infectious diseases   93
    primary health care   28
disability-adjusted life year (DALY)   10, 96
disadvantaged groups as stakeholders   108–9
disease
    definition   5–6
    global burden of   97
    infectious   93, 96–7
    and occupation   18

socio-economic determinants   15
zoonotic   96
displaced persons   95

ecological model of health behaviour   40–1
economic determinants   110
ecosystems   93, 100
effectiveness   277
efficiency   276
enabling (facilitating) factors   142, 143
education
   health   12–14
   and socio-economic status   18–19
   and training   165–6
empowerment
   community   226–7
   definition   216
   evaluating   224–7
   group   226
   and health   216–19
   monitoring   224–7
   organisational   226
   personal   225–6
   psychological   225–6
   spectrum of   218
   structural   226–7
environment and health   99–102
environmental factors and epidemiological assessment   140–1
environmental tobacco smoke (ETS) project   241
equity in health   70, 277–8
essential public health services   107
evaluating a housing program (case study)   262–4
evaluation   254
   formative   261, 269
   health promotion program   268–78
   impact   269
   models   259–61, 279
   parameters   276–8
   and planning   258–9
   process   269
   steps in   261–2
   strategies   243, 258–9, 269–71
   study design   271–8
   summative   261, 269
   theory-driven   260
   types of   261
   utilisation   278

evaluation of a school-based stop-smoking campaign (case study)   282–3
evidence-informed policy   257–8
evidence-informed practice   257
experimental study design   271–2

Family Wellbeing (FWB) empowerment program   221, 222–4
Fiji
   clinical governance   161, 164, 165, 166, 167, 168–70
   community capacity   207–8
'First Aid for Scalds' campaign   244–5
formative evaluation   261, 269
formative investigation   241, 243, 248
Freeman, H.E.   254
Funnell, S.   280, 281–2

Gambrill, E.   257
gap analysis   107
genetic factors and epidemiological assessment   141
geographic characteristics and health   20–1
Germov, J.   7, 8
Gibbs, L.   257
Gladwell, M.   188–9
global burden of disease   97
Global Commission on International Migration   95
global ecological changes   93
Global Outbreak Alert and Response Network (GOARN)   99
GOTME   186
government
   decision-making   183
   relations and advocacy   183–5
   services   235–6
Gray, D.   85
group empowerment   226
groups and health promotion   286

Haglund, B.J.A.   205
Health21 initiatives   31, 32
health
   assessment, culturally inclusive   237–8
   definition   5
   and demographics   19–20, 240
   determinants of   9–10

education   12–14
and empowerment   216–19
and environment   99–102
equity   70, 277–8
interventions   240
issues   240
issues, research on   16
issues and travel   93–6
measurement   10–12
models of   6–9, 259–61, 279
and population mobility   95–6
public   14, 15
socio-economic determinants   15
and society   97–9
and travel   93–5
see also population health
health adjusted life expectancy (HALE)   10, 12
health belief model (HBM) of behaviour change   36
health care costs   13, 125
health education, multicultural community   233–48
Health for All Policy Framework   31
'Health is Gold'   246–8
health professionals   105–8
assessing the needs of   106–8
Health Promoting Hospital project   32, 33, 38
Health Promoting Universities project   33
health promotion   12–14, 135
advocacy   174–5, 187, 188–90
behaviour change theories   36–41
coalition building   187–8
and communities   22–3
current issues   23–4
definition   13, 135
evaluation   268–78
healthy population groups   33–4
healthy settings   32–3
Indigenous Australians   70–1, 73, 77–88
international   31–2
interventions   22–3, 240
local level   31–2
and media advocacy   185–7
models   34–41, 239, 279, 286–7
multicultural community   233–48
national   31–2
organisational levels   35
Ottawa Charter   13, 15, 28, 29–31, 79

and population health   23–4
practitioners   71, 73, 77–8, 200
projects   174
program, cross-cultural population-based   239–44
program evaluation   268–78
program planning   140, 141–2
stakeholders   181, 278
theories   34–41, 126, 239, 286–7
health services, reorientating   31
Healthy Cities program   32–3
healthy population groups   33–4
heart disease   11
HIV/AIDS   58, 96, 105, 236
home ownership   76
Huff, R.M.   235
human needs   229
human resources, planning   160–71
case studies   168–70
definition   160
key stakeholders   161–3
leadership   160–1
local champions   161–3
mentoring   166–7
partnership, collaboration and sponsors   163–4
roles and responsibilities   164–5
rural Australia   170
supervising   166–7
sustainability   167–8
training   165–6
human resources needs   105
Human Rights and Equal Opportunity Commission (HREOC)   72, 75, 77

ill health, measurements of   11
illness
definition   5–6
Indigenous Australians   76
immunisation   13, 16, 23, 82, 115, 125, 276
impact evaluation   269
improved-focus model   260–1
income
Indigenous Australians   76
distribution and mortality   18
in-depth interviewing method   57
indicators, cultural relevance of   243

Indigenous Australians   70–88
    community development   220–1
    definition   70
    diversity   73–5
    health   217
    health, historical context   71–3
    health indicators   75–7
    health initiatives   86–7
    health promotion   70–1, 87–8
    health promotion literature   79–86
    health promotion practitioners   71, 73, 77–8
    needs assessment   65–6
Index of Relative Socio-Economic Status (ISRD)   18
individual and health promotion   287
infectious diseases   93, 96–7
infections and travel   93–6
influenza   93–4
innovation   38–9
interest groups   109–11
International Council of Nurses (ICN)   161
International Health Regulations (IHR)   98
International Union for Health Promotion and Education (IUHPE)   31
interrupted time series   273
interview, focus group   57–9
interviewing method, in-depth   57–9

key informants   108
Kildea, Sue   85
Kline, M.V.   235
KSAs   107

labour force participation   76
leadership   160–1
    local   198
Leadership for Change (LCF) program   161
life expectancy   19, 76
life styles   17
Likert scale   107
Lipsey, M.W.   254
literacy level of migrants   243
literature searches and health promotion   240
lobbying and advocacy   183–5

McCashen, Wayne   218
McMichael, A.J.   97
Mark, M.M.   258

Marmot, M.   15, 80, 82
media advocacy   185–7
media and communication   39–40
mental illness   7, 11, 20
mentoring   166–7
messages
    multicultural   243
    targeting and framing advocacy   182
migrant populations   22, 233–48
mixed methods   51
Mobilizing Action through Planning and Partnership (MAPP)   107, 108, 109
mortality   11
    and age groups   19–20
    and income distribution   18
    Indigenous Australians   76
Muller, F.   205
multicultural community, health promotion/education   233–48
    acculturation   240–1
    community-based services   236–7
    cross-cultural communication   234–5, 238
    cross-cultural competency training   238–9
    cultural diversity   238
    evaluation strategies   243–4
    formative investigation   241
    government services   235–6
    health assessment   237–8
    health interventions   240
    health issues   240
    health promotion   239–44
    migration context   233–4
    project team   242
    promotional resources   242
Multiple Risk Factor Intervention Trial (MRFIT)   271
Municipal Public Health Plan (MPHP) in Victoria   114–16

National Aboriginal Community Controlled Health Organisation (NACCHO)   91, 220, 231
National Accreditation Authority for Translators & Interpreters (NAATI)   242
National Association of Country and City Health Officials   107, 119
National Better Health Program   29, 32

National Health and Medical Research Council
    (NH&MRC)   16, 70, 86
National Public Health Partnership   29, 32
National Public Health Performance Standards
    Program (NPHPSP)   106–8
needs assessment   46–67
    community-based methods   61–2
    community groups   63–4
    data collection   46, 48, 50, 51, 52, 125
    definition   46
    Delphi method   54–5, 59
    in-depth interviewing method   57
    Indigenous Australians   65–6
    focus group interview   57–9
    of health professionals   106–8
    and health promotion interventions   240
    methods   50–2, 53–5
    need for   48–9
    nominal group technique   59–60
    observation   55–6
    photovoice method   62, 65–6
    population characteristics   62–4
    prioritising health needs, community
        groups   63–4
    prioritising identified needs   111–14
    and problem identification   52, 125
    processes   49–62
    rapid appraisal method   60–1
    questionnaire method   53–4
    St Ives, Sydney   64–5
    strategies for   50–2
    survey method   53–4
    use of existing data   52
    vulnerable target group   62–3
new public health model   7
nominal group technique   59–60
non-experimental study design   271, 272,
    274–6

obesity in children   131–2
observation and needs assessment   55–6
occupation and disease   18
organisational empowerment   226
organisational links in communities   200
organisational structures in communities   198–9
Ottawa Charter of Health Promotion   13, 15, 28,
    29–31, 79, 174, 217
outcome hierarchy   281

outcomes   108
outside agents   200

paradigms   255–6
participatory learning action (PLA)   109
Patton, M.Q.   262
Pauwels, A.   234
Pearson, Noel   72, 81, 221
personal empowerment   225–6
Personal Wellbeing Index   10
Penrith Food Project   190–1
philosophy   254–5
photovoice method, needs assessment   62, 65–6
policy
    advocacy for health   176–9
    definition   174
    objectives   177–8
    public health   32, 174, 187
population health
    Australia   16–17
    and communities   17–23
    cultural characteristics   212
    current issues   23–4
    demographic characteristics   19–20
    evolution of   14–16
    geographic characteristics   20–1
    physical characteristics   19
    social characteristics   17–19
population mobility and health   95–6
positive paradigm   255
Posavac, E.J.   261
poverty   17–18
power   218
PRECEDE model   135–43
    change processes   37
PRECEDE–PROCEED model   135–43, 295–8
    administrative/policy assessment   154–6
    behavioural factors   140
    environmental factors   140–1
    epidemiological assessment   139–40
    etiological factors   140–2
    genetic factors   141
    goals and objectives   149–51
    implementation   156
    intervention alignment   154–6
    re-defining the target group   148–9
    relevance to planning health promotion
        programs   141–2

types of factors   142–3
predisposing (motivating) factors   142
prescribed influentials   110
prevalence   111
primary health care
   Alma-Ata Declaration   27, 29, 163
   developed countries   28–9
   developing countries   28
   development   27–9
   philosophy   254–5
problem assessment of communities   199
problem identification   125
process evaluation   269
process objectives   108
program cost   276
program cycle   269–71
program goals   124
program logic   279
program logic matrix   281
program planning   135
   administrative/policy assessment   154–6
   epidemiological assessment   139–40
   evaluation strategies   243, 258–9
   goals and objectives   149–51
   health promotion   140, 141–2
   identification of etiological factors   140–2
   implementation   156
   intervention alignment   154–6
   PRECEDE–PROCEED model   135–43
   re-defining the target group   148–9
program quality   276
program theory   279
project design   241
project manual   128–30
project objectives   124
project planning   288–94
project team   242, 243
projects, prerequisites for developing   125–31
   checklist   130–1
   design   127
   feasibility   125
   forms   129
   identifying a problem   125
   induction or intuition   126
   is the problem soluble?   126
   project manual   128–30
   protocol   128

   quality control and monitoring   130
   schedules   129
   significance of the problem   125–6
promotional materials   243
promotional resources   242
protective factors   135
psychological empowerment   225–6
public health   14, 15
   project, planning stage   160
   program   108, 110, 112
   policy   32, 174, 187, 188–90
Public Health Workforce Questionnaire (PHWQ)   107

qualitative methods   50–1, 127, 205, 227, 241, 275
quality of life   10, 13, 16, 27, 31, 34, 47, 55, 93, 125, 138, 141, 142, 227, 276
quality of life (QOL) index   10
quantitative methods   50, 51, 127, 275
quasi-experimental study design   272–4
questionnaires, translation of   244

randomised controlled trial (RCT)   255, 271, 272
rapid appraisal method   60–1
reinforcing (maintaining or rewarding) factors   142
resource mobilisation in communities   199–200
Rifkin, S.   205
risk factors   141
Ross, N.A.   17
Rossi, P.H.   259, 260
Roughan, J.J.   205
rural and remote areas   20–1, 170–1
Rycroft-Malone, J.   257

60 and Better Program   16, 34
sampling   244
self-assessed health status   10, 12
Seniors Pedestrian Injury Prevention Program (SIPP)   152–3
severe acute respiratory syndrome (SARS)   93, 96, 98
Smith, M.F.   281
smoking   241, 246–8
social integration   38
social marketing   39, 185, 242, 279, 287
social network   5, 37, 38, 39, 141
social science program model   259–60

social support   38
social skeleton: health, illness and structure–agency model   7, 8–9
socio-economic determinants, health and disease   15
socio-economic status   17–19, 22
society and health   97–9
St Ives, Sydney (health needs assessment)   64–5
stakeholders   105–9
  and community participation   197
  control over program management   201
  definition   161
  disadvantaged and vulnerable groups   108–9
  health promotion   181
  key   161–3
  management strategy   181
  and program evaluation   278
structural empowerment   226–7
Suchman, E.A.   280, 281
summative evaluation   261, 269
supervising   166–7
sustainability   160, 167–8
SWOT analysis   114

Task Force of the American Evaluation Association   258
Thayer-Bacon, B.   256, 261
theory of reasoned action   36–7
theory-driven evaluation   260
Tokbai-Talaa village   206

translating and interpreting service (TIS)   235
transtheoretical model (TTM) of change   37
travel and health issues   93–6

University of the Third Age (U3A)   34
US National Environmental Health Association   100
utilitarianism   111

value   233
Vietnam veterans   100
visual representation of community capacity   205–6
vulnerable groups as stakeholders   108–9
vulnerable target group, needs assessment   62–3

Wallack, L.   186
Weiss, C.H.   254, 255, 258
wellness
  issues, research on   16
  measurements of   1112
Wholey, J.S.   261
windshield tours   61
women's health   16, 22
World Health Organization (WHO)   5, 27, 31, 47, 94, 96, 98, 99, 217, 227, 254, 257

Yeatman, H.   190

zoonotic diseases   96

Printed in Australia
17 Dec 2013
OUP001H7